Case Studies in Epilepsy

Case Studies in Epilepsy

Editor: Leonardo Roberts

AMERICAN
MEDICAL PUBLISHERS
www.americanmedicalpublishers.com

AMERICAN
MEDICAL PUBLISHERS
www.americanmedicalpublishers.com

Cataloging-in-Publication Data

Case studies in epilepsy / edited by Leonardo Roberts.
p. cm.
Includes bibliographical references and index.
ISBN 979-8-88740-597-1
1. Epilepsy. 2. Epilepsy--Research. 3. Epilepsy--Research--Methodology
4. Epileptics. 5. Brain--Diseases. 6. Developmental disabilities. I. Roberts, Leonardo.
RC372 .R43 2023
616.853--dc23

American Medical Publishers,
41 Flatbush Avenue,
1st Floor, New York,
NY 11217, USA

ISBN 979-8-88740-597-1 (Hardback)

Contents

Preface

This book has been an outcome of determined endeavour from a group of educationists in the field. The primary objective was to involve a broad spectrum of professionals from diverse cultural background involved in the field for developing new researches. The book not only targets students but also scholars pursuing higher research for further enhancement of the theoretical and practical applications of the subject.

Epilepsy is a neurological disorder which is characterized by recurrent seizures that are caused by abnormal electrical activity in the brain. It can affect people of all ages, and the severity of its impact can range from mild to severe. The diagnosis of this disease involves critical examinations of medical history, physical examinations, and various diagnostic tests such as electroencephalogram (EEG), magnetic resonance imaging (MRI), and blood tests. The diagnosis helps in determining the type of epilepsy, identify its potential underlying causes, and rule out other conditions that may mimic seizures. It can be managed through antiepileptic medications, which aim to reduce the frequency and severity of seizures. Some of the other treatment options are ketogenic diet, vagus nerve stimulation, and epilepsy surgery. This book unravels the recent studies on epilepsy. Those in search of information to further their knowledge will be greatly assisted by it.

It was an honour to edit such a profound book and also a challenging task to compile and examine all the relevant data for accuracy and originality. I wish to acknowledge the efforts of the contributors for submitting such brilliant and diverse chapters in the field and for endlessly working for the completion of the book. Last, but not the least; I thank my family for being a constant source of support in all my research endeavours.

Editor

1

Phenotypic and Genotypic Characterization of *NPRL2*-Related Epilepsy: Two Case Reports

Yulin Sun [1,2†], *Lin Wan* [1,2†], *Huimin Yan* [1,2], *Zhichao Li* [1,2] *and Guang Yang* [1,2,3*]

[1] *Department of Pediatrics, Chinese PLA General Hospital, Beijing, China,* [2] *Department of Pediatrics, The First Medical Center, Chinese PLA General Hospital, Beijing, China,* [3] *The Second School of Clinical Medicine, Southern Medical University, Guangzhou, China*

***Correspondence:**
Guang Yang
yangg301@126.com

† *These authors have contributed equally to this work*

The phenotype of nitrogen permease regulator-like 2 (*NPRL2*) gene-related epilepsy clinically manifests as a range of epilepsy syndromes, including familial focal epilepsy with variable foci (FFEVF), sleep-related hypermotor epilepsy (SHE), temporal lobe epilepsy (TLE), frontal lobe epilepsy (FLE), and infantile spasms (IS). The association between phenotype and genotype of *NPRL2* variants has not been widely explored. This study aimed to explore the phenotype and genotype spectrum of *NPRL2*-related epilepsy. Here, we presented two clinical cases with *NPRL2*-related epilepsy, and discussed the characteristics, diagnosis, and treatment processes in the context of existing literature. Two novel *NPRL2* likely pathogenic variants were identified by next-generation sequencing, including one splicing mutation (c.933-1G>A), and one frameshift mutation (c.257delG). The results of literature review showed that there were a total of 20 patients with *NPRL2*-related epilepsy whose mutations were mostly missense and hereditary. These findings indicate that the possibility of *NPRL2* gene mutations in focal epilepsy should be considered for patients with family history, and that patients carrying different *NPRL2* variants have different clinical manifestations. Our study expanded the genotype spectrum of *NPRL2* and suggested that the type of *NPRL2* variants might provide important information for the prognosis evaluation.

Keywords: focal epilepsy, genotype, phenotype, *NPRL2*, case report

INTRODUCTION

Nitrogen permease regulator-like 2 (*NPRL2*), part of the GATOR1 complex that negatively regulates the mechanistic target of rapamycin (mTOR), reportedly affects brain development and function (1). The *NPRL2* gene, which is located on chromosome 3p21.3 and encodes a protein containing 380 amino acids, plays a key role of connecting the DEP domain-containing protein 5 (DEPDC5) and the nitrogen permease regulator-like 3 (NPRL3) of the GATOR1 complex (2). Pathogenic variants in the *NPRL2* gene can cause loss of function of the GATOR1 complex, thereby abnormally enhancing activity of the mTOR signaling pathway (3, 4). The phenotypic spectrum of *NPRL2*-related epilepsy ranges from sporadic early onset epilepsy, which is accompanied by cognitive impairment, to familial focal epilepsy, especially in the familial focal epilepsy with variable foci (FFEVF). These manifestations are similar to clinical phenotypes observed in patients with pathogenic variants in the *DEPDC5* and *NRPL3* genes (5). Here, we described the clinical characteristics of two cases with different novel likely pathogenic variants in *NPRL2*. Furthermore, we reviewed the advanced publications and summarized the associations between phenotype and genotype in *NPRL2*-related epilepsy.

METHODS

Research Subjects

All procedures of this study were approved by the Ethics Committee of the Chinese PLA General Hospital (reference numbers: 2021-98). Written informed consent to participate in this study was provided by the legal guardian of the participants. Extracted patient data and medical records was deidentified and coded without identifiers. Our study involved one Chinese family clinically diagnosed with familial focal epilepsy (FFE) and one child clinically diagnosed with infantile spasms (IS). All participants were admitted to Chinese PLA General Hospital. Our inclusion criteria included (1) confirmed diagnosis of focal epilepsy and infantile spasms based on the criteria of the International League Against Epilepsy (ILAE) (6); (2) family history of epilepsy; and (3) pathogenic or likely pathogenic *NPRL2* mutation in the affected family members. All the probands received comprehensive clinical evaluations by experienced neurologists in our hospital. MRI (1.5T) and EEG were performed on these participants. Auxiliary examinations, including liver and kidney function, blood and urine organic acids, and electrolytes, were performed.

Genetic Study

Two milliliters of venous blood of patient and parents were collected and DNA was extracted from the samples. Using Trio Whole-exome sequencing (WES) technology, it sequenced exons of nearly 20,000 human genes and about 20 bp upstream and downstream through targeted probe capture and high-throughput second generation sequencing (tested by Shenzhen Anji Kang Medical Inspection Laboratory). Bioinformatics analysis and mutation screening were based on original data from the sequencer, converted from.bcl to.fastq using bcl2fastq, and files were aligned with Human Reference Genome GRCH37/hg19 using BWA, SAMtools, and Picard software. The frequency of variation in the population was annotated by the international 1000 Genome Project, Genome Aggregation Database and Exome Aggregation Consortium. Online Mendelian Inheritance in Man (OMIM), Human Gene Mutation Database (HGMD), and disease-related human genome variation database (ClinVar) were used to annotate diseases. We used PolyPhen 2, SIFT, MutationTaster, and other software to predict and analyze protein function damage.

Pathogenic or likely pathogenic variants were screened according to the American College of Medical Genetics and Genomics (ACMG) classification guidelines and the clinical phenotypes of the patients (7). All clinically significant variations were validated by first-generation Sanger sequencing.

Literature Search

A systematic literature search in PubMed and OMIM was performed. MeSH and title or abstract were used for all eligible studies that mainly focus on the *NPRL2* variants in FFE. The research strategy was as follows: "NPRL2" AND ("familial focal epilepsy" or "hereditary focal epilepsy" or "familial focal epilepsy with variable foci" or "familial epilepsy" or "infantile spasms"). Data from all eligible studies were analyzed and discussed by two reviewers.

RESULTS

Case Presentation

Family A

A girl, aged 3 years and 11 months, presented with intermittent seizures mainly manifested by intermittent focal motor in the left limb or presented with generalized tonic-clonic seizure, with or without loss of consciousness. The seizures, which occurred during night sleep, mostly between 5 and 7 am, lasted for 15–20 s at a frequency of two to three times a week. The child was born of natural birth and had no history of asphyxia or hypoxia. Her intelligence, language, and movement were generally normal. Notably, her father had a history of focal epilepsy, which was diagnosed when he was 6 years old. His focal motor seizures have been under control with carbamazepine, although sensory auras may be triggered by drowsiness or fatigue. The grandfather of our index case also had a history of epilepsy, although the exact type of seizure was unknown. We found no evidence of abnormalities in the girl after comprehensive physical examination, which also included blood and urine organic acids, blood sugar, electrolyte, along with liver, and kidney function analysis. Moreover, head MRI showed no obvious signal abnormalities. However, EEG demonstrated medium and equal amount, short segment, paroxysmal, medium high potential, 2.2–2.9 HZ spike-slow wave, and sharp-slow wave discharges in the right anterior temporal region during sleep. The final diagnosis was temporal lobe epilepsy (TLE). She was orally administered with oxcarbazepine (32 mg/kg/d). The seizures were controlled, and she had acquired seizure freedom for 24 months by the end of June 2021.

Family B

A 4-month-old male infant had multiple unprovoked seizures 10 days after birth. The seizures were predominantly focal to generalized tonic-clonic seizures in semiology. These occurred more than 10 times a day and lasted for 10 s each. After oral phenobarbital treatment, the seizures were under control. During the drug reduction period, he developed epileptic spasms, presenting with sudden nodding with limbs extension. These occurred more than 10 times a day in clusters and, most often, shortly after waking. The child was born of natural birth and had no history of asphyxia or hypoxia. Family history was also normal. He could look up and turn over. There was no obvious developmental delay. After admission, we found no evidence of abnormalities in the auxiliary examinations. His head MRI showed no obvious signal abnormalities except that bilateral ventricles were enlarged. EEG demonstrated the

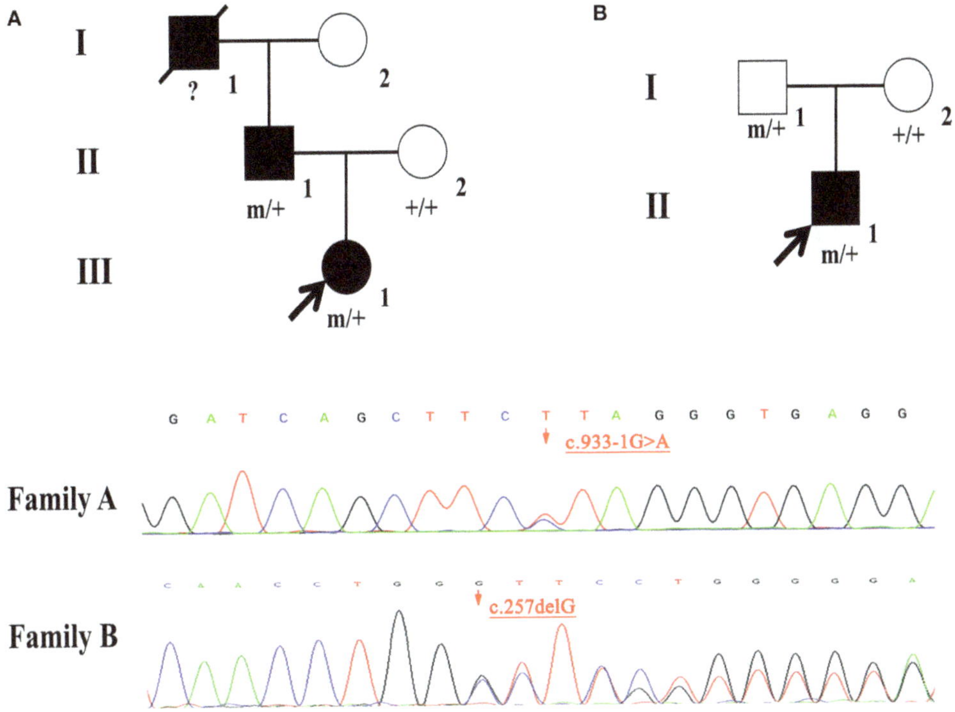

FIGURE 1 | (A,B) Individuals carrying the NPRL2 mutation are indicated by "m/+". Individuals with negative mutation are indicated by "+/+", and individuals without blood samples are indicated by "?".

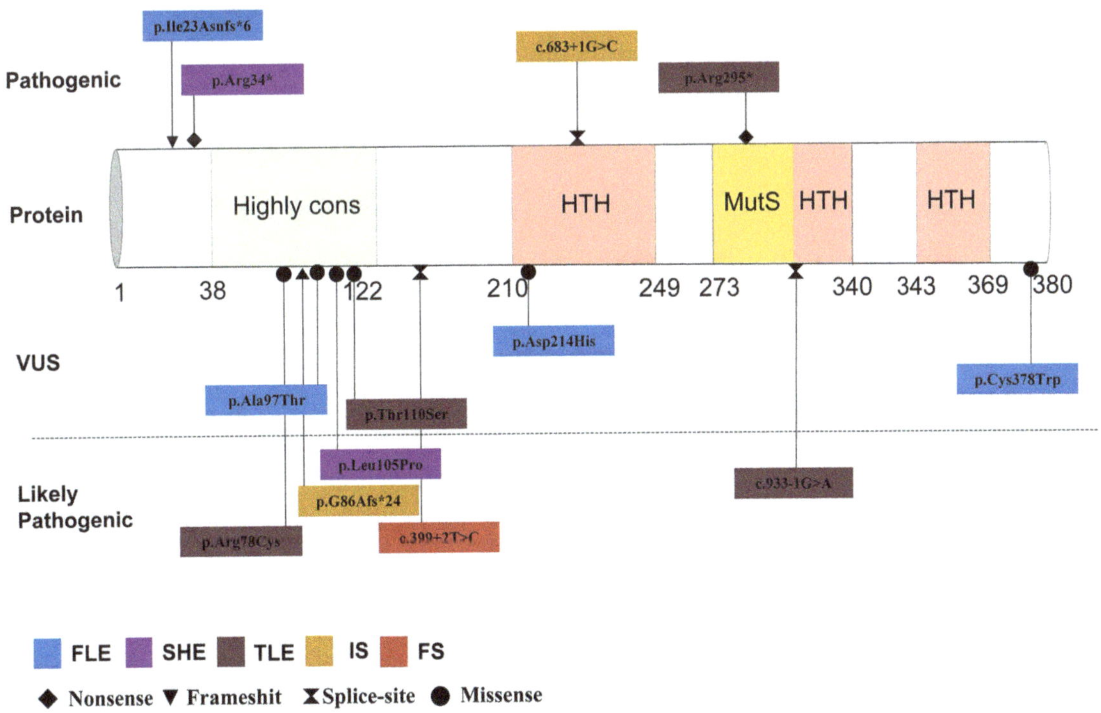

FIGURE 2 | Mutation site and phenotype spectrum of NPRL2 gene.

TABLE 1 | Genotypic and phenotypic characteristics of *NPRL2*-related epilepsy from previous literature identified to the present.

References	Number of cases	cDNA variant	Protein alteration	Variant class	MRI	EEG discharge region	Phenotype	Number of AEDs used	Other treatments	Outcome
Weckhuysen et al.	3	c.68_69delCT	p.Ile23Asnfs*6	Frameshift	N; PET: right frontoinsular hypometabolism/N/–	Right frontal island lobe and frontal orbital/left temporal region/–	FLE/TLE/UE/	8/1/-	Right-frontal orbitotomy/none/–	Controlled/ controlled/–
Ricos et al.	2	c.100C>T	p.Arg34*	Nonsense	–	–	SHE	–	–	–
	1	c.883C>T	p.Arg295*	Nonsense	–	–	TLE	–	–	–
	1	c.329C>G	p.Thr110Ser	Missense	–	–	TLE	–	–	–
	1	c.640G>C	p.Asp214His	Missense	–	–	FLE	–	–	–
	5	c.314T>C	p.Leu105Pro	Missense	–	–	2SHE/1FE/2UE	–	–	–
Perucca et al.	2	c.232C>T	p.Arg78Cys	Missense	N/–	Left temporal region/–	TLE/UE	2/–	None/–	Uncontrolled/–
Baldassari et al.	1	c.100C>T	p.Arg34*	Nonsense	FCD in right frontal lobe	Right cingulate gyrus	SHE	8	Surgery, VNS	Controlled
	1	c.1134C>G	p.Cys378Trp	Missense	N; PET: N	Right frontal lobe	FLE	9	Ketogenic diet	Improved
	1	c.683+1G>C	p.(?)	Splice-site	FCD in left parieto-temporal	Hypsarrhythmia	IS	4	ACTH, surgery	Controlled
Deng et al.	1	c.289G>A	p.Ala97Thr	Missense	–	–	FLE	1	None	Controlled
Licchetta et al.	1	c.314T>C	p.Leu105Pro	Missense	–	–	SHE	–	–	–
Zhang et al.	2	c.399+2T>C	p.(?)	Splice-site	N/N	Left frontal and central regions/ left frontal region	FE; F to G T-C; IS/FS	2/–	–	Controlled/–
Our study	2	c.933-1G>A	p.(?)	Splice-site	N	Right anterior temporal region/–	TLE/FE	1/1	None	Controlled/ controlled
	1	c.257delG	p.G86Afs*24	Frameshift	N	Hypsarrhythmia	IS	2	ACTH	Uncontrolled

N, normal; –, not applicable or without information; FCD, focal cortical dysplasia; VNS, vagus nerve stimulation; ACTH, adrenocorticotropic hormone; SHE, sleep-related hypermotor epilepsy; TLE, temporal lobe epilepsy; FLE, frontal lobe epilepsy; IS, infantile spasm; FE, focal epilepsy; UE, unclassified epilepsy; FGTC, focal to generalized tonic-clonic; FS, febrile seizures.

typical findings of hypsarrhythmia. Disorganized, asymmetric, and asynchronous 150–200 μV slow waves could be seen in both wakefulness and sleep stages. Despite appropriate treatment with adrenocorticotropic hormone and topiramate (8 mg/kg/d), seizures remained uncontrolled by the end of September 2021.

Novel Mutation in *NPRL2* Gene

Two novel mutations in the *NPRL2* (NM_006545.4), including c.933-1G>A and c.257delG, were identified by WES. Results from Sanger sequencing validated these findings and confirmed that both the father and child carried the same variant with a wild-type mother in Family A and B (**Figure 1**). The variant c.933-1G>A is a splicing mutation found in family A, which affects the structure of mRNA and results in loss of function mutation (LoF), meeting a highly pathogenic evidence (PVS1). This variant has neither been previously recorded in the reference population gene frequency database nor reported in the ClinVar and HGMD databases, meeting moderate intensity pathogenic evidence (PM2). The splicing variant c.933-1G>A was classified as likely pathogenic according to the ACMG criteria and guidelines (7). The variant c.257delG is a frameshift mutation found in family B, which can cause protein truncation or activate nonsense mediated mRNA degradation, thus affecting the function of coding protein products. Similarly, the variant c.257delG rating was described as PVS1 + PM2 and was classified as likely pathogenic.

DISCUSSION

The *NPRL2* gene, which is located on chromosome 3p21.3, with a transcript that is highly expressed in the brain frontal, temporal, parietal, and occipital lobes, has a similar distribution pattern to that of *DEPDC5* and *NPRL3* transcriptions (3, 8). *NPRL2* forms the GATOR1 complex together with DEPDC5 and NPRL3. *NPRL2* plays a crucial role in connecting DEPDC5 and NPRL3 and has also been implicated in development of hereditary focal epilepsy (8). GATOR1 dysfunction caused by any gene mutation of the above components can promotes activity of the mTOR signaling pathway, thereby causing hereditary focal epilepsy (9, 10). Other studies have proved that the Arg78 residue of *NPRL2* is a catalytic residue on GATOR1, and plays a role in regulating cell proliferation, differentiation, and death, as well as development and function of the brain by Rag GTPases-mediated activation of mTORC1 (11).

By September 2021, a total of 22 patients with *NPRL2*-related epilepsy had been reported. Combined with our study, there were a total of 25 patients with *NPRL2*-related epilepsy, of which 11 were male and 13 were female, respectively, while the gender of one case was unknown (3, 8, 12–16). Among the cases whose specific clinical details could be obtained by manual screening, we found no evidence of abnormalities in their personal history, with all of them having normal development prior to seizure onset. Except for three cases of *de novo* variants and one case of unknown source of variant, the rest were familial genetic variation. Previous studies have shown that distribution of mutation types in the *GATORl* complex gene is mainly LoF mutations (nonsense and frameshift variants), and these account for 67% of all the cases (3). Combined with the reported cases, 13 *NPRL2* gene variants were detected, of which missense variants were the most common (46.2%), followed by splice (23.1%), nonsense (15.4%), and frameshift (15.4%) variants. Details of these variants and the corresponding phenotypes are shown in **Figure 2** and **Table 1**.

A total of 11 cases with age of onset can be obtained, which revealed that *NPRL2*-related epilepsy can occur from infancy to adulthood. Previous studies have found no significant relationship between the phenotype of epilepsy with affected components in the GATORl complex, which may be attributed to the co-performing function of the three protein composition complexes (2). Focal seizure was the most common type of seizure, although tonic seizures and epileptic spasms were also observed. The most common epileptic phenotype was SHE, which was observed in six cases, followed by TLE (five cases), FLE (four cases), and IS (two cases). Two cases of unclassified focal epilepsy (FE) and four cases of unclassified epilepsy (UE) were also included. One case presented multiple seizure types (FE, IS, and focal to generalized tonic-clonic seizures) and one case presented febrile seizures (FS) in the latest study (16).

Notably, a majority of *NPRL2* gene-associated epilepsy exhibited no structural damage, suggesting that the epileptogenic mechanisms may generate a relatively wide range of neurofunctional abnormalities and epileptogenic network formation (14). Eleven cases described the findings of MRI, of which eight patients with normal brain MRI. All three children with definite epileptogenic foci were surgically treated, with post-operative histological examination revealing focal cortical dysplasia (FCD) Ia, FCD IIa, and FCD Ia. On the other hand, brain MRI of one case showed no abnormalities, but head positron emission tomography (PET) demonstrated right frontoinsular hypometabolism. It suggested that PET may be helpful to detect focal structural abnormalities in patients with MRI-negative hereditary focal epilepsy.

Of the 25 patients included in this study, we obtained information about antiseizure medications in 11 cases, of which 6 (54.5%) were drug-resistant epilepsy. Among the five patients with drug-controlled seizures, two were treated with oxcarbazepine, one with sodium valproate, and one with a combination of topiramate and vitamin B6 therapy. Another case was controlled by carbamazepine, but there were obvious onset precursors in case of fatigue, insufficient sleep, and continuous missed medication. The underlying molecular mechanism suggests that mTOR inhibitors, such as rapamycin, may be promising drugs for *NPRL2* gene-related epilepsy, due to the abnormal activation of the mTOR signaling pathway caused by *NPRL2* gene variation, although further explorations are still needed to ascertain the stage of disease treatment (5, 17, 18).

CONCLUSION

We reported two novel *NPRL2* likely pathogenic variants identified in two Chinese families. In patients with a family history of focal epilepsy, *NPRL2* variants should be considered. Combined with the reported cases, we found that patients harboring LoF mutations tend to suffer from refractory epilepsy and other severe comorbidities. Our study might provide significant information to physician for the treatment and prognosis evaluation of patients with *NPRL2*-related epilepsy.

ETHICS STATEMENT

The studies involving human participants were reviewed and approved by the Ethics Committee of the Chinese PLA General Hospital. Written informed consent to participate in this study was provided by the participant's legal guardian/next of kin. Written informed consent was obtained from the individuals and/or minor's legal guardian/next of kin for the publication of any potentially identifiable images or data included in this article.

AUTHOR CONTRIBUTIONS

YS and LW wrote the first draft. HY and ZL revised the manuscript. GY drafted the manuscript and the final approval version to be published. All authors contributed to the article and approved the submitted version.

REFERENCES

1. Baldassari S, Licchetta L, Tinuper P, Bisulli F, Pippucci T. GATOR1 complex: the common genetic actor in focal epilepsies. *J Med Genet.* (2016) 53:503–10. doi: 10.1136/jmedgenet-2016-103883
2. Dokudovskaya S, Rout MP. SEA you later alli-GATOR–a dynamic regulator of the TORC1 stress response pathway. *J Cell Sci.* (2015) 128:2219–28. doi: 10.1242/jcs.168922
3. Baldassari S, Picard F, Verbeek NE, van Kempen M, Brilstra EH, Lesca G, et al. The landscape of epilepsy-related GATOR1 variants. *Genet Med.* (2019) 21:398–408. doi: 10.1038/s41436-018-0060-2
4. Dawson RE, Nieto Guil AF, Robertson LJ, Piltz SG, Hughes JN, Thomas PQ. Functional screening of GATOR1 complex variants reveals a role for mTORC1 deregulation in FCD and focal epilepsy. *Neurobiol Dis.* (2020) 134:104640. doi: 10.1016/j.nbd.2019.104640
5. Iffland PH II, Carson V, Bordey A, Crino PB. GATORopathies: the role of amino acid regulatory gene mutations in epilepsy and cortical malformations. *Epilepsia.* (2019) 60:2163–73. doi: 10.1111/epi.16370
6. Fisher RS, Cross JH, D'Souza C, French JA, Haut SR, Higurashi N, et al. Instruction manual for the ILAE 2017 operational classification of seizure types. *Epilepsia.* (2017) 58:531–42. doi: 10.1111/epi.13671
7. Richards S, Aziz N, Bale S, Bick D, Das S, Gastier-Foster J, et al. Standards and guidelines for the interpretation of sequence variants: a joint consensus recommendation of the American College of Medical Genetics and Genomics and the Association for Molecular Pathology. *Genet Med.* (2015) 17:405–24. doi: 10.1038/gim.2015.30
8. Weckhuysen S, Marsan E, Lambrecq V, Marchal C, Morin-Brureau M, An-Gourfinkel I, et al. Involvement of GATOR complex genes in familial focal epilepsies and focal cortical dysplasia. *Epilepsia.* (2016) 57:994–1003. doi: 10.1111/epi.13391
9. Dibbens LM, de Vries B, Donatello S, Heron SE, Hodgson BL, Chintawar S, et al. Mutations in DEPDC5 cause familial focal epilepsy with variable foci. *Nat Genet.* (2013) 45:546–51. doi: 10.1038/ng.2599
10. Ishida S, Picard F, Rudolf G, Noé E, Achaz G, Thomas P, et al. Mutations of DEPDC5 cause autosomal dominant focal epilepsies. *Nat Genet.* (2013) 45:552–5. doi: 10.1038/ng.2601
11. Shen K, Valenstein ML, Gu X, Sabatini DM. Arg-78 of Nprl2 catalyzes GATOR1-stimulated GTP hydrolysis by the Rag GTPases. *J Biol Chem.* (2019) 294:2970–5. doi: 10.1074/jbc.AC119.007382
12. Ricos MG, Hodgson BL, Pippucci T, Saidin A, Ong YS, Heron SE, et al. Mutations in the mammalian target of rapamycin pathway regulators NPRL2 and NPRL3 cause focal epilepsy. *Ann Neurol.* (2016) 79:120–31. doi: 10.1002/ana.24547
13. Perucca P, Scheffer IE, Harvey AS, James PA, Lunke S, Thorne N, et al. Real-world utility of whole exome sequencing with targeted gene analysis for focal epilepsy. *Epilepsy Res.* (2017) 131:1–8. doi: 10.1016/j.eplepsyres.2017.02.001
14. Deng J, Fang F, Wang XH, Dai LF, Tian XJ, Chen CH. [Clinical and genetic characteristics of focal epilepsy in children caused by GATOR1 complex gene variation]. *Zhonghua Er Ke Za Zhi.* (2019) 57:780–5. doi: 10.3760/cma.j.issn.0578-1310.2019.10.010
15. Licchetta L, Pippucci T, Baldassari S, Minardi R, Provini F, Mostacci B, et al. Sleep-related hypermotor epilepsy (SHE): contribution of known genes in 103 patients. *Seizure.* (2020) 74:60–4. doi: 10.1016/j.seizure.2019.11.009
16. Zhang J, Shen Y, Yang Z, Yang F, Li Y, Yu B, et al. A splicing variation in NPRL2 causing familial focal epilepsy with variable foci: additional cases and literature review. *J Hum Genet.* (2021). doi: 10.1038/s10038-021-00969-z. [Epub ahead of print].
17. Ishida S. [DEPDC5, a new key to understand various epilepsies]. *Nihon Yakurigaku Zasshi.* (2018) 152:281–5. doi: 10.1254/fpj.152.281
18. Yuskaitis CJ, Rossitto LA, Gurnani S, Bainbridge E, Poduri A, Sahin M. Chronic mTORC1 inhibition rescues behavioral and biochemical deficits resulting from neuronal Depdc5 loss in mice. *Hum Mol Genet.* (2019) 28:2952–64. doi: 10.1093/hmg/ddz123

2

Case Report: Hemispherotomy in the First Days of Life to Treat Drug-Resistant Lesional Epilepsy

Konstantin L. Makridis [1,2,3], *Christine Prager* [1,2], *Anna Tietze* [4], *Deniz A. Atalay* [1,2], *Sebastian Triller* [1,2], *Christian E. Elger* [1,2,5], *Ulrich-Wilhelm Thomale* [6] *and Angela M. Kaindl* [1,2,3*]

[1] Department of Pediatric Neurology, Charité – Universitätsmedizin Berlin, Berlin, Germany, [2] Center for Chronically Sick Children, Charité – Universitätsmedizin Berlin, Berlin, Germany, [3] Institute of Cell- and Neurobiology, Charité – Universitätsmedizin Berlin, Berlin, Germany, [4] Neuroradiology, Charité – Universitätsmedizin Berlin, Berlin, Germany, [5] Beta Neurologie – Kompetenzzentrum für Epilepsie, Beta Klinik GmbH, Bonn, Germany, [6] Pediatric Neurosurgery, Charité – Universitätsmedizin Berlin, Berlin, Germany

***Correspondence:**
Angela M. Kaindl
angela.kaindl@charite.de

Background: Neonatal drug-resistant epilepsy is often caused by perinatal epileptogenic insults such as stroke, ischemia, hemorrhage, and/or genetic defects. Rapid seizure control is particularly important for cognitive development. Since early surgical intervention and thus a short duration of epilepsy should lead to an optimal developmental outcome, we present our experience with hemispherotomy in an infant at the corrected age of 1 week.

Methods: We report successful hemispherotomy for drug-resistant epilepsy in an infant with hemimegalencephaly at a corrected age of 1 week.

Results: The infant was diagnosed with drug-resistant lesional epilepsy due to hemimegalencephaly affecting the left hemisphere. Given congruent electroclinical findings, we performed a left vertical parasagittal transventricular hemispherotomy after critical interdisciplinary discussion. No complications occurred during the surgery. Intraoperatively; 118 ml of red blood cells (30 ml/kg) and 80 ml of plasma were transfused. The patient has been seizure-free since discharge without further neurological deficits.

Conclusion: We demonstrate that early epilepsy surgery is a safe procedure in very young infants if performed in a specialized center experienced with age-specific surgical conditions and perioperative management. The specific surgical difficulties should be weighed against the risk of life-long developmental drawbacks of ongoing detrimental epilepsy.

Keywords: hemispherotomy, epilepsy surgery, epilepsy, drug-resistant epilepsy, infant, pediatrics, EEG

INTRODUCTION

Neonatal-onset drug-resistant epilepsy results from perinatal epileptogenic insults such as stroke, ischemia, hemorrhage, and/or genetic defects. Rapid seizure control is key for the cognitive developmental outcome of affected young individuals. Initial treatment always involves antiseizure medication (ASM), complemented sometimes later by medical diets to inhibit seizure activity. In about a third of all patients with epilepsy, however, two concomitantly or subsequently applied ASM fail to control seizure activity (1). The chance of achieving seizure freedom with additional ASM in these so-called drug-resistant patients is estimated to be as low as <5% (2). While epilepsy surgery can cure epilepsy in a subset of drug-resistant patients and contribute to a better development (3), the operative risk due to low weight, low blood volume and a different texture of the developing brain discourages most epilepsy centers from offering surgery in the 1st months of life. So far, there are few reports of infants aged 2–6 months or younger undergoing epilepsy surgery. The studies published so far are very heterogeneous in terms of type of surgery, surgical technique as well as age range (4–6). Given that an early surgical intervention and thus short duration of epilepsy should result in an optimal developmental outcome, we have focused on such epilepsy surgery cases. Here, we present our experience with hemispherotomy in an infant at a corrected age of 1 week.

CASE REPORT

A premature infant born at 33 weeks of gestation to non-consanguineous, healthy parents was referred to our center at the age of corrected 39 weeks (chronological age 6 weeks) for drug-resistant epilepsy. The child presented with apnea and bilateral facial clonic seizures 10 min post-partum provoking intubation and mechanical ventilation for 2 days. Focal-onset seizures affecting mainly the right-sided face and lower extremities were noted on the 7th day of life but did not respond to vitamin B6, phenobarbital, levetiracetam, and phenytoin. At the time of transfer to our intensive care unit the boy had a left-hemispheric electro-clinical status epilepticus on 55 mg/kg/d levetiracetam and 5 mg/kg/d phenobarbital, with persistent epileptic discharges over the left hemisphere with clinically visible grimacing, fasciculations, hyperextension and torsion of the upper body, and concomitant hypotension and tachycardia. An adjustment of the

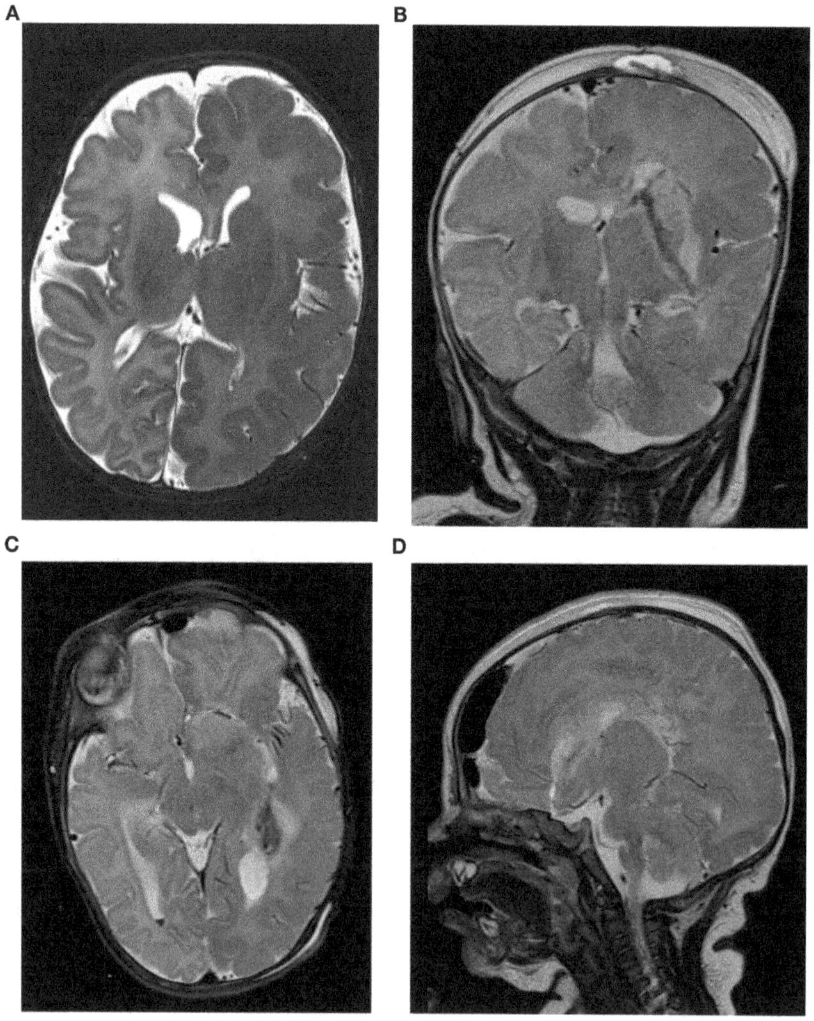

FIGURE 1 | Cranial MRI of the patient. **(A)** The presurgical axial T2-weighted image shows left hemimegalencephaly with thickened cortex, an irregular gyral pattern and abnormal T2w hypointensity of the white msatter suggestive of accelerated myelination in the entire left hemisphere. Postsurgical coronal **(B)**, axial **(C)**, and sagittal **(D)** T2-weighted images demonstrate the left sided hemispherotomy.

anticonvulsive therapy to levetiracetam (60 mg/kg/d), clobazam (0.5 mg/kg/d), lacosamide (5 mg/kg/d), and a discontinuation of phenobarbital had no sustained effect. The patient continued to have at least three seizures per day. In several VEEGs recorded over time the seizure onset could be clearly lateralized to the left hemisphere. The seizures usually start in the centroparietal and occipital region on the left side. No ictal EEG and epilepsy-typical potentials could be demarcated on the right side. Cranial MRI revealed a left-sided hemimegalencephaly with extensive gyration abnormalities, myelination abnormalities, and minor intraventricular and cortical cerebellar hemorrhage (**Figure 1A**). Standardized developmental assessment revealed age appropriate cognitive (DQ 105), language and fine and gross motor skills, using the Bayley Scales of Infant and Toddler Development 3rd ED.

Based on the above results, the infant was diagnosed with drug-resistant lesional epilepsy due to a hemimegalencephaly affecting the left hemisphere with congruent electroclinical findings. Following a critical discussion in our interdisciplinary pediatric epilepsy surgery board and with the parents, a left vertical parasagittal transventricular hemispherotomy (modified from Delalande technique) (7) under navigation and intraoperative ultrasound guidance was performed, at a corrected age of 1 week (chronological age 60 days) and a body weight of 3,920 g. Given the anatomical circumstances of narrow ventricles and a moderate midline shift due to the hemimegalencephaly surgery was particularly challenging to work in narrow corridors of dissecting the ipsilateral corpus callosum, fornix, insular, and anterior basal white matter tissue and not harming either central venous and middle cerebral arterial vasculatures. As standard in our epilepsy surgery program, an external ventricular drainage was not placed. However, no complications occurred during the surgical procedure that lasted 3 h and 48 min from incision to suture; 118 ml red blood cells (RBC) (30 ml/kg) and 80 ml plasma were transfused intraoperatively. No signs of mass occupying intracranial bleeding or edema were seen in a cranial MRI performed as part of the routine follow-up 24 h postoperatively (**Figures 1B–D**). Similarly, cranial ultrasound follow-ups performed routinely in infants post-hemispherotomy did not reveal any cerebrospinal fluid circulation problems. Postresection electrocorticography showed no epileptiform discharges on the right hemisphere. Postoperatively, the infant showed vivid bilateral movements with only a discrete right-sided muscle weakness. The patient has been seizure-free since discharge without any additional neurologic deficits at 2-month follow-up visit. The case study was approved by the Local Ethics Committee (approval no. EA2/084/18).

DISCUSSION

We demonstrate that epilepsy surgery in early infancy is a safe approach in very young infants if performed in a specialized center experienced with the age-specific surgical conditions and perisurgical management. The overall hemispherotomy-linked mortality has been reported to be 1.1% for the general epilepsy surgery population (8), and complications range from bleeding to meningoencephalitis to thrombosis and edema. Hydrocephalus occurs in 14% following hemisperotomy (8). Neurosurgery in infants is complicated by the immature brain texture and fragile vessels, the limited space in case of edema, the impact of blood loss considering the low total blood volume in infants and potential hemodynamic and coagulation problems due to RBC administration (9). However, only few cases have been reported and there is a lack of knowledge in this age group. Putative and largely unknown complications of an early intervention should be weighed against the risk of life-long developmental drawbacks of ongoing detrimental epilepsy and/or anticonvulsant therapy. However, early epilepsy surgery in infancy is receiving increased attention (10, 11). First results are promising with seizure freedom ranging from 66 to 82.7%. In a large proportion of patients, ASM can be discontinued. However, data on cognitive and functional outcome are lacking. Therefore, there is a need for prospective studies to determine the minimal requirements for epilepsy surgery in young infants to target and provide better care for these patients and to improve neurosurgical techniques for this special age group.

ETHICS STATEMENT

The studies involving human participants were reviewed and approved by the Ethics Committee at Charité - Universitätsmedizin Berlin (approval no. EA2/084/18). Written informed consent from the participants' legal guardian/next of kin was not required to participate in this study in accordance with the national legislation and the institutional requirements.

AUTHOR CONTRIBUTIONS

KM and AK contributed to conception and design of the study. KM organized the database and wrote the first draft of the manuscript. All authors discussed the results, revised the first draft, and contributed to the final manuscript.

REFERENCES

1. Kwan P, Brodie MJ. Early identification of refractory epilepsy. *N Engl J Med.* (2000) 342:314–9. doi: 10.1056/NEJM200002033420503
2. Blond BN, Hirsch LJ, Mattson RH. Misperceptions on the chance of seizure freedom with antiseizure medications after two failed trials. *Epilepsia.* (2020) 61:1789–90. doi: 10.1111/epi.16594
3. Loddenkemper T, Holland KD, Stanford LD, Kotagal P, Bingaman W, Wyllie E. Developmental outcome after epilepsy surgery in infancy. *Pediatrics.* (2007) 119:930–5. doi: 10.1542/peds.2006-2530
4. Kumar RM, Koh S, Knupp K, Handler MH, O'Neill BR. Surgery for infants with catastrophic epilepsy: an analysis of complications and efficacy. *Child's Nerv Syst.* (2015) 31:1479–91. doi: 10.1007/s00381-015-2759-6
5. Gowda S, Salazar F, Bingaman WE, Kotagal P, Lachhwani DL, Gupta A, et al. Surgery for catastrophic epilepsy in infants 6 months of age and younger. *J Neurosurg Pediatr.* (2010) 5:603–7. doi: 10.3171/2010.1.PEDS08301
6. González-Martínez JA, Gupta A, Kotagal P, Lachhwani D, Wyllie E, Lüders HO, et al. Hemispherectomy for catastrophic epilepsy in infants. *Epilepsia.* (2005) 46:1518–25. doi: 10.1111/j.1528-1167.2005.53704.x

7. Delalande O, Bulteau C, Dellatolas G, Fohlen M, Jalin C, Buret V, et al. Vertical parasagittal hemispherotomy: surgical procedures and clinical long-term outcomes in a population of 83 children. *Neurosurgery.* (2007) 60(2Suppl.1):ONS19–32. doi: 10.1227/01.NEU.0000249246.48299.12
8. Griessenauer CJ, Salam S, Hendrix P, Patel DM, Tubbs RS, Blount JP, et al. Hemispherectomy for treatment of refractory epilepsy in the pediatric age group: a systematic review. *J Neurosurg Pediatr.* (2015) 15:34–44. doi: 10.3171/2014.10.PEDS14155
9. Sood S, Asano E, Luat A. Minimizing blood loss in hemispherectomy for hemimegalencephaly in low-weight infants: technical note. *Childs Nerv Syst.* (2020) 36:841–5. doi: 10.1007/s00381-020-04534-5
10. Roth J, Constantini S, Ekstein M, Weiner HL, Tripathi M, Chandra PS, et al. Epilepsy surgery in infants up to 3 months of age: safety, feasibility, and outcomes: a multicenter, multinational study. *Epilepsia.* (2021) 62:1897–906. doi: 10.1111/epi.16959
11. Iwasaki M, Iijima K, Kawashima T, Tachimori H, Takayama Y, Kimura Y, et al. Epilepsy surgery in children under 3 years of age: surgical and developmental outcomes. *J Neurosurg Pediatr.* (2021) 28:395–403. doi: 10.3171/2021.4.PEDS21123

3

Case Report: A Case of Concomitant Paroxysmal Kinesigenic Dyskinesia and Epilepsy: Can we Treat Two Birds with One Stone?

*Jun-Hong Geng, Yang Zheng, Quan-Fu Li, Qun Hou, Xiao-Hang Wang and Yan Jiang**

Department of Neurology, The First Affiliated Hospital of Zhejiang Chinese Medical University, Hangzhou, China

Correspondence:
Yan Jiang
jiangyan@zcmu.edu.cn

Background: Paroxysmal kinesigenic dyskinesia (PKD) is characterized by recurrent episodes of movement-induced motor attacks. PKD patients may have concomitant epilepsy. Differentiation between the two disorders and effective control of both diseases remain challenging.

Case Presentation: We present a Chinese girl with typical manifestations of PKD, who also suffered from generalized tonic-clonic seizure attacks at the same time. Genetic testing confirmed a *PRRT2* mutation (c.649dupC). Oxcarbazepine was initially used, but withdrawn due to a hypersensitivity reaction. Levetiracetam was initiated afterwards, which was effective for seizures but failed to control her PKD symptoms. The addition of lacosamide (LCM) completely controlled her PKD symptoms.

Conclusion: This is the first case reporting the effectiveness of LCM for concomitant PKD and epilepsy. Our case proposes a novel alternative for such patients who are resistant or cannot tolerate conventional anti-sodium antiepileptics.

Keywords: lacosamide, paroxysmal kinesigenic dyskinesia, epilepsy, movement disorder, PRRT2

INTRODUCTION

Paroxysmal Kinesigenic Dyskinesia (PKD) is a rare disease characterized by recurrent, sudden attacks of dystonia, chorea, ballistic, and athetoid involuntary movements, which are triggered by sudden voluntary movements (1). The diagnosis of PKD is mainly based on features including movement-induced attacks with a short duration, reserved consciousness, a dramatic antiepileptic drug (AED) responsiveness and a positive family history or proline-rich transmembrane protein 2 (*PRRT2*) mutation (2). It has been reported that 8% of PKD had concomitant epilepsy (3). Despite its rarity, patients with concomitant PKD and epilepsy remain the biggest challenge, since a correct diagnosis remain difficult and a proportion were reported to be resistant to AEDs treatment (4, 5).

The first challenge in managing patients with both PKD and epilepsy lie in the diagnosis, given the similar presentations as paroxysmal recurrent motor attacks. Two-thirds of patients with PKD was misdiagnosed with epilepsy (3). The other challenge is treatment. Effective drugs remain unknown for patients with both PKD and epilepsy. Previous reports mostly use a trial-and-error strategy when choosing drugs, which might bring extra stress and economic burdens.

In this study, we described a 15-year-old Chinese girl, who carried a *PRRT2* gene mutation, presenting with concomitant PKD and epilepsy. Her movement symptoms had an excellent response to LCM. We also summarized previous reports on concomitant PKD and epilepsy, hoping to address the diagnostic and therapeutic challenges in such patients.

CASE REPORT

The 15-year-old girl was born at 38 weeks of gestation by vaginal delivery to a pair of non-consanguineous Chinese parents. She was the only child and her prenatal period was uneventful. Her growth and developmental milestones were normal.

At age of 5, she suffered from a seizure at sleep in the early morning, characterized by limb twitching and jerking, with loss of consciousness, which lasted for 3 min. She complained of weakness and headache after the attack. She was subsequently sent to the hospital where the electroencephalogram (EEG) and magnetic resonance imaging (MRI) were both non-revealing. At the age of 8, she presented with paroxysms of abnormal involuntary posturing of both hands, ranging from a few seconds to 1 min. The episodes were mostly triggered by sudden movement or emotional stress. Her consciousness was fully preserved during the attacks. Her family history was negative for seizures. However, her mother had dyskinesia after sudden movements when she was young, such as suddenly standing up or running. Her mother's symptoms completely disappeared after the age of 16. Additionally, her mother's younger sister and cousin had similar dyskinesia.

The girl went to a tertiary hospital and was diagnosed with PKD at the age of 10. She was initially treated with oxcarbazepine, which unfortunately, caused an allergic reaction in the form of skin rashes. Levetiracetam was initiated, with an initial dose of

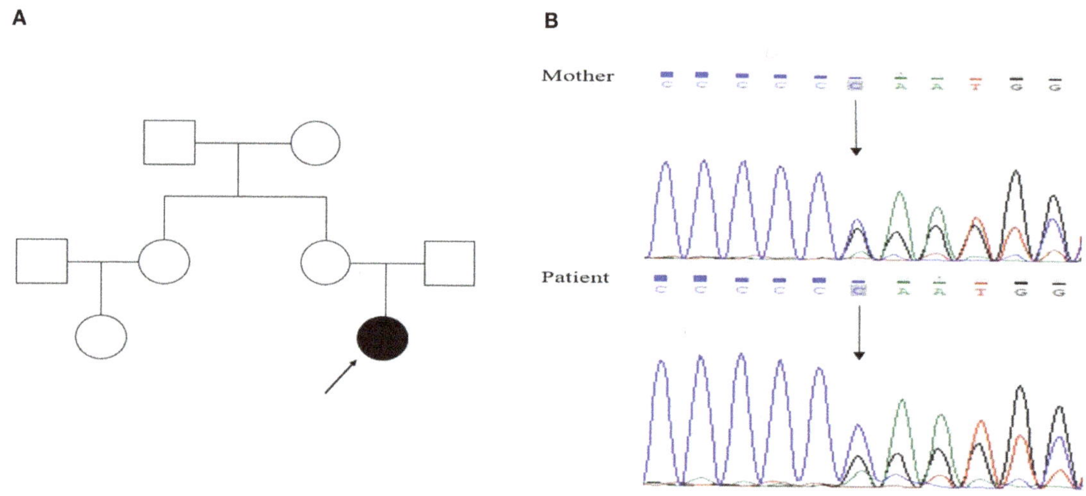

FIGURE 1 | (A) Family pedigree of the proband (filled symbols represent the patient, open symbols normal persons, index case indicated by arrow); **(B)** genetic analysis showed that both the patient and her mother had a heterozygous mutation, c.649dupC, in the *PRRT2* gene.

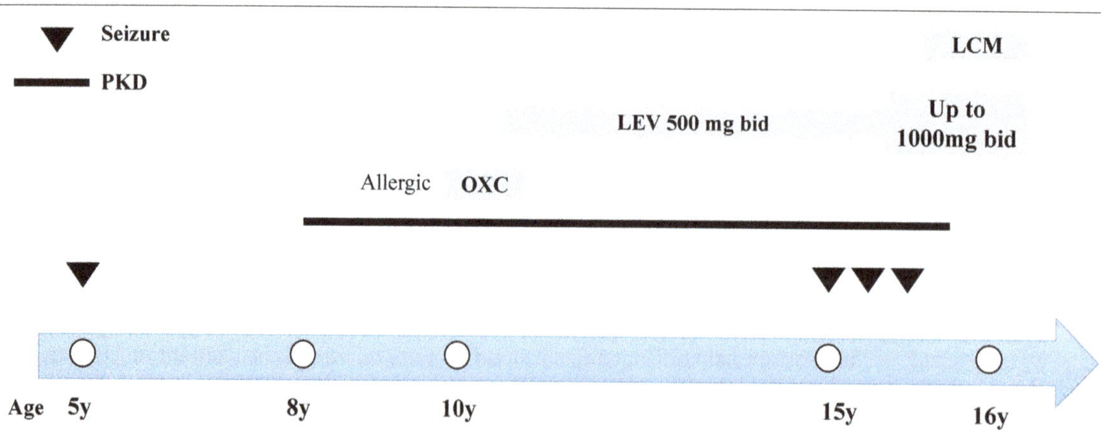

FIGURE 2 | Clinical course and treatment of the case. The x-axis indicates the age of patient at each attack. Epileptic seizures are indicated by inverted triangles. The course of PKD is denoted by the black line. The name, dosage and timing of drug treatment are shown at the top of the diagram. bid, twice daily; LCM, lacosamide; LEV, levetiracetam; OXC, oxcarbazepine.

500 mg twice daily. However, she still had paroxysmal dystonia despite the levetiracetam treatment, with a frequency of about once per week.

At the age of 15, she suffered from another seizure at sleep in the early morning, characterized by limb twitching and jerking with loss of consciousness, which lasted for around 3 min. Weakness and headache were reported after the attack. EEG at an outside institute showed the presence of scattered theta waves, sharp waves and sharp slow waves induced by hyperventilation. Long-term EEG showed intermittent bilateral frontal slowing. Neurologic examinations and brain MRI were normal at that time. Similarly, she experienced two grand mal seizures in the next month, both at sleep in the early morning. Dosage of levetiracetam was increased to 1,000 mg twice daily. However, the paroxysmal dystonia persisted. The diagnosis of concomitant PKD and epilepsy was considered. Genetic testing revealed a heterozygous frameshift mutation of c.649dupC (p.Arg217Profs*8) (**Figure 1**). LCM, at a dose of 50 mg twice daily, was added to the previous treatment. The patient responded excellently to the treatment. Neither dystonia nor seizures recurred after the LCM treatment (**Figure 2**). No adverse effects such as cardiac abnormalities and mental disorders were observed. The patient remained free of both PKD and seizures at the last follow-up 10 months after the initiation of LCM.

DISCUSSION

Herein, we report a case of an adolescent female who had concomitant PKD and epilepsy with a *PRRT2* mutation (c.649dupC). The diagnostic pearls for patients with episodic motor attacks are listed. We also discuss managements for patients with concomitant PKD and epilepsy. The excellent efficacy of even low-dose LCM highlights a new therapeutic option for such patients.

The first challenge in our case lies in the correct diagnosis of PKD and epilepsy. Both disorders can present with recurrent movements and both have a good initial response to anti-sodium-channel AEDs, though epilepsy patients would develop drug resistance later in disease course (6). To differentiate PKD and epilepsy, a careful history taking is vital. Certain ancillary testing including EEG, MRI and genetic testing would be helpful as well. PKD has an age of onset between 1 and 20 years of age with attacks consistently triggered by sudden movements, sometimes in the context of emotional, or physiologic stress (7). Kinesigenic paroxysmal movements in PKD are short and frequent. The patient has a reserved consciousness during attacks. Neurological examination and EEG are always normal (1). Epileptic seizures can mimic PKD as well, though seizure attacks are highly stereotyped and may occur during sleep. Mutations in *SCN8A*, *CHRNA4*, *KCNT1*, and *DEPDC5* were associated with epilepsy (8, 9), while *PRRT2* mutation was frequently related to PKD. In this patient, the movement-induced motor attacks are diagnosed with PKD, given the presence of triggers like sudden movements or emotional stress, the normal results on repeated MRI, a positive family history and the presence of *PRRT2* mutation.

TABLE 1 | Clinical characteristics of previously-reported patients with concomitant PKD and epilepsy.

References	Sex	Age at onset of epilepsy	Age at onset of PKD	Symptomatology	Family history of PKD	Brain CT or MRI	Scalp EEG	Causative gene	Ineffective drugs	Effective drugs
Whitty et al. (4)	Male	12y	13y	GTCS	No	–	Sharp wave	–	PMD+ PB	PMD+PHT
Hudgins et al. (13)	Female	13y	Infancy	GTCS	–	–	Normal	–	–	MPB+PHT
	Male	5y	8m	GTCS	Yes	–	Normal	–	–	MPB+PHT
	Female	11y	2y	GTCS	Yes	–	Normal	–	–	MPB+PHT
Jung et al. (14)	Male	8y	3y	GTCS	Yes	–	Normal	–	–	PHT+PB
Tan et al. (3)	Male	12y	12y	GTCS	Yes	Normal	Normal	–	–	PHT
	Male	16y	4.5y	GTCS	No	–	Spike-and-wave	–	–	PB
Guerrini et al. (5)	Female	2y6m	3m	Absence	No	Normal	Spike-and-wave	–	VPA, CBZ,	LTG+ESM
Cuenca et al. (15)	Female	4m	–	GTCS	Yes	Normal	Normal	–	BZDs,	PB
	Male	–	–	GTCS	Yes	Normal	Normal	–	LTG+TPM	CBZ
Prashantha et al. (16)	Male	23y	18y	GTCS	No	Calcifications	Normal	–	–	Ca, Vit D, CBZ
Seo SY et al. (17)	Female	7y	6m	Hypotonic	Yes	Normal	CTS	*PRRT2*	–	
Tanabe Y et al. (18)	Female	–	14y	GTCS	No	Normal	Slow wave	*PRRT2*	PHT	
Zhang et al. (19)	Male	8y	9y	GTCS	No	Calcifications	Sharp wave, sharp slow wave	–	–	OXC
									CZP, LEV	CBZ
									–	Ca, Vit D, CBZ

GTCS, generalized tonic-clonic seizures; PMD, primidone; PB, phenobarbital; PHT, phenytoin; MPB, mephobarbital; VPA, valproate; CBZ, carbamazepine; BZDs, benzodiazepines; LTG, lamotrigine; TPM, topiramate; ESM, ethosuximide; OXC, oxcarbazepine; CZP, clonazepam; Ca, calcium; Vit D, vitamin D; LEV, levetiracetam; CTS, centrotemporal spike.

The recurrent generalized tonic-clonic attacks all at night and presence of post-attack headache pointed toward the diagnosis of epilepsy. However, we did not further investigate the etiology of epilepsy considering the financial burdens of the patient. Herein, given a thorough history taking and evidence from EEG and genetic evidence, we diagnose the patient with concomitant PKD and epilepsy.

PKD is characterized by an exquisite response to antiepileptic drugs. First line treatments are carbamazepine, oxcarbazepine and phenytoin (1, 10). A dramatic response to antiepileptic drugs is seen in 98.4% of *PRRT2*-PKD patients (7). Treatment failure was mainly reported in homozygous or compound heterozygous *PRRT2* mutation carriers (11, 12). Importantly, effective treatments to control both PKD and epilepsy remain undetermined, as shown in **Table 1** (3–5, 13–19). Allergic reactions to certain AEDs like carbamazepine or oxcarbazepine further limited their use in such patients. Therapeutic options, both safe and efficacious, are urgently needed for those with concomitant PKD and epilepsy.

LCM is a third-generation antiepileptic drug, with unique mechanisms of enhancing the slow inactivation of voltage-gated sodium channels. Unlike other traditional sodium channel blockers such as phenytoin and carbamazepine which inhibit the fast inactivation of the channels, LCM mainly reduces the long-term availability of sodium channels for activation, resulting in the normalization of activation thresholds (20). Mathew et al. reported a 19-year-old boy with PKD, who was responsive to LCM treatment (at a dose of 50 mg twice daily) after a hypersensitivity reaction of oxcarbazepine (21). Another recent retrospective study included four children with PKD, one of them had a *PRRT2* mutation (c.649dupC). The low dose of LCM showed an excellent efficacy in all children, regardless of the status of *PRRT2* mutations (22). However, large sampled studies on the correlation between *PRRT2* mutations and LCM response is lacking. Our patient with concomitant *PRRT2*-positive PKD and epilepsy had a good response to even low-dose LCM after an allergic reaction to oxcarbazepine and treatment failure with levetiracetam. Our case further demonstrated the efficacy of low-dose LCM in patients with concomitant PKD and epilepsy, offering an optimal and safe therapeutic option for such patients.

To our knowledge, this is the first case using LCM for concomitant *PRRT2* PKD and epilepsy. We suggest that the use of low-dose LCM might be an efficacious, safe and tolerable option for such patients. Further studies with a large cohort are needed to confirm our findings, especially those who are allergic or unresponsive to carbamazepine and oxcarbazepine.

ETHICS STATEMENT

The studies involving human participants were reviewed and approved by Ethics Committee of the First Affiliated Hospital of Zhejiang Chinese Medical University. Written informed consent to participate in this study was provided by the participants' legal guardian/next of kin.

AUTHOR CONTRIBUTIONS

J-HG drafting of the article, clinical examination of the patient, and bibliographic search. YZ and YJ conceptualized and designed the study, coordinated and supervised data collection and analyzation, and critically reviewed and revised the manuscript. Q-FL, QH, and X-HW contributed to conception and design of the study. All authors contributed to the article and approved the submitted version.

ACKNOWLEDGMENTS

We warmly thank the patient and her family. J-HG wants to thank, in particular, the care and support from Yi-Kang Sun over passed years.

REFERENCES

1. Bruno MK, Hallett M, Gwinn-Hardy K, Sorensen B, Considine E, Tucker S, et al. Clinical evaluation of idiopathic paroxysmal kinesigenic dyskinesia: new diagnostic criteria. *Neurology.* (2004) 63:2280–7. doi: 10.1212/01.wnl.0000147298.05983.50
2. Huang XJ, Wang SG, Guo XN, Tian WT, Zhan FX, Zhu ZY, et al. The phenotypic and genetic spectrum of paroxysmal kinesigenic dyskinesia in China. *Mov Disord.* (2020) 35:1428–37. doi: 10.1002/mds.28061
3. Tan LC, Tan AK, Tjia H. Paroxysmal kinesigenic choreoathetosis in Singapore and its relationship to epilepsy. *Clin Neurol Neurosurg.* (1998) 100:187–92. doi: 10.1016/s0303-8467(98)00038-9
4. Whitty CW, Lishman WA, Fitzgibbon JP. Seizures induced by movement:a form of reflex epilepsy. *Lancet.* (1964) 2:1403–6. doi: 10.1016/s0140-6736(64)91980-4
5. Guerrini R, Sanchez-Carpintero R, Deonna T, Santucci M, Bhatia KP, Moreno T, et al. Early-onset absence epilepsy and paroxysmal dyskinesia. *Epilepsia.* (2002) 43:1224–9. doi: 10.1046/j.1528-1157.2002.13802.x
6. Löscher W, Potschka H, Sisodiya SM, Vezzani A. Drug resistance in epilepsy: clinical impact, potential mechanisms, and new innovative treatment options. *Pharmacol Rev.* (2020) 72:606–38. doi: 10.1124/pr.120.019539
7. Huang XJ, Wang T, Wang JL, Liu XL, Che XQ, Li J, et al. Paroxysmal kinesigenic dyskinesia: clinical and genetic analyses of 110 patients. *Neurology.* (2015) 85:1546–53. doi: 10.1212/wnl.0000000000002079
8. de Gusmão CM, Garcia L, Mikati MA, Su S, Silveira-Moriyama L. Paroxysmal genetic movement disorders and epilepsy. *Front Neurol.* (2021) 12:648031. doi: 10.3389/fneur.2021.648031
9. Freitas ME, Ruiz-Lopez M, Dalmau J, Erro R, Privitera M, Andrade D, et al. Seizures and movement disorders: phenomenology, diagnostic challenges and therapeutic approaches. *J Neurol Neurosurg Psychiatry.* (2019) 90:920–8. doi: 10.1136/jnnp-2018-320039
10. Yang Y, Su Y, Guo Y, Ding Y, Xu S, Jiang Y, et al. Oxcarbazepine versus carbamazepine in the treatment of paroxysmal kinesigenic dyskinesia. *Int J Neurosci.* (2012) 122:719–22. doi: 10.3109/00207454.2012.715109
11. Labate A, Tarantino P, Viri M, Mumoli L, Gagliardi M, Romeo A, et al. Homozygous c.649dupC mutation in PRRT2 worsens the BFIS/PKD phenotype with mental retardation, episodic ataxia, and absences. *Epilepsia.* (2012) 53:e196–9. doi: 10.1111/epi.12009
12. Delcourt M, Riant F, Mancini J, Milh M, Navarro V, Roze E, et al. Severe phenotypic spectrum of biallelic mutations in PRRT2 gene. *J Neurol Neurosurg Psychiatry.* (2015) 86:782–5. doi: 10.1136/jnnp-2014-309025
13. Hudgins RL, Corbin KB. An uncommon seizure disorder: familial paroxysmal choreoathetosis. *Brain.* (1966) 89:199–204. doi: 10.1093/brain/89.2.199

14. Jung SS, Chen KM, Brody KA. Paroxysmal choreoathetosis. Report of Chinese cases. *Neurology.* (1973) 23:749–55. doi: 10.1212/wnl.23.7.749
15. Cuenca-Leon E, Cormand B, Thomson T, Macaya A. Paroxysmal kinesigenic dyskinesia and generalized seizures: clinical and genetic analysis in a Spanish pedigree. *Neuropediatrics.* (2002) 33:288–93. doi: 10.1055/s-2002-37079
16. Prashantha DK, Pal PK. Pseudohypoparathyroidism manifesting with paroxysmal dyskinesias and seizures. *Mov Disord.* (2009) 24:623–4. doi: 10.1002/mds.22382
17. Seo SY, You SJ. Paroxysmal kinesigenic dyskinesia in a patient with a PRRT2 mutation and centrotemporal spike discharges on electroencephalogram: case report of a 10-year-old girl. *Korean J Pediatr.* (2016) 59:S157–60. doi: 10.3345/kjp.2016.59.11.S157
18. Tanabe Y, Taira T, Shimotake A, Inoue T, Awaya T, Kato T, et al. An adult female with proline-rich transmembrane protein 2 related paroxysmal disorders manifesting paroxysmal kinesigenic choreoathetosis and epileptic seizures. *Rinsho Shinkeigaku.* (2019) 59:144–8. doi: 10.5692/clinicalneurol.cn-001228
19. Zhang C, Zhou X, Feng M, Yue W. Paroxysmal dyskinesia and epilepsy in pseudohypoparathyroidism. *Mol Genet Genomic Med.* (2020) 8:e1423. doi: 10.1002/mgg3.1423
20. Rogawski MA, Tofighy A, White HS, Matagne A, Wolff C. Current understanding of the mechanism of action of the antiepileptic drug lacosamide. *Epilepsy Res.* (2015) 110:189–205. doi: 10.1016/j.eplepsyres.2014.11.021
21. Mathew T, Aroor S, Nadig R, Sarma GR. Lacosamide in paroxysmal kinesigenic dyskinesia. *Mov Disord.* (2012) 27:801–2. doi: 10.1002/mds.24928
22. Furukawa G, Negishi Y, Takeuchi T, Ishihara N, Okumura A. Important aspects to consider for patients with episodic motor attacks are listed. *Brain Dev.* (2020) 42:617–20. doi: 10.1016/j.braindev.2020.04.009

4

Case Report: Stereoelectroencephalography and Stereoelectroencephalography-Guided Radiofrequency Thermocoagulation in Familial Lateral Temporal Lobe Epilepsy

Ziqi Wei[1], *Xiaolai Ye*[2,3], *Changquan Wang*[3], *Jiwen Xu*[2,3], *Puming Zhang*[1]*, *Qiangqiang Liu*[2,3]* *and Jun Zhao*[1]

[1] School of Biomedical Engineering, Shanghai Jiao Tong University, Shanghai, China, [2] Department of Neurosurgery, Clinical Neuroscience Center Comprehensive Epilepsy Unit, Ruijin Hospital, Shanghai Jiao Tong University School of Medicine, Shanghai, China, [3] Clinical Neuroscience Center, Ruijin Hospital Luwan Branch, Shanghai Jiao Tong University School of Medicine, Shanghai, China

***Correspondence:**
Puming Zhang
pmzhang@sjtu.edu.cn
Qiangqiang Liu
windsto@163.com

Familial lateral temporal lobe epilepsy (FLTLE) is genetic focal epilepsy usually characterised by auditory symptoms. Most FLTLE cases can be controlled by anti-seizure medications, and to our best knowledge, there are no previous reports about stereoelectroencephalography (SEEG) used for patients with FLTLE. In this report, we present two patients with FLTLE in one family and their SEEG performances, together with ^{18}F-fluorodeoxyglucose (^{18}F-FDG) PET and MRI results. In case 1, fast activities originated from the right superior temporal gyrus and spread rapidly to the right anterior insular lobe and hippocampus. In case 2, there were two seizure patterns: (1) The fast activities or sharp slow waves were identified at the left superior temporal gyrus, then, sharp waves and spike waves spread in the left superior temporal gyrus; (2) There were fast activities and slow-wave oscillation originated in the left superior temporal gyrus, then, the fast activities spread in the left superior temporal gyrus and finally spread to the other sites. An SEEG-guided radiofrequency thermocoagulation was performed for both patients and one of them underwent resection surgery. Seizures are well-controlled and the patients are very satisfied with the therapeutic effects.

Keywords: superior temporal gyrus, stereoelectroencephalography-guided radiofrequency thermocoagulation, stereoelectroencephalography, familial lateral temporal lobe epilepsy, case report

INTRODUCTION

Familial lateral temporal lobe epilepsy (FLTLE) is genetic focal epilepsy usually characterised by auditory symptoms. Despite the complexity of FLTLE, it is generally considered as a benign epilepsy syndrome and routinely used anti-seizure medications can usually control seizures (1).

Stereoelectroencephalography (SEEG) is a methodology for presurgical invasive evaluation and SEEG-guided radiofrequency thermocoagulation (RFTC) can be used as an alternative to resection surgery. Using stereotactically implanted electrodes, SEEG provides neuronal electrical activities recordings in the deep brain (2) and helps locate epileptogenic zone for thermocoagulation or resection surgery (3). Most FLTLE seizures can be controlled by anti-seizure medications, and there are no previous reports about SEEG being used in the treatment of patients with FLTLE. Here we report two refractory FLTLE cases in one family. SEEG and SEEG-guided RFTC were performed for both patients and one of them underwent resection surgery. Seizures are well-controlled and the patients are very satisfied with the therapeutic effects.

CASE REPORT

Case 1

A 47-year-old woman, with her grandmother and her son, was diagnosed with FLTLE. Seizures firstly occurred when she was 22, with the symptoms of a sudden loss of consciousness, daze, delayed movements, chewing, and hand groping-like movements. Genetic tests were refused.

In scalp electroencephalogram (EEG), interictal spikes and intermittent slow waves were observed in the bilateral anterior temporal region and sphenoidal electrode. Seizures were characterised by initial attenuation of background activity followed by low-voltage fast activity in the right temporal-occipital lobe, then, quickly spread to the right and left temporal lobe.

No abnormality was found in 3.0T T1-weighted (voxel space $= 2 \times 2 \times 2$ mm^3, TR $=$ 381 ms, TE $=$ 2.3 ms), T2-weighted (voxel space $= 2 \times 2 \times 2$ mm^3, TR $=$ 3,000 ms, TE $=$ 100 ms) or fluid-attenuated inversion recovery (FLAIR) (voxel space$=2 \times 2 \times 2$ mm^3, TR $=$ 4,800 ms, TE $=$ 411.7 ms) MRI. The ^{18}F-fluorodeoxyglucose (^{18}F-FDG) PET results were characterised by hypometabolism in the right superior temporal gyrus, right medial temporal lobe (**Figure 1**), and right insular lobe. The SEEG was performed, and the positions of electrodes were shown in **Figure 2**.

The SEEG in the interictal period showed obvious fast activities in the right superior temporal gyrus and the right anterior insular lobe. In the ictal period, fast activities originated from the right superior temporal gyrus (N1-8) and spread rapidly to the right anterior insular lobe (I3-8) and hippocampus (H1-3, B1-3) (**Figure 1B**).

The SEEG-guided RFTC was performed at electrodes N1-8 (**Figure 1B**), but there was no significant seizure decrease after the RFTC. She underwent the right anteromedial temporal lobe and insular lobe resection. The postoperative T1-weighted MRI results are shown in **Figure 3A**. Follow-up results showed that in the next 2 years, only one seizure occurred in 3 months after the operation.

Case 2

Case 2 was a son of case 1, with normal delivery and no nervous system injury. The first seizure occurred at the age of 19, with limb tonic seizures at the frequency of about once a month. When he came to our hospital at 24, he felt dizzy and cannot understand other people's language, then, he experienced consciousness loss, bilateral upper limbs flexion, and elicited mouth movements. Genetic tests showed an abnormality in the microtubule-associated protein tau (MAPT) gene and linked it to chr17:44060593.

Scalp EEG showed that the epileptiform activities mainly occurred in the left sphenoidal electrode and frontotemporal region. Ictal EEG was characterised by initial attenuation, followed by rhythmic 5–6 Hz activities in the left sphenoidal electrode and frontotemporal region.

No abnormality was found in MRI results with the same scanning parameters as in case 1. The PET results suggested hypometabolism in the left superior temporal gyrus, left supramarginal gyrus, and inferior central gyrus (**Figure 4A**).

The SEEG in the interictal period showed obvious abnormal discharges in the left superior temporal gyrus, which then affected the lateral temporal lobe. Two types of seizure patterns were identified.

In the first seizure pattern, the patient felt dizzy and had auditory hallucinations. The seizures were then followed by daze, wink, and chewing. During this pattern, fast activities or sharp slow waves were identified at the left superior temporal gyrus (N'3-5), then, sharp waves and spike waves spread in the left superior temporal gyrus (N'2-8, W'5-10, X'4-8), as shown in **Figure 4B**.

The second seizure pattern was characterised by feeling uncomfortable, groaning, right and then both upper limbs tonic seizures, right-turning head, and, finally, secondarily generalised tonic-clonic seizures. There were fast activities and slow-wave oscillation at the left superior temporal gyrus (N'3-5), then, the fast activities spread in the left superior temporal gyrus (W'2-9, N'2-6) and, finally, spread to the other sites (**Figure 4C**).

The RFTC was performed at electrodes W'1-10, N'1-8, and X'1-10. The T1-weighted MRI results after the RFTC are shown in **Figure 3B**. According to the last follow-up at 18 months after the RFTC, he remained seizure-free (Engel 1A).

DISCUSSION

Familial temporal lobe epilepsy (FTLE) can be subdivided into lateral and mesial forms by clinical and genetic characteristics, and FLTLE is characterised by auditory auras (1). Several protein mutations were considered to be associated with temporal lobe epilepsy, such as axon guidance proteins, leucine-rich glioma inactivated 1 protein, microtubular protein, pore-forming, chromatin remodelling, and chemokine proteins (4). Hyperphosphorylated tau protein has been identified in patients with refractory temporal lobe epilepsy and might be the cause of the cognitive decline in these patients (5). Given that there were no other genetic abnormalities detected in case 2, we suppose that MAPT mutation played a role in the case of FLTLE. However, such supposition still needs further verification.

For patients with FTLE, most of the reports mentioned that they had a good response to anti-seizure medications, and the disease would be gradually controlled with the increase of age. Cendes et al. (6) reported 36 FTLE cases, including eight with refractory epilepsy who underwent surgery. Fabera et al. (7) also reported two FTLE cases that underwent left

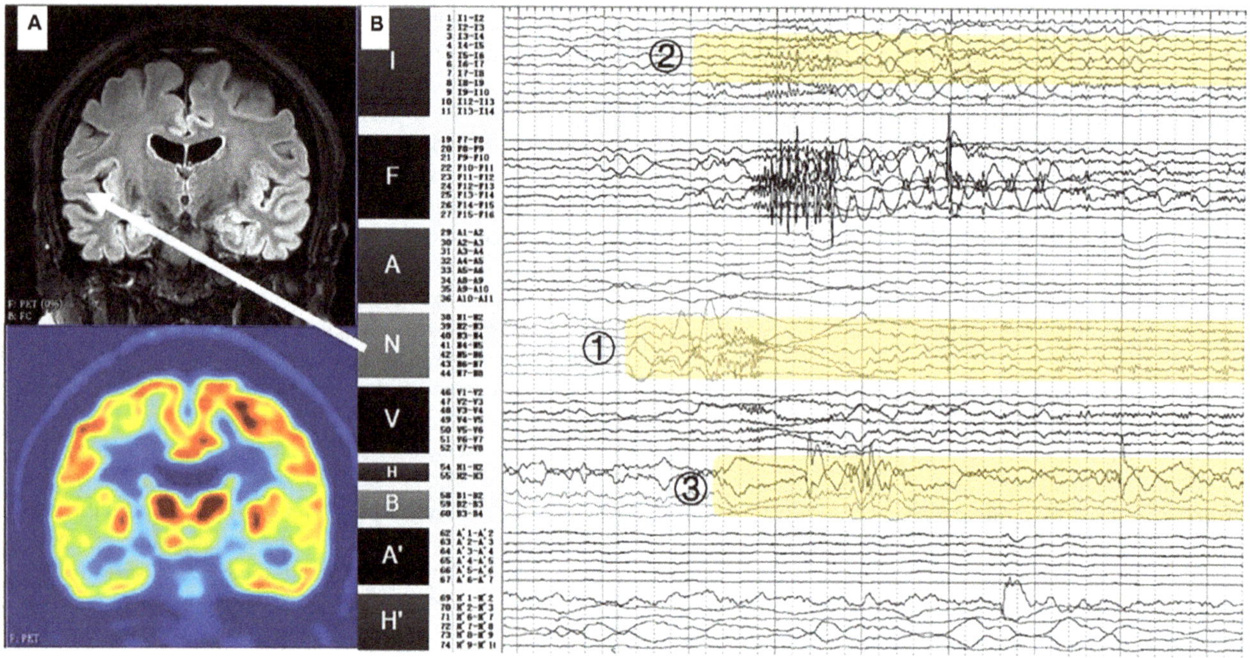

FIGURE 1 | (A) T1-weighted MRI and PET results of case 1. No abnormality was found in MRI, while hypometabolism was identified in the right superior temporal gyrus. **(B)** Stereoelectroencephalography (SEEG) signals in the ictal period. Fast activities originated from the right superior temporal gyrus ① (N1-8) and spread rapidly to the right insular lobe ② (I3-8) and hippocampus ③ (H1-3, B1-3). White arrow: the location of the electrodes N in MRI (right superior temporal gyrus).

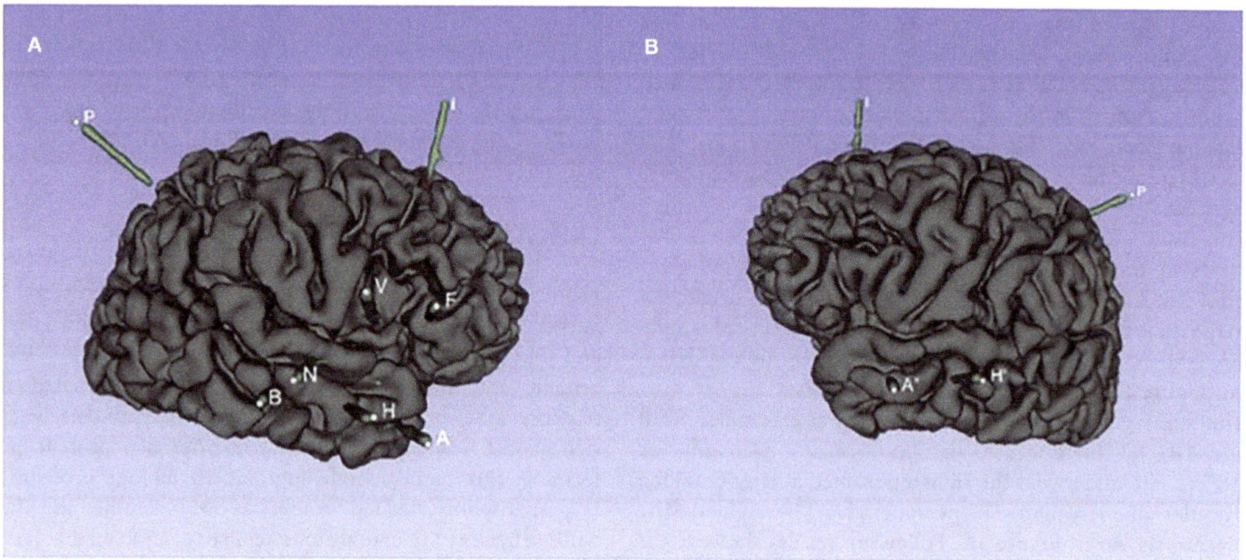

FIGURE 2 | The spatial position of SEEG electrodes of case 1. **(A)** Right hemisphere. Entry points to target points: A: the middle temporal gyrus to the amygdala; H: the middle temporal gyrus to the head of the hippocampus; B: the middle temporal gyrus to the middle of the hippocampus; N: the superior temporal gyrus to the posterior insular gyrus; V: opercular partis to the short gyri of insula; F: pars triangularis to anterior cingulated cortex; I: the middle frontal gyrus to the accessory gyrus; P: the supramarginal gyrus to the anterior insular gyrus. **(B)** Left hemisphere. Entry points to target points: A′: the middle temporal gyrus to the amygdala; H′: the middle temporal gyrus to the head of the hippocampus.

anteromedial temporal lobectomy. Koizumi et al. (8) reported five refractory epilepsy cases in one family. Among them, four patients underwent bilateral subdural electrode implantation and resection, two patients underwent standard anterior temporal lobectomy and two underwent lateral temporal lobectomy, and all of them were rated as Engel 1 after the operation. The cases

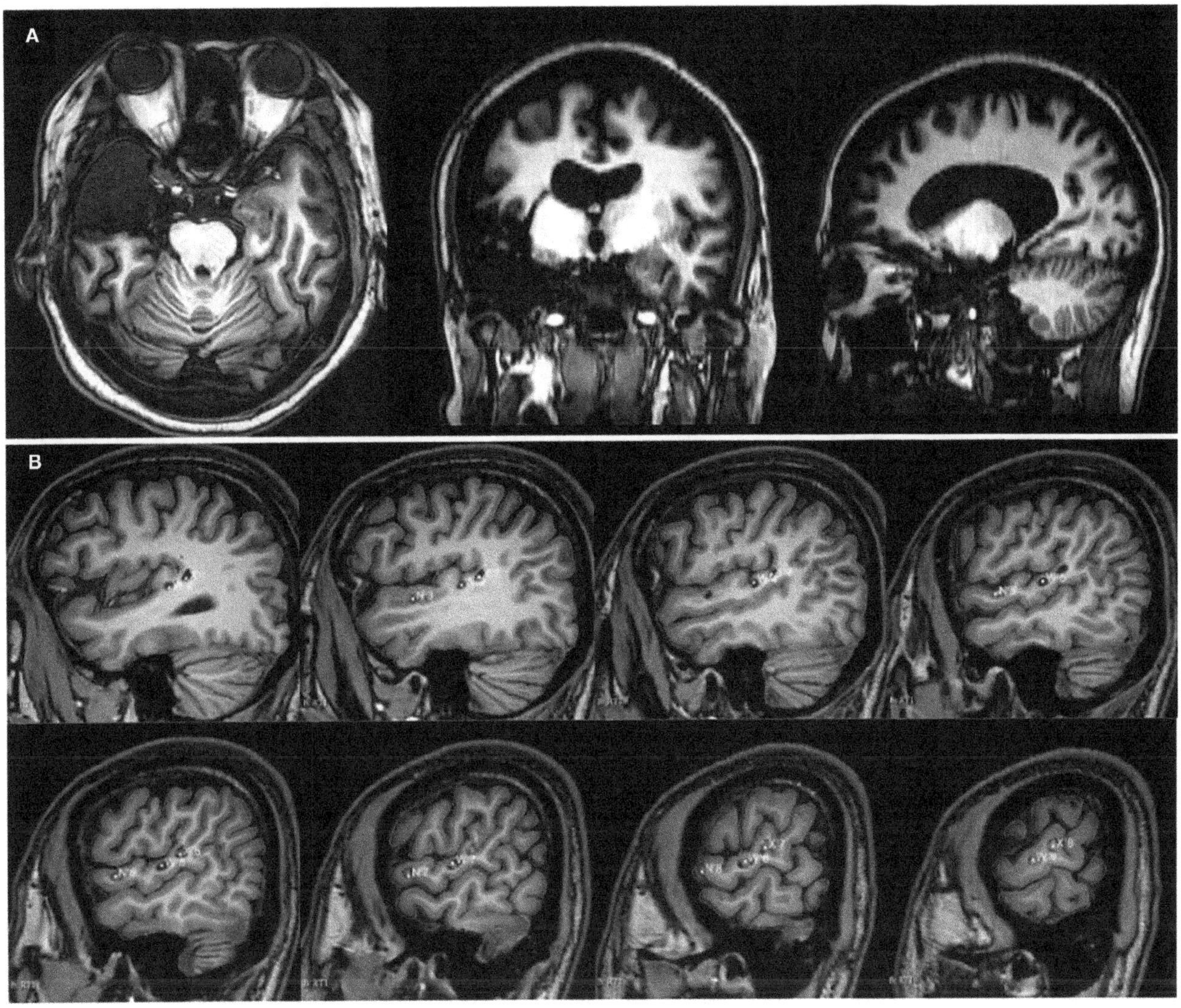

FIGURE 3 | Postoperative T1-weighted MRI results. **(A)** T1-weighted MRI results of case 1 after the right anteromedial temporal lobe and insular lobe resection. **(B)** T1-weighted MRI results of case 2 after SEEG-guided radiofrequency thermocoagulation (RFTC). The locations and labels of the electrodes for the thermocoagulation were marked in blue.

reported in this paper also showed that surgery has a good effect on patients with refractory FLTLE.

According to the results of SEEG and clinical information, the superior temporal gyrus was confirmed as the onset area, and SEEG-guided RFTC was performed. However, only case 2 had a significant curative effect. The SEEG signal can provide effective information to locate the epileptogenic zone, but by the limited number of electrodes and the range of thermocoagulation, SEEG-guided RFTC may easily miss the epileptogenic zone. Koizumi et al. (8) reported two cases, whose epileptic focuses were located in the superior temporal gyrus by electrocorticographic results, one case in the lateral temporal lobe (including the superior temporal gyrus) and the other in the inferior temporal gyrus and fusiform gyrus. Whether these results suggest that the epileptic focus of FLTLE located in the superior temporal lobe still needs more clinical results to confirm. We identified three different seizure spreading patterns: (1) pure superior temporal gyrus with auditory symptoms; (2) mesial temporal lobe with automatisms; and (3) frontal lobe with movement symptoms.

Interestingly, the epileptic focus in case 1 is located in the right superior temporal gyrus, whereas the one in case 2 is located in the left superior temporal gyrus. In the FLTLE family reported by Koizumi et al., the three patients' epilepsy focuses were located on the left side and one on the right (8). The invasive EEG monitoring results suggest that, although FLTLE is an autosomal dominant genetic disease, the side of epileptic focus is not fixed.

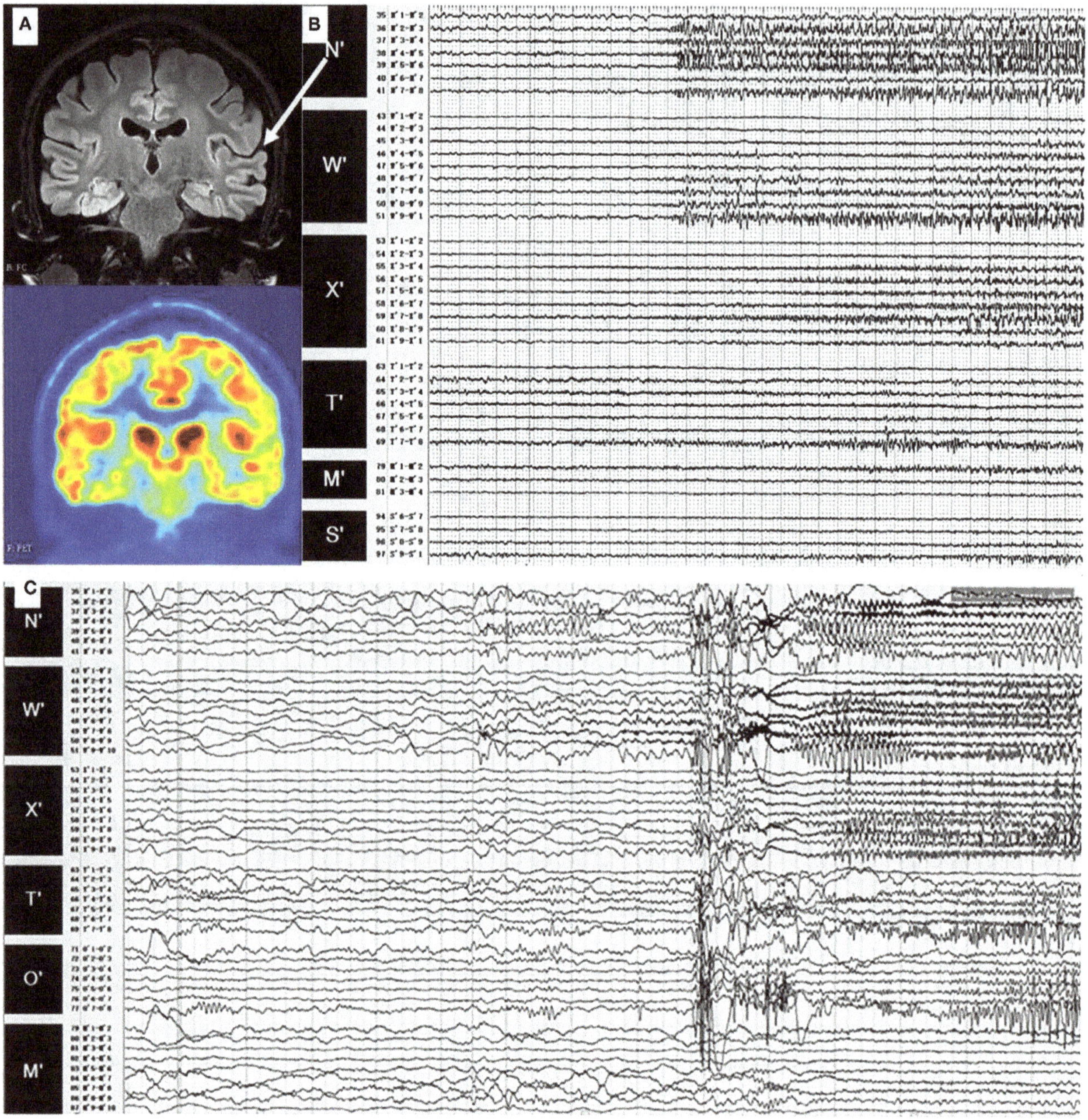

FIGURE 4 | (A) Preoperative T1-weighted MRI and PET results of case 2. No abnormality was found in MRI, while hypometabolism was identified in the left superior temporal gyrus. **(B)** SEEG signals of the first seizure pattern. During this pattern, fast activities or sharp slow waves were identified at the left superior temporal gyrus (N′3-5), then sharp waves and spike waves spread in the left superior temporal gyrus (N′2-8, W′5-10, X′4-8). **(C)** SEEG signals of the second seizure pattern. There were fast activities and slow-wave oscillation at the left superior temporal gyrus (N′3-5), then the fast activities spread in the left superior temporal gyrus (W′2-9, N′2-6), and finally, spread to the other sites. White arrow: the location of the electrodes N′ in MRI (left superior temporal gyrus).

ETHICS STATEMENT

The studies involving human participants were reviewed and approved by the Ruijin Hospital Luwan Branch Ethics Committee, Shanghai Jiao Tong University School of Medicine. The patients/participants provided their written informed consent to participate in this study. Written informed consent was obtained from the individual(s) for the publication of any potentially identifiable images or data included in this article.

AUTHOR CONTRIBUTIONS

QL, XY, CW, and JX designed and implemented the treatment and provided clinical information. ZW, PZ, and JZ summarised relevant researches and wrote and revised the case report. All authors contributed to the article and approved the submitted version.

REFERENCES

1. Andermann F, Kobayashi E, Andermann E. Genetic focal epilepsies: state of the art and paths to the future. *Epilepsia.* (2005) 46:61–7. doi: 10.1111/j.1528-1167.2005.00361.x
2. Mullin J P, Shriver M, Alomar S, Najm I, Bulacio J, Chauvel P, et al. Is SEEG safe? A systematic review and meta-analysis of stereo-electroencephalography-related complications. *Epilepsia.* (2016) 57:386–401. doi: 10.1111/epi.13298
3. An N, Ye X, Liu Q, Xu J, Zhang P. Localization of the epileptogenic zone based on ictal stereo-electroencephalogram: brain network and single-channel signal feature analysis. *Epilepsy Res.* (2020) 167:106475. doi: 10.1016/j.eplepsyres.2020.106475
4. Perveen N, Ashraf W, Alqahtani F, Rasool M F, Samad N, Imran I. Temporal lobe epilepsy: what do we understand about protein alterations? *Chem Biol Drug Des.* (2021) 98:377–94. doi: 10.1111/cbdd.13858
5. Tai X Y, Koepp M, Duncan J S, Fox N, Thompson P, Baxendale S, et al. Hyperphosphorylated tau in patients with refractory epilepsy correlates with cognitive decline: a study of temporal lobe resections. *Brain.* (2016) 139:2441–55. doi: 10.1093/brain/aww187
6. Cendes F, Cendes IL, Andermann E, Andermann F. Familial temporal lobe epilepsy: a clinically heterogeneous syndrome. *Neurology.* (1998) 50:554–7. doi: 10.1212/WNL.50.2.554
7. Fabera P, Krijtova H, Tomasek M, Krysl D, Zamecnik J, Mohapl M, et al. Familial temporal lobe epilepsy due to focal cortical dysplasia type IIIa. *Seizure.* (2015) 31:120–3. doi: 10.1016/j.seizure.2015.07.014
8. Koizumi S, Kawai K, Asano S, Ueki K, Suzuki I, Saito N. Familial lateral temporal lobe epilepsy confirmed with intracranial electroencephalography and successfully treated by surgery. *Neurologia Medico-Chirurgica.* (2011) 51:604–10. doi: 10.2176/nmc.51.604

5

Macroglossia Associated with Clobazam Administration: A Case Report and Literature Review

Jeff F. Zhang[1*], *Kevin Nickerson*[1], *Ravi Piryani*[2], *Osman Farooq*[3] *and Anil K. Swayampakula*[2]

[1] *Jacobs School of Medicine and Biomedical Sciences, University at Buffalo, Buffalo, NY, United States,* [2] *Division of Critical Care Medicine, Department of Pediatrics, John R. Oishei Children's Hospital, Buffalo, NY, United States,* [3] *Division of Pediatric Neurology, John R. Oishei Children's Hospital, Buffalo, NY, United States*

***Correspondence:**
Jeff F. Zhang
jeffzhan@buffalo.edu

Clobazam is a benzodiazepine derivative used as an antiepileptic agent for the treatment of focal and generalized seizures and drug-resistant epilepsy associated with Lennox-Gastaut Syndrome. While somnolence and mood-related side effects are commonly observed, acute macroglossia following initiation of Clobazam therapy has not been previously reported in the medical literature. In this case report, we present a female pediatric patient who developed significant tongue swelling with protrusion beyond the oral cavity after initiation of Clobazam for treatment-resistant epilepsy. Symptoms were unresponsive to antihistamines and steroids but resolved gradually in the days following discontinuation of Clobazam with no lingering sequelae.

Keywords: antiseizure drug, Clobazam, epilepsy, macroglossia, pediatric neurology

INTRODUCTION

Macroglossia is defined as a painless enlargement of the tongue that presents either congenitally in association with a wide variety of inherited disorders (e.g., Down Syndrome, Hunter and Hurler Syndromes, Beckwith-Wiedemann Syndrome) or acquired as a result of inflammation, amyloidosis, and endocrine and metabolic disorders. In rare cases, severe tongue swelling causing upper airway obstruction presents as a medical emergency requiring reduction glossectomy, which is indicated in an estimated maximum of 10% of cases of macroglossia (1). Frequently, acquired macroglossia resolves spontaneously with treatment of the underlying cause, and corticosteroids have also shown effectiveness in reducing glossal edema associated with trauma and mechanical injury (2).

Macroglossia secondary to angioedema is commonly observed in the setting of drug hypersensitivity reactions, in which drug-antigen presentation causes crosslinking of IgE immunoglobulins on the surface of mast cells with subsequent degranulation of intracellular contents. The release of vasoactive substances such as histamine and bradykinin leads to increases in the permeability of submucosal and subcutaneous capillaries, resulting in fluid shifts into the interstitial environment that cause localized tissue swelling. The onset of glossal swelling following the administration of Clobazam therapy for refractory epilepsy has not been previously reported in the literature and the pathophysiology by which these symptoms occur is currently unknown. In this case report, we present a pediatric patient who developed significant tongue swelling with protrusion beyond the oral cavity in the days after initiating Clobazam therapy for treatment-resistant epilepsy and whose symptoms resolved gradually following discontinuation of the drug.

Day 1	Lorazepam and Fosphenytoin doses given in ED. Midazolam drip started in PICU
Day 2	Clobazam administered
Day 3	
Day 4	Antibiotics discontinued
Day 5	Tongue swelling first noted. Furosemide given
Day 6	Tongue swelling worsens. Diphenhydramine given
Day 7	
Day 8	Tongue swelling continues to worsen. Clobazam discontinued
Day 9	Dexamethasone started
Day 10	
Day 11	Dexamethasone discontinued due to lack of improvement
Day 12	Tongue swelling unchanged. patient intubated due to concern of airway loss
Day 13	Tongue swelling improves. patient extubated
Day 14	Tongue swelling continues to improve
Day 15	Complete resolution of symptoms

FIGURE 1 | Timeline of patient hospitalization events.

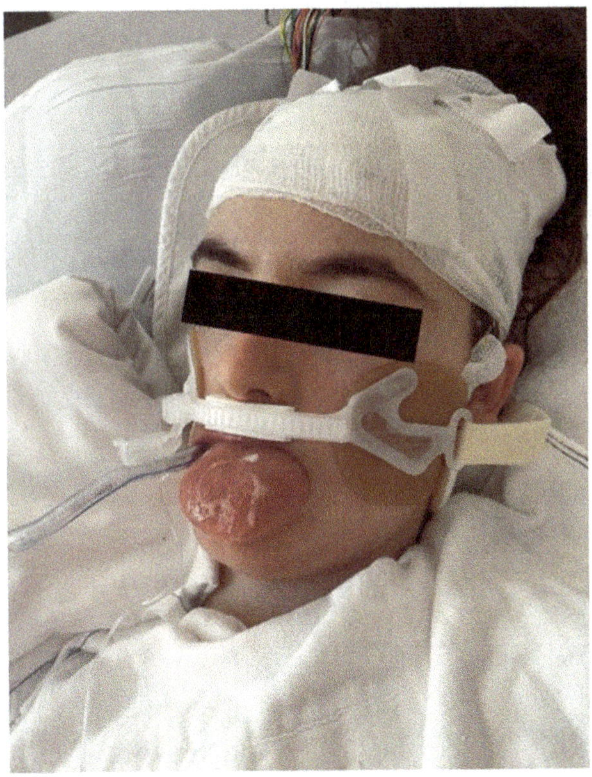

FIGURE 2 | Patient with notable tongue enlargement and protrusion from oral cavity.

CASE PRESENTATION

A 17-year-old Caucasian female, born at 34 weeks *via* Cesarean section, presented to the emergency department (ED) with status epilepticus. Her past medical history was significant for unbalanced chromosome 6 and 21 translocation, gross developmental delay, polymicrogyria, low-lying cerebellar tonsils, arachnoid cyst, micrognathia, scoliosis, and multifocal drug-resistant epilepsy since age 5 (managed on Levetiracetam, Lacosamide, and rectal Diazepam as needed). At baseline, the patient experiences four seizures per day lasting between 30 and 60 s and the parents report the patient maintains good compliance with her antiseizure drug regimen. In the 24 h prior to admission, the father estimated that she had ~80 breakthrough seizures with episodes of head deviation and whole body stiffening and shaking each lasting between 30 and 120 s in duration. No significant improvement was observed after giving extra doses of Levetiracetam and Lacosamide. The family denied any recent history of fever, upper respiratory infection, nausea, vomiting, urinary symptoms, trauma, or travel. Previous attempts to control the patient's seizures using Topiramate, Sodium Valproate, Oxcarbazepine, Zonisamide, and Lamotrigine were ineffective. **Figure 1** represents the timing of events in the patient's hospital course by day of admission.

Lab results showed leukocytosis (WBC, 15.1×10^9/L) with neutrophils 59.9% and lymphocytes 32.0%, and reactive thrombophilia (482×10^9/L). Comprehensive metabolic panel was significant only for anion gap elevation (16 mmol/L) and low bicarbonate (15 mmol/L) which resolved over the following days. Ceftriaxone was started for empiric coverage; initial blood cultures grew Staphylococcal species and Vancomycin was added. The patient's seizures were terminated by Lorazepam and Fosphenytoin loading in the ED. She was continued on her home antiseizure medications and continuous video electroencephalography (EEG) was started. The patient was stabilized in the ED and transferred to the pediatric floor. Overnight, the patient began to have seizures again and EEG detected epileptogenic sharp waves over the left hemisphere. Due to continued seizures, the patient was subsequently transferred to the pediatric intensive care unit (PICU), started on a Midazolam drip, and required endotracheal intubation for airway protection. Clobazam 5 mg BID was initiated on Day 2 of hospital admission for further seizure control. Head CT and brain MRI were negative for acute intracranial pathology. Antibiotics were discontinued on Day 4 following negative blood, urine, and cerebrospinal fluid cultures, and the patient's seizures were reported to be adequately controlled at this time. On Day 5 of PICU admission, the patient was noted to have mild tongue swelling; this was initially thought to be secondary to fluid overload and the patient was started on Furosemide given her overall volume status. While her volume status notably improved, her tongue swelling continued to worsen, with inability to manually retract the tongue and protrusion beyond the oral cavity over the following day (**Figure 2**). No signs of infection or trauma were noted within the oral cavity on inspection. Trial of Diphenhydramine did not improve the tongue swelling. Given that Clobazam was the only new medication that she had not previously received, it was suspected to be the offending agent and replaced with Clonazepam on Day 8 of hospitalization. No recurrence of seizures were noted and EEG was discontinued. On the following day, a steroid course with Dexamethasone was initiated for the patient's macroglossia. Serum complement panel demonstrated normal C4 levels (39.6 mg/dL) and elevated C1 esterase inhibitor (53 mg/dL). Further inquiry into family history was also negative for angioedema. On Day 12, following 72 h of steroid administration, the patient's tongue was noted to still be edematous and protruding. Intubation and mechanical ventilation had been maintained due to concern of airway loss from macroglossia. On Day 13, she started to show improvement with tongue swelling and was successfully extubated with no complications. Complete resolution of macroglossia was observed on Day 15 of hospitalization, seven days following the discontinuation of Clobazam.

DISCUSSION

Clobazam is a benzodiazepine antiepileptic agent used to treat a range of focal and generalized seizure disorders, as well as drug-resistant seizures associated with syndromes such as Lennox-Gastaut Syndrome and Dravet Syndrome. Its mechanism of action is through its binding to γ-aminobutyric acid-A (GABA-A) receptors and potentiation of GABA action by increasing the channel conduction of chloride ions in response to ligand binding, thereby increasing the seizure threshold (3). Clobazam differs from typical benzodiazepines due to placement of its two

Naranjo Adverse Drug Reaction Probability Scale

Question	Yes	No	Do Not Know	Score
1. Are there previous conclusive reports on this reaction?	+1	0	0	0
2. Did the adverse event appear after the suspected drug was administered?	+2	-1	0	+2
3. Did the adverse reaction improve when the drug was discontinued or a specific antagonist was administered?	+1	0	0	+1
4. Did the adverse event reappear when the drug was re-administered?	+2	-1	0	0
5. Are there alternative causes (other than the drug) that could on their own have caused the reaction?	-1	+2	0	+2
6. Did the reaction reappear when a placebo was given?	-1	+1	0	0
7. Was the drug detected in blood (or other fluids) in concentrations known to be toxic?	+1	0	0	0
8. Was the reaction more severe when the dose was increased or less severe when the dose was decreased?	+1	0	0	0
9. Did the patient have a similar reaction to the same or similar drugs in any previous exposure?	+1	0	0	0
10. Was the adverse event confirmed by any objective evidence?	+1	0	0	+1
TOTAL SCORE:				+6

FIGURE 3 | Naranjo adverse drug reaction probability scale (9). Score was calculated as "+6" due to the patient's adverse event appearing following administration of Clobazam, improvement of symptoms following discontinuation of the drug, other causes for the patient's tongue edema ruled out, and the results of the patient's presentation and work-up confirmed with neurology, immunology, and otolaryngology consults.

nitrogen atoms at the 1st and 5th positions of the diazepine ring resulting in partial agonism of the GABA-A receptor, rather than the 1st and 4th ring positions of other benzodiazepines which act as full agonists (3). This structural variation confers an improved side effect profile and also increases its anxiolytic and antiepileptic properties due to improved binding affinity for the GABA-A $\alpha 2\beta 3\gamma 2$ subtype (4). Common side effects noted in up to 80% of patients during Phase III drug trials included somnolence, pyrexia, lethargy, drooling, and constipation (5). While side effects are generally mild, increased severity has been observed in patients prescribed Clobazam along with cannabinoid agents such as Epidiolex for the treatment of refractory epilepsy (6). Serological studies show cannabidiol use in combination with Clobazam was correlated with a five-fold increase in concentration of N-desmethylclobazam, the active metabolite of Clobazam, due to shared metabolism by the hepatic cytochrome P450 enzyme CYP2C19 (7). Patients with "poor metabolizer" phenotypes due to high rates of polymorphism in the CYP2C19 gene have also been noted to be at a higher risk of adverse drug effects (8). However, the patient described in our case report did not have a history of cannabinoid use and CYP2C19 genotyping had not been conducted.

Our report presents the first published case of acute tongue enlargement in the context of naïve Clobazam exposure. While the patient had also been treated with antibiotics, Lorazepam' Fosphenytoin, and Midazolam during her inpatient course, the patient's previous exposure to these medications, lack of rash or pruritus, and minimal response to Diphenhydramine and corticosteroid therapy likely rule out allergic or inflammatory etiologies. In addition, our findings of elevated C1-esterase inhibitor levels, normal C4 complement levels, and negative family history for angioedema accounted for any possible pathologies related to bradykinin-mediated angioedema. Improvements in macroglossia observed while the patient was still intubated and lack of similar symptoms following previous intubations also make a traumatic cause for the patient's acute tongue swelling less likely. However, calculation of the Naranjo adverse drug reaction probability scale (9) for our patient (represented in **Figure 3**) yielded a score of "+6," which determined a "Probable" drug-related cause for the patient's macroglossia, and it had been noted that Clobazam was the only new medication that the patient had been exposed to during this hospital stay. While isolated tongue swelling has not previously been described in the literature following Clobazam administration, two reports have presented four adult patients (10) and one pediatric patient (11) who developed distal extremity edema associated with chronic Clobazam use (within 1-3 months of therapy) that spontaneously resolved within 2–6 weeks following discontinuation of the drug. In both cases, the pathophysiology was speculated to be due to the disruption of autonomic signaling in the myocardium and peripheral vasculature due to benzodiazepine-mediated increases in chloride channel conduction (12). However, no reports of macroglossia or extremity edema have been reported in the acute setting in the days following initiation of Clobazam therapy.

Notably, acute tongue swelling has been reported in patients receiving barbiturates for sedation. Darshan et al. reported a patient who developed severe tongue swelling with protrusion after placement into a drug-induced coma using Pentobarbital (13). The patient was weaned off Pentobarbital with improvement of his tongue swelling over the following week; however, later in his hospital course, he was administered Pentobarbital again and three days later developed similar symptoms of macroglossia, which again resolved in a few days following discontinuation of Pentobarbital (13). In another report, Parthvi et al. reported a patient who was administered Phenobarbital for agitation related to alcohol withdrawal and also developed isolated tongue swelling that was ruled to not be related to anaphylaxis or angioedema (14). In a similar mechanism of action to benzodiazepines, barbiturates act as positive allosteric modulators of GABA-A receptors by binding to a distinct site from benzodiazepines and increasing GABA-mediated activity. Phenobarbital and Pentobarbital have also been found to be mainly metabolized by hepatic CYP2C19 (15), and patients with genetic polymorphisms resulting in decreased enzymatic activity have been noted to be at higher risk of developing side effects related to barbiturate intake (16). We would hypothesize that in patients with a poor metabolizer phenotype characterized by reduced CYP2C19 activity, elevated drug metabolite levels disrupt autonomic vasoconstriction in the tongue (a highly neurovascular structure) and produce the characteristic macroglossia observed in these patients, though further serological and genotyping studies are required to draw definitive conclusions in this susceptible patient population.

Unresolved macroglossia poses a significant risk for unsuccessful extubation, resulting in obstructive symptoms post-extubation or possible cardiac arrest due to an inability to pass an oral or nasotracheal tube and necessitating emergency tracheostomy. Fortunately, as in the case of our patient, drug-related symptoms of macroglossia have been observed to resolve quickly and spontaneously following discontinuation of the offending agent without any lingering sequelae. In this case report, we hope to increase awareness among clinicians for this possible side effect of Clobazam therapy in order to avoid unnecessary testing and treatment which may prolong a patient's length of stay.

CONCLUSIONS

Macroglossia is a previously unreported side effect associated with initiation of Clobazam therapy for drug-resistant epilepsy. Early recognition of this symptom and discontinuing the offending agent may to lead to spontaneous resolution of macroglossia and can reduce hospital length of stay.

AUTHOR CONTRIBUTIONS

JZ: drafting the manuscript, editing the manuscript, approving the manuscript, and accountable for manuscript integrity. KN and RP: editing the manuscript and approving the manuscript. OF and AS: project conception, editing the manuscript, and approving the manuscript. All authors contributed to the article and approved the submitted version.

REFERENCES

1. Topouzelis N, Iliopoulos C, Kolokitha OE. Macroglossia. *Int Dent J.* (2011) 61:63–9. doi: 10.1111/j.1875-595X.2011.00015.x
2. Alarfaj AA, AlHayek AR, Alghanim R, Al-Jazan NA. Self-induced traumatic macroglossia: case report and literature review. *Case Rep Otolaryngol.* (2019) 2019:6040354. doi: 10.1155/2019/6040354
3. Humayun MJ, Samanta D, Carson RP. *Clobazam.* Treasure Island, FL: StatPearls (2021).
4. Jensen HS, Nichol K, Lee D, Ebert B. Clobazam and its active metabolite N-desmethylclobazam display significantly greater affinities for alpha- versus alpha-GABA(A)-receptor complexes. *PLoS ONE.* (2014) 9:e88456. doi: 10.1371/journal.pone.0088456
5. Ng YT, Conry JA, Drummond R, Stolle J, Weinberg MA, Investigators OVS. Randomized, phase III study results of clobazam in Lennox-Gastaut syndrome. *Neurology.* (2011) 77:1473–81. doi: 10.1212/WNL.0b013e318232de76
6. Abu-Sawwa R, Scutt B, Park Y. Emerging use of epidiolex (cannabidiol) in epilepsy. *J Pediatr Pharmacol Ther.* (2020) 25:485–99. doi: 10.5863/1551-6776-25.6.485
7. Devinsky O, Patel AD, Thiele EA, et al. Randomized, dose-ranging safety trial of cannabidiol in Dravet syndrome. *Neurology.* (2018) 90:e1204–11. doi: 10.1212/WNL.0000000000005254
8. Dean L. Clobazam therapy and CYP2C19 Genotype. In: Pratt VM, Scott SA, Pirmohamed M, Esquivel B, Kane MS, Kattman BL, Malheiro AJ, editors. *Medical Genetics Summaries. Bethesda, MD: National Center for Biotechnology Information* (2012).
9. *LiverTox*: Clinical and Research Information on Drug-Induced Liver Injury. Bethesda, MD: National Institute of Diabetes and Digestive and Kidney Diseases (2012).
10. Mathew T, D'Souza D, Nadimpally US, Nadig R. Clobazam-induced pedal edema: "An unrecognized side effect of a common antiepileptic drug". *Epilepsia. Mar.* (2016) 57:524–5. doi: 10.1111/epi.13316
11. Incecik F, Ozcanyüz DG. Unusual side effects due to clobazam: a case report with edema of the extremities. *Acta Neurol Belg.* (2018) 118:521–2. doi: 10.1007/s13760-018-0901-4
12. Agelink MW, Majewski TB, Andrich J, Mueck-Weymann M. Short-term effects of intravenous benzodiazepines on autonomic neurocardiac regulation in humans: a comparison between midazolam, diazepam, and lorazepam. *Crit Care Med. May.* (2002) 30:997–1006. doi: 10.1097/00003246-200205000-00008
13. Darshan P, Gurpreet J, Justin R. A case of acute tongue enlargement. *Chest.* (2013) 144:909A. doi: 10.1378/chest.1698580
14. Parthvi R, Lewandowski E, Fuhrer G. Phenobarbital-associated macroglossia. *Am J Ther.* (2021) 28:e265–6. doi: 10.1097/MJT.0000000000001094
15. Wishart DS, Knox C, Guo AC, et al. DrugBank: a comprehensive resource for in silico drug discovery and exploration. *Nucleic Acids Res.* (2006) 34:D668–72. doi: 10.1093/nar/gkj067
16. Yukawa E, Mamiya K. Effect of CYP2C19 genetic polymorphism on pharmacokinetics of phenytoin and phenobarbital in Japanese epileptic patients using non-linear mixed effects model approach. *J Clin Pharm Ther.* (2006) 31:275–82. doi: 10.1111/j.1365-2710.2006.00712.x

6

Case Report: Cognitive Assessment before an Amnesic Seizure in Transient Epileptic Amnesia Syndrome

Coline Bouyer[1*] *and Bertrand de Toffol*[1,2]

[1] *Service de neurologie Centre Hospitalier de Cayenne, Cayenne, France,* [2] *CIC Inserm 1424 CH Cayenne, Cayenne, France*

***Correspondence:**
Coline Bouyer
coline.bouyer@ch-cayenne.fr

A patient with transient epileptic amnesia syndrome presented a clinically observable amnesic seizure immediately after a neuropsychological assessment. An hour and a half before the onset of the seizure, the patient progressively developed an isolated alteration of episodic memory. These data question the ictal/interictal distinction in this syndrome as well as the speed of propagation of an epileptic activity.

Keywords: epilepsy, memory, neuropsychology, transient epileptic amnesia (TEA), amnesic seizure

INTRODUCTION

Transient epileptic amnesia (TEA) is a mesial temporal epileptic syndrome for which the diagnostic criteria, defined by Zeman et al. (1), are: (1) A history of recurrent witnessed episodes of transient amnesia; (2) Cognitive functions other than memory judged to be intact during typical episodes by a reliable witness; (3) Evidence for a diagnosis of epilepsy based on one or more of the following: (a) Epileptiform abnormalities on electroencephalography; (b) The concurrent onset of other clinical features of epilepsy (e.g., lip-smacking, olfactory hallucinations); (c) A clear-cut response to anticonvulsant therapy.

A recent general review (2), based on a substantial patient cohort, concluded that TEA is a distinctive form of late-onset limbic epilepsy. Patients have recurrent episodes of transient amnesia, typically lasting for around 30 min, often when waking, frequently occurring at intervals of around 1 month. Other symptoms can occur, such as olfactory hallucinations (43% of the patients), repetitive questioning (57%) or motor automatisms (41%) (2). During the amnesic attacks, patients remain able to carry on a conversation and act appropriately (3), which suggests the preservation of cognitive functions (other than memory) such as attention, perception, language, and executive functions. Standard interictal neuropsychological assessments (NPA), which evaluate episodic memory on a short temporality, generally show normal performance (3, 4). The majority of patients report interictal memory impairment, specifically an accelerated long-term forgetting (ALF) and autobiographical amnesia (AbA). Thirty % of the patients mention a distinctive form of emotional lability (2). Specific NPA objectify patients' subjective complaint. They evaluate the ALF with a 1 h-delayed recall (5–7), a 24 h-delayed recall (8), a 1 week (or more) delayed recall (4, 9, 10). They test AbA with semi-structured interviews (11, 12). The condition of TEA syndrome is most often of unknown etiology and has a benign prognosis.

We report here the exceptional case of a well-characterized TEA patient who presented an amnesic attack in the immediate aftermath of an NPA. We can thus detail the appearance and progression of subtle cognitive impairments 1 h and a half before the clinical seizure.

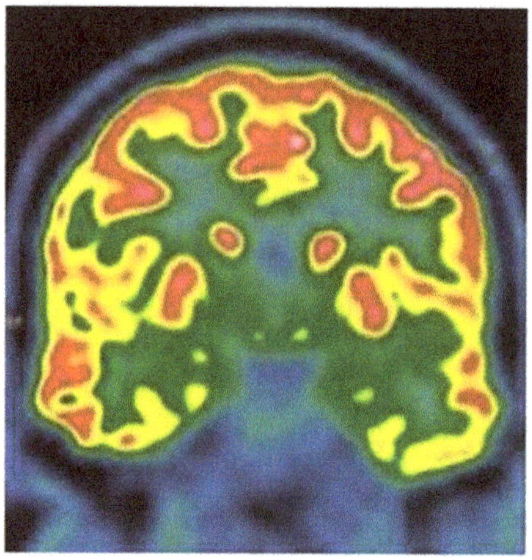

FIGURE 1 | 18 FDG PET scan coronal cut showing bilateral mesial temporal hypometabolism more pronounced on the left temporal lobe.

CASE DESCRIPTION

We report the case of a man who was 60 years old at the time of the diagnosis. He had been retired for 7 months and was house painter.

The patient came to see a neurologist for recurrent attacks:

- The first one happened four months before his retirement, during a period of overwork. While he was working, he suddenly felt disorientated, didn't know what he was doing.
- Two months later, he had a second attack when waking up. The patient describes the sensation of having a gray veil in front of his face. He felt lost, didn't know what he had to do or where he wanted to go.
- One month later, also while waking up, he had a third attack. Once again, he felt like having a gray veil in front of him and didn't know what he had to do. During the morning, while he was driving, his wife observed that he seemed haggard without any loss of contact or difficulty for driving.
- The next month, when waking up the day after Christmas, the patient felt disorientated and couldn't remember what had happened the day before.

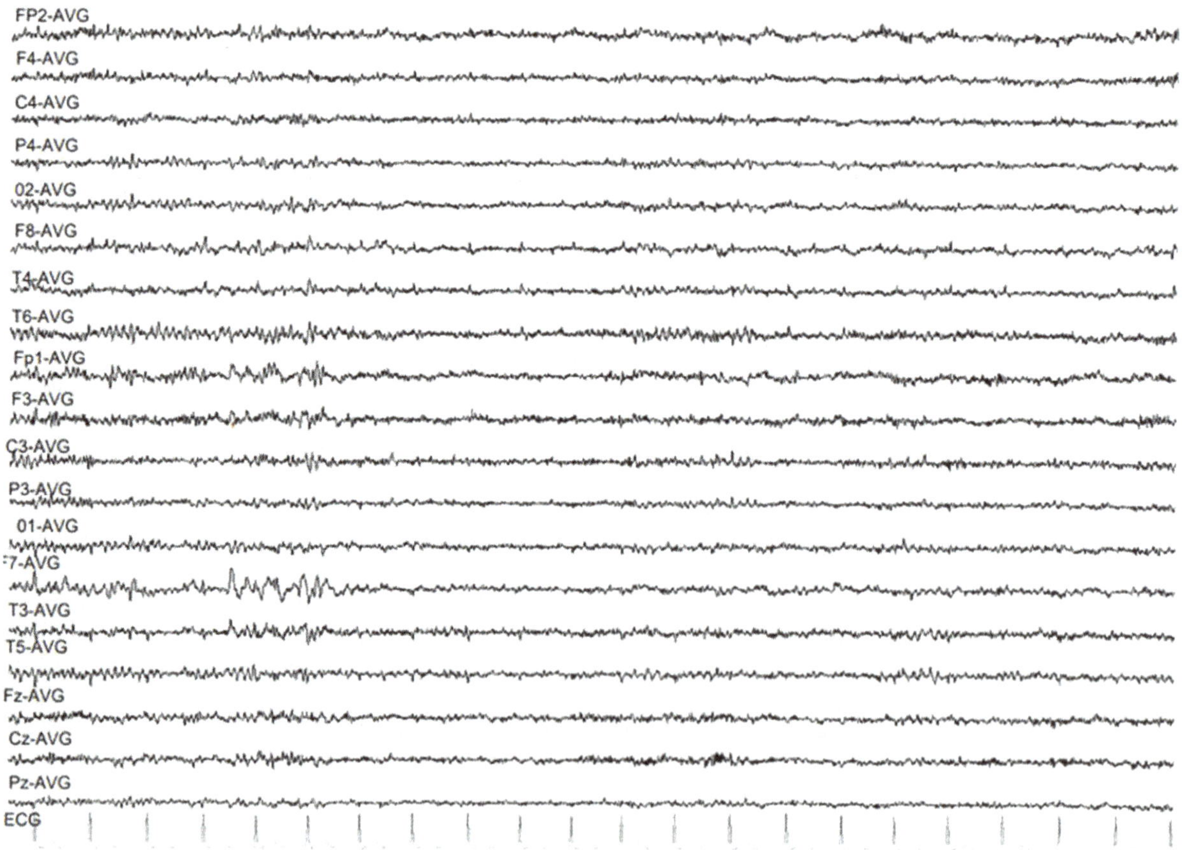

FIGURE 2 | EEG showing slow wave focus associated with spikes on the left temporal lobe.

TABLE 1 | Neuropsychological assessments.

		NPA 1	NPA 2	NPA 3	Cut off
		Score	**Score**	**Score**	
Mental status					
MMSE (13)		29/30	28/30	30/30	27
Memory					
Working memory					
Digit Span Recall (WAIS IV) (19)	Total	11/19	14/19	13/19	5
Anterograde memory					
- Verbal memory					
RL/RI-16 (15)		List A	List B	List C	
	Immediate Recall	16/16	16/16	16/16	13
	1st Free Recall	6/16	4/16**	8/16	5.16
	2nd Free Recall	6/16*	7/16	6/16*	6.42
	3rd Free Recall	8/16	3/16**	10/16	7.93
	1st Total Recall	12/16*	8/16**	12/16*	12
	2nd Total Recall	15/16	9/16**	13/16*	13
	3rd Total Recall	15/16	11/16**	14/16*	14
	Recognition	16/16	13/16*	16/16	
	20′ delayed Free Recall	9/16	6/16**	8/16*	8.16
	20′ delayed Total Recall	16/16	10/16**	15/16	14
	1 week DFR	0/16		2/16	
	1 week DTR	7/16		5/16	
	FR	0	0	0	
	Intrusions	free recall: 0 induced recall: 2	free recall: 5 induced recall: 14	free recall: 2 Induced recall: 5	
	Intrusions at 1 week	free recall: 0 induced recall: 7		free recall: 2 induced recall: 2	
Logical memory (MEM III) (14)	Immediate recall	7/19	1/19**	7/19	5
	Delayed recall	4/19*	1/19**	3/19**	5
	Recognition	22/30 C17-C25	19/30 C3-C9	15/30 ≤C2	C5
- Visual memory					
10/36 (18)	Total immediate recalls	24/30	15/30	22/30	9
	Delayed recall	9/10	3/10*	8/10	3
Face recognition (MEM III) (14)	Immediate recognition	9/19			5
	Delayed recognition	10/19			5
Rey complex figure		9/36*	7/36*	12/36*	15
Autobiographical memory					
TEMPau (12, 23)					
Episodic Score	0–17 years old	4			0
	18–30 years old	0**			1.69
	Over 30 years old	0*			0.15
	5 last years	0*			0.19
	12 last months	4			2.29
Global Score	0–17 years old	7**			9.09
	18–30 years old	7**			9.11
	Over 30 years old	9*			8.275
	5 last years	6**			7.09
	12 last months	11			9.88
Language					
Denomination (21)	DO 80	80/80	79/80	80/80	

(Continued)

TABLE 1 | Continued

		NPA 1 Score	NPA 2 Score	NPA 3 Score	Cut off
Executive functions					
GREFEX Version (20)					
Fluency	Animals (2′)	32	25	33	18
	Letter P (2′)	23	26	23	10
Stroop	Interference—Denomination (sec)	95	60	47	90
TMT	B-A (sec)	34	26	17	120
Visuoconstruction					
Rey complex figure (17)	Type	I	IV	IV	
	Score	27/36*	26/36*	30/36	29
Emotional state					
HADS (22)	Anxiety	8/21*	3/21	11/21*	8–10
	Depression	1/21	7/21	4/21	8–10

*Score below the pathological threshold or below −1.65 standard deviation; **score below −2 standard deviation.
NPA, Neuropsychological Assessment; MMSE, Mini Mental State Examination; RL/RI-16, Rappel libre/rappel indicé à 16 items; DFR, Delayed Free Recall; DTR, Delayed Total Recall; FR, False Recognition; C, Centile; TMT, Trail Making Test; HADS, Hospital Anxiety and Depression Scale.

- A fifth episode happened 2 months later, he was shopping with his wife when he felt disorientated and didn't know what he had to do.

Three attacks appeared when the patient was waking up. During the attacks, the patient systematically had a confused look, as if he was lost, iterative questioned the people around him, but he was able to perform motor acts without error. There were no other temporal lobe epilepsy symptoms (such as olfactory hallucinations or motor automatisms) described by the patient or his wife. All these episodes lasted around 5 min with a post critical phase which could last from a few minutes to 1 h. During the post critical phase, the patient had memory impairment which seemed both retrograde—for example, after the acute phase of the first attack, he didn't remember if he had called his client the day before or not—and anterograde — his wife noted that he didn't correctly memorize information at post critical phase but she didn't notice any element of aphasia. The patient could remember that he had had a seizure because he did not feel well but he could not describe what he had done or said. Between the attacks, his wife observed some disturbance of autobiographical memory and an unusual emotionality. The patient had no more complaint.

Brain MRI, TEP-scan, video-EEG, spinal tap and NPA were performed. Clinical seizures were controlled with 100 mg lamotrigine per day.

Brain MRI was normal. PET scan showed bilateral hippocampal and parahippocampal hypometabolism (**Figure 1**) and video-EEG showed a slow wave focus associated with spikes under the left anterior and middle temporal electrodes especially during sleep (**Figure 2**). The spinal tap was normal. All known autoimmune antibodies were negative.

NEUROPSYCHOLOGICAL ASSESSMENTS

During each NPA, we evaluated the global cognitive efficiency with the MMSE (13). Anterograde verbal memory was evaluated using the logical memory from Weschler Memory Scale III (WMS—III, immediate and 30-min delayed recall, and recognition) (14) and the RL/RI-16 (immediate and 20-min delayed recall) (15). For logical memory subtest, the same two stories were presented to the patient for each NPA but we used three different lists of words to assess the RL/RI-16. These three lists are validated and considered as comparable (15, 16). Anterograde visual memory was assessed with the recall of the Rey-Osterrieth Complex Figure (17), the 10/36 spatial recall test (18) and the faces recognition test from the WMS-III. Verbal working memory was tested with the WAIS-IV digit span subtest (19). Executive functions were tested with Subtests from GREFEX battery (20). Visuoconstruction was assessed with the copy of Rey-Osterrieth Complex Figure. Language was evaluated with the DO 80 denomination test (21). Emotional state was controlled with the HADS (22). In addition, we assessed the Autobiographical memory with the TEMPau task (12, 23) during a second appointment for the first NPA. We also examined long-term consolidation with asking a 1-week delayed recall of the RL/RI-16 list of words to research an ALF. This evaluation is only a clinical observation because there are no norms for this task. We did not ask a 1-week delayed-recall for Logical Memory because of the impaired performance on 20-min delayed recall.

Three NPA were performed (summarized in **Table 1**). The tests were proposed in the same order during the three NPA (**Table 2**).

1. First NPA

The first NPA revealed a global preservation of cognitive functions on the standard evaluation, as it has been described in literature except for episodic memory. The RL/RI-16 showed an encoding impairment on the first total recall, and a slight retrieval difficulty but the middle term storage appeared normal. Delayed recall of the logical memory subtest, which requires recalling two stories presented only once, was impaired but delayed recognition remained normal. The patient said that this type of exercise had always been difficult for him. Visual memory appeared efficient except when the test required incident learning.

Furthermore, according to his complaint, the results suggest an ALF: the patient could not spontaneously recall any item of the RL/RI-16 list of words after 1 week, retrieved seven with help and proposed seven intrusions. The patient also presented an AbA. The impairment was more important for episodic memories which aligns with the literature data. We observed a U-distribution with a better performance for childhood episodic memories and for the past year (**Figure 3**). The detailed study of the profile showed that the past year episodic memories evoked by the patient concerned the last months and the last days before the evaluation. The patient could not report any episodic memory for the three interim periods (**Table 1**).

The score of Rey-Orsterrieth Complex Figure was impaired by slight disproportions and one omission but it did not constitute real visuoconstruction impairment.

Emotional state evaluation indicated anxiety manifestations.

In the end, we asked the patient to come again a year later for a new NPA.

2. Second NPA: during an acute phase

As agreed, the patient came 1 year later. He was still taking 100mg of lamotrigine per day. He only had one seizure since the first NPA. It had occurred 2 months before the second NPA, when waking up, and his wife observed the same disorientation and iterative questioning associated with some iterative deglutition movements.

During the interview, the patient was perfectly coherent and gave an informative speech. He did not mention any new complaint. He still reported an unusual emotionality and an AbA. These features did not disturb his daily functioning. There was no autonomy loss and he still managed his rental houses without difficulty. His wife agreed with this information.

The assessment revealed a preservation of global cognitive efficiency. Language, executive functions and working memory were maintained. In contrast, verbal episodic memory was significantly impaired on the RL/RI-16, more than during the first NPA: all the scores were impaired and below two standard deviations. The repetition of immediate recalls, during which the missing items are recalled by the examiner, didn't significantly improve the scores so we could notice an encoding impairment. Furthermore, the patient gave 19 intrusions. Immediate recognition was also impaired. Immediate recall of logical memory subtest was substantially impaired whereas

TABLE 2 | Order of tests administration.

Order	Test	Estimated duration (minutes)
1.	MMSE	10
2.	RL/RI-16: - Immédiate recall - 1st, 2nd, and 3rd recall - Immediate recognition	25
3.	Rey-osterrieth complex figure: - Copy	3
4.	Digit span subtest (WAIS-IV)	12
5.	Rey-osterrieth complex figure: - Recall	5
6.	RL/RI-16: - 20 min delayed recall	5
7.	Logical memory - Immediate recall	10
8.	10/36: - 1st, 2nd, and 3rd recall	10
9.	TMT	5
10.	Stroop	5
11.	10/36: - Delayed recall	5
12.	Logical memory: - Delayed recall - Recognition	10
13.	Fluency	5
14.	DO 80	5
15.	HADS	10

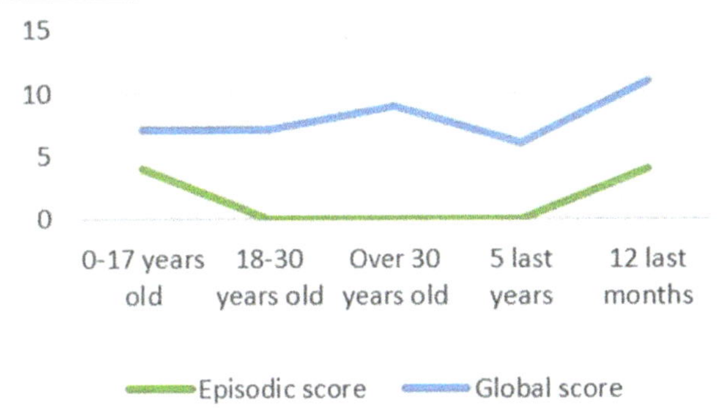

FIGURE 3 | The TEMPau shows a U-distribution with a better performance for childhood episodic memories and for the past year.

it was normal during the first NPA. Visual episodic memory evaluation objectified an encoding difficulty and a storage impairment of visuospatial information during the 10/36 task. This time visuoconstruction was impaired by deformations and a planning trouble that was not present during the first NPA. However, the HADS did not show anxiety or depression symptoms.

We therefore observed, from this second NPA, an isolated encoding and storage impairment in verbal and visual episodic

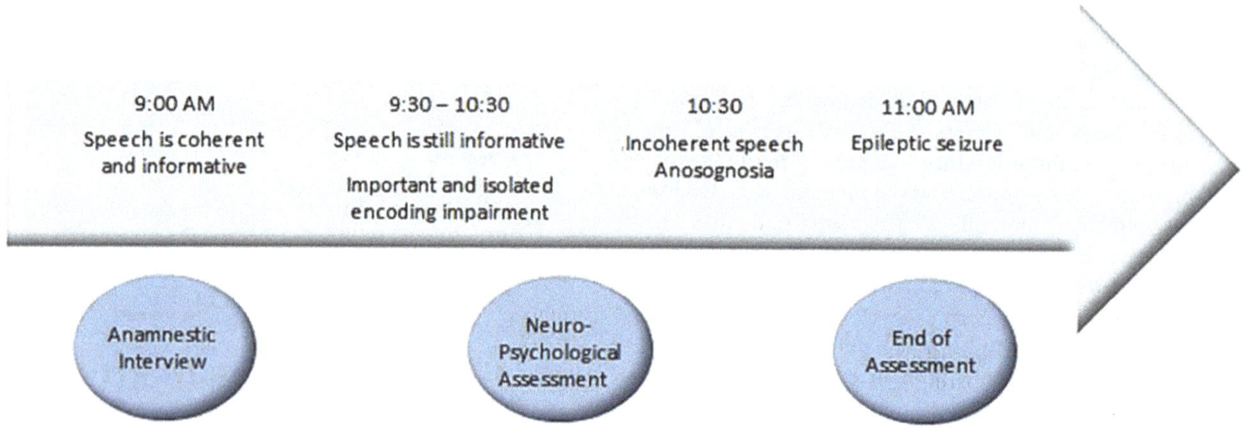

FIGURE 4 | Unfolding facts.

memory with only an associated visuoconstruction difficulty and a diminution of anxiety.

During the last part of the examination, the patient began to justify his results, saying that he had never been good for memory tasks. At the end of the tests assessment, the psychologist took some time to discuss the results. That is when the patient began to give unclear answers during the conversation. He gave repetitive justifications. When the psychologist asked questions about the daily life, he gave irrelevant responses. When the psychologist said that the NPA was complete and that he was going to call his wife, the patient had a clinically observable seizure with pallor of the face, repetitive swallowing movements, disorientation and comprehension disorder. He repeated "I don't understand what you are saying". He then repeated what the psychologist said by echolalia. The episode lasted 5 min then the patient could speak normally and said that he didn't feel well during the seizure but did not remember that he was repeating the same sentences. **Figure 4** sums up the unfolding facts.

Thus, more than an hour and a half before the observation of a clinical seizure, a significant and isolated impairment of verbal and visual episodic memory encoding and storage was measured, followed by some degree of anosognosia (patient attempted to justify the difficulties). Anxiety was reduced on the mood self-assessment questionnaire. Given the occurrence of an amnesic seizure at the end of the second NPA, the patient was asked to come back 1 month later to reassess the tests.

The appointment was set up during the afternoon, to avoid stressing the patient on awakening.

3. Third NPA

When the patient came back 1 month later, he had not had any seizure. His complaint was still the same. He remembered that he came for the NPA 2 one month before and that he had a seizure.

The third NPA revealed a preservation of global cognitive efficiency, language, executive functions and working memory. Visuoconstruction was normalized. The assessment of verbal episodic memory showed an encoding and consolidation difficulty but the 20-min delayed recall showed a normal storage. As on the first NPA, logical memory subtest showed impaired delayed recall, and the recognition was also impaired. Emotional state evaluation indicated anxiety manifestations.

An ALF was observed 1 week later: only two words of the RL/RI-16 list were spontaneously recalled and three more with the indication of the category, with four intrusions.

Overall, the third NPA showed substantially the same clinical profile than during the first NPA (**Table 1**). One year after the first evaluation, the cognitive profile was stable; the patient was still independent in daily life and managed his finances without any difficulty.

COMMENTS

This patient with TEA syndrome, characterized by amnesic episodes subjectively controlled by 100 mg lamotrigine, had a normal standard neuropsychological assessment on two occasions (NPA 1 and 3) but showed an accelerated forgetting and autobiographical memory impairment, as described in literature (2). The progressive occurrence of an encoding impairment an hour and a half before a clinical seizure requires reconsideration of the classical ictal/interictal distinction on the one hand and the speed of propagation of an epileptic discharge on the other. A clinically observable seizure is only "the tip of the iceberg". Subtle cognitive symptoms can set in within several minutes. Our observation shows that, in an apparently asymptomatic subject, there may be a reversible prolonged encoding impairment of epileptic origin. Ten cases of surface EEG recording during an amnesic seizure were reported; 8/10 cases showed bilateral temporal seizure activity, and the others had unilateral temporal seizure activity (one left sided and one right sided). Amnesia was observed as an ictal phenomenon in six cases and as postictal in four cases (24). The precise temporal relationship between seizure onset and offset and the associated amnesia is, however, uncertain in the majority of cases of TEA (2). Epileptiform abnormalities on the EEG are rarely seen on a standard waking EEG but often on a nocturnal prolonged sleep EEG (25). Hippocampal interictal spikes recorded on S-EEG during sleep have been shown to disrupt consolidation due to transfer interference between the hippocampus and neocortex (26). It can be suggested that accelerated forgetting and impaired autobiographical memory are the consequence of insufficiently controlled epileptic activity. Some authors consider that ALF results from a consolidation and/or reconsolidation disorder and is consistent with a mesial temporal dysfunction. Encoding process remains preserved (7, 10). ALF could result from a subclinical epileptic activity, impacting the memory-related brain areas (3), which would disturb a long-term stabilization (27).

Our case report raises an important practical question: Should treatment be given to suppress observable seizures or should treatment be enhanced to reduce interictal memory impairment? Should one try to suppress the spikes seen on the sleep EEG in TEA syndrome?

AUTHOR CONTRIBUTIONS

CB performed the neuropsychological assessment and drafted the paper. BT shared his theoretical knowledge and drafted the paper. Both authors contributed to the article and approved the submitted version.

ACKNOWLEDGMENTS

We thank Dr. Stal, Dr. Julian, and Prof. Nacher.

REFERENCES

1. Zeman AZJ, Boniface SJ, Hodges JR. Transient epileptic amnesia: a description of the clinical and neuropsychological features in 10 cases and a review of the literature. *J Neurol Neurosurg Psychiatry.* (1998) 64:435–43. doi: 10.1136/jnnp.64.4.435
2. Baker J, Savage S, Milton F, Butler C, Kapur N, Hodges J, et al. The syndrome of transient epileptic amnesia: a combined series of 115 cases and literature review. *Brain Commun.* (2021) 3:fcab038. doi: 10.1093/braincomms/fcab038
3. Butler C, Zeman A. Syndromes of Transient Amnesia. In: *The Neurology of Conciousness.* (Amsterdam, Netherlands: Elsevier) (2016). p. 365–78.
4. Mosbah A, Tramoni E, Guedj E, Aubert S, Daquin G, Ceccaldi M, et al. Clinical, neuropsychological, and metabolic characteristics of transient epileptic amnesia syndrome. *Epilepsia.* (2014) 55:699–706. doi: 10.1111/epi.12565
5. Atherton KE, Nobre AC, Zeman AZ, Butler CR. Sleep-dependent memory consolidation and accelerated forgetting. *Cortex.* (2014) 54:92–105. doi: 10.1016/j.cortex.2014.02.009
6. Hoefeijzers S, Dewar M, Della Sala S, Butler C, Zeman A. Accelerated long-term forgetting can become apparent within 3–8 hours of wakefulness in patients with transient epileptic amnesia. *Neuropsychology.* (2015) 29:117–25. doi: 10.1037/neu0000114
7. Jansari AS, Davis K, McGibbon T, Firminger S, Kapur N. When "long-term memory" no longer means "forever": analysis of accelerated long-term forgetting in a patient with temporal lobe epilepsy. *Neuropsychologia.* (2010) 48:1707–15. doi: 10.1016/j.neuropsychologia.2010.02.018
8. Martin RC, Loring D, Meador KJ, Lee GP, Thrash N, Arena JG. Impaires long-term retention despite normal verbal learning in patients with temporal lobe dysfunction. *Neuropsychology.* (1991) 5:3–12. doi: 10.1037/0894-4105.5.1.3
9. Muhlert N, Milton F, Butler CR, Kapur N, Zeman AZ. Accelerated forgetting of real-life events in Transient Epileptic Amnesia. *Neuropsychologia.* (2010) 48:3235–44. doi: 10.1016/j.neuropsychologia.2010.07.001
10. Tramoni E, Felician O, Barbeau EJ, Guedj E, Guye M, Bartolomei F, et al. Long-term consolidation of declarative memory: insight from temporal lobe epilepsy. *Brain.* (2011) 134:816–31. doi: 10.1093/brain/awr002
11. Kopelman MD, Wilson BA, Baddeley AD. The autobiographical memory interview: a new assessment of autobiographical and personal semantic memory in amnesic patients. *J Clin Exp Neuropsychol.* (1989) 11:724–44. doi: 10.1080/01688638908400928
12. Piolino P, Desgranges B, Eustache F. La mémoire autobiographique: théorie et pratique. *Marseille: Solal.* (2000).
13. Derouesne C, Poitreneau J, Hugonot L, Kalafat M, Dubois B, Laurent B. Mini-mental state examination: a useful method for the evaluation of the cognitive status of patients by the clinician. Consensual French version. *Presse Medicale Paris Fr 1983.* (1999) 28:1141–8.
14. Wechsler D. MEM-III, Echelle clinique de mémoire, 3ème édition. *ECPA.* (2001).
15. Van der Linden M. *L'évaluation des troubles de la mémoire: présentation de quatre tests de mémoire épisodique (avec leur étalonnage).* Marseille: SOLAL. (2004).
16. Stoykova R, Matharan F, Raoux N, Amieva H. An alternative word-list for the Free and cued selective reminding test (FCSRT): list presentation and reliability study. *Gériatrie Psychol Neuropsychiatr Viellissement.* (2013) 11:317–22. doi: 10.1684/pnv.2013.0416
17. Rey A. *Manuel du Test de copie et de reproduction de mémoire de figure géométriques complexes.* Paris: ECPA (1959).
18. Bever C, Grattan L, Panitch H, Johnson K. The brief repeatable battery of neuropsychological tests for multiple sclerosis: a preliminary serial study. *Mult Scler J.* (1995) 1:165–9. doi: 10.1177/135245859500100306
19. Wechsler D. WAIS-IV, *Echelle d'Intelligence de Wechsler pour Adultes, 4ème édition.* Paris: ECPA (2011).
20. Godefroy O. *Fonctions exécutives et pathologies neurologiques et psychia: évaluation en pratique clinique.* Marseille: Ed Solal (2008).
21. Deloche G, Metz-Lutz MM, Kremin H, Hannequin D, Ferrand L, Perrier D, et al. *Test de dénomination orale de 80 images : DO 80.* Paris: ECPA (1989).
22. Zigmond AS, Snaith RP. The Hospital Anxiety and Depression Scale. *Acta Psychiatr Scand.* (1983) 67:361–70. doi: 10.1111/j.1600-0447.1983.tb09716.x
23. Piolino, P. La mémoire autobiographique : théorie et pratique en neuropsychologie. *Revue Québécoise de Psychologie.* (2006) 3:1–20.
24. Butler CR, Zeman AZ. Recent insights into the impairment of memory in epilepsy: transient epileptic amnesia, accelerated long-term forgetting and remote memory impairment. *Brain.* (2008) 131:2243–63. doi: 10.1093/brain/awn127
25. Ramanan VK, Morris KA, Graff-Radford J, Jones DT, Burkholder DB, Britton JW, et al. Transient Epileptic Amnesia: A Treatable Cause of Spells Associated With Persistent Cognitive Symptoms. *Front Neurol.* (2019) 10:939. doi: 10.3389/fneur.2019.00939
26. Lambert I, Tramoni-Negre E, Lagarde S, Roehri N, Giusiano B, Trebuchon-Da Fonseca A, et al. Hippocampal Interictal Spikes during Sleep Impact Long-Term Memory Consolidation. *Ann Neurol.* (2020) 87:976–87. doi: 10.1002/ana.25744
27. McGaugh JL. Memory—A century of consolidation. *Science.* (2000) 287:248–51. doi: 10.1126/science.287.5451.248

7

Seizures and Consciousness Disorder Secondary to Intracranial Hypotension after Spinal Surgery: A Case Report and Literature Review

Yuqing Lv[1] *and Hui Xiang*[2*]

[1] *Department of Gastroenterology, Zhongnan Hospital of Wuhan University, Wuhan, China,* [2] *Department of Critical Care Medicine, Zhongnan Hospital of Wuhan University, Wuhan, China*

***Correspondence:**
Hui Xiang
xianghuisky@163.com

Rationale: Cerebrospinal fluid (CSF) leakage is a common condition after spinal surgery and is also the most common cause of intracranial hypotension. Intracranial hypotension (IH) is typically characterized by an orthostatic headache with associated nausea, vomiting, tinnitus, vertigo, hypoacusis, neck stiffness, and photophobia. There have been limited case reports describing surgery-associated IH presenting with seizures and disorder of consciousness. Due to the atypia of symptoms, these clinical manifestations are usually ignored or even misdiagnosed. As a result, clinicians face a significant challenge in detecting IH early and understanding its various clinical presentations. Meanwhile, we summarize the cases of IH presenting as seizures in recent years, including its clinical characteristics and effective treatment, which will be very helpful for the early diagnosis of IH.

Patient concerns: A 72-year-old Chinese male patient developed status epilepticus, a disorder of consciousness, and quadriplegia when he finished spinal surgery, although he had no previous seizures or any seizure risk factors.

Diagnosis: After MRI and CT examination, subdural hygromas were found under both sides of the skull, and combined with the clinical manifestations of the patient, intracranial hypotension due to cerebrospinal fluid leakage was diagnosed.

Interventions: In the early stage, we carried out strict perioperative critical care for the patient. Trendelenburg position was conducted to relieve intracranial hypotension. The dural repair surgery was performed after the diagnosis of CSF leakage.

Outcomes: Seizures in the patient were resolved. Three months after discharge, he was gradually returning to normal life.

Lessons: One possible cause of unexplained seizures and disorder of consciousness after spinal surgery is cerebrospinal fluid leakage associated with intracranial hypotension syndrome. Trendelenburg position and dural repair surgery are effective ways to relieve intracranial hypotension and associated symptoms. Better awareness of the association between IH (intracranial hypotension) and seizures may help us improve early recognition of the syndrome.

Keywords: seizure, intracranial hypotension, status epilepticus, cerebrospinal fluid leakage, spinal surgery, critical care

INTRODUCTION

The syndrome of intracranial hypotension has been increasingly diagnosed since the introduction of magnetic resonance imaging (MRI), and its incidence is now about 5 per 1,00,000 of the population (1). Cerebrospinal fluid (CSF) leakage is the most common cause of intracranial hypotension. Defects along the dura (including tears and fistulas), leading to CSF leakage, can be congenital and traumatic in etiology (2), with surgery being the most common traumatic cause. Intracranial hypotension (IH) typically presents with a postural headache with associated nausea, vomiting, tinnitus, vertigo, hypoacusis, neck stiffness, and photophobia (2–5), while seizures and the disorder of consciousness are rare. Therefore, the disorder of consciousness and seizures after spinal surgery are of concern because they may be associated with intracranial hypotension caused by cerebrospinal fluid leakage.

ETHICS STATEMENTS

Informed written consent was obtained from the patient's son after the nature of the study had been fully explained to them. The patient's son provided informed consent for the publication of the case.

CASE PRESENTATION

A 72-year-old Chinese male patient developed seizures, disorder of consciousness, and quadriplegia when he finished spinal surgery. Due to 3 years of pain and numbness in both lower limbs, he underwent spinal surgery, including L3/4/5 posterior decompression, interbody fusion, and internal fixation, plus L2/3 left lamina decompression. His medical history was significant hypertension for about 8 years and he usually took amlodipine, an oral antihypertensive drug. Therefore, his blood pressure was well-controlled. He had no previous seizures or any seizure risk factors.

The operation went smoothly and the patient soon regained consciousness. Then, the endotracheal tube was safely removed. In the surgical resuscitation room, the patient complained of itchy skin and generalized clonic seizures, which became progressively worse, characterized by bilateral clonic movements in the upper and lower limbs. Profound tachycardia and hypertension accompanied the spell. Therefore, the patient was transferred to the intensive care unit (ICU) immediately and tracheal intubation was performed instantly. Subsequently, consciousness disturbance occurred with blood oxygen saturation declining, and the ECG (electrocardiograph) monitor displayed that there was an atrial fibrillation rhythm and it quickly developed into ventricular fibrillation. He was given timely shock defibrillation, after which sinus rhythm was regained, with Norepinephrine maintaining blood pressure. Meanwhile, the emergency blood gas analysis suggested a pH of 6.9 and a pCO_2 of 95 mmHg. For emergency seizure control, intravenous midazolam was given. In addition, an extremely high level of creatine kinase and myohemoglobin was found in his blood test, which was thought to be the result of a violent convulsion. We gave the patient rocuronium bromide, a muscle relaxant, to prevent further muscle damage.

An emergency brain CT (computerized tomography) was conducted, suggesting that the space under the inner plate of the skull was widened on both sides, which was considered a subdural effusion (**Figure 1**). No obvious signs of cerebral hemorrhage and cerebral infarction were found. After first aid, we conducted target temperature management for the patient and implemented a hypothermia strategy to maintain its core temperature between 32 and 34°C. Levetiracetam and midazolam were added to abort seizures as the disorder of consciousness and seizures persisted. Norepinephrine and dopamine were used to achieve a mean arterial pressure >65 mmHg, with a maximum of 1 μg/kg/min for norepinephrine and 15 μg/kg/min for dopamine. Blood oxygen saturation fluctuated around 85% at pure oxygen concentration due to the presence of refractory hypoxemia. On the second day of ICU admission, he was given a tracheostomy and ventilator-assisted ventilation to maintain oxygen saturation >94% and pCO_2 between 35 and 45 mmHg. Given his lack of gastrointestinal hemorrhage and intestinal dysfunction, enteral nutrition was administered within 48 h, along with insulin to keep his blood sugar at 8–10 mmol/L.

Three days after the symptom onset, the use of vasoactive agents and sedatives such as midazolam were suspended, and a significant improvement in convulsions was observed, as well as blood oxygen saturation was maintained above 94% at 35 oxygen concentration, which was an indication that respiration and epilepsy were getting better. Simultaneously, blood pressure also returned to normal, at around 140/60 mmHg, thus the use of epinephrine was interrupted. As the patient's condition stabilized, we performed an EEG for 24 h, which revealed a diffuse slow waves background with a large number of fast waves, but we did not pick up the epileptic waves. Whereas, we observed that more than 350 ml of hemorrhagic fluid could be drained from the drainage tube of the patient's waist wound every day, and he was still in a comatose state without an obvious response to pain stimuli. We reviewed the blood concentration of valproate and it was in the normal range. A CT scan of the brain was also reviewed, indicating there was mild cerebral edema and ventricular shrinkage. The existence of cerebrospinal fluid leakage was highly suspected and it was considered that the patient's consciousness disturbance and epileptic seizure might be related to it because it can lead to intracranial hypotension. We adopted a Trendelenburg position to prevent the excessive outflow of cerebrospinal fluid. Sure enough, after changing the patient's position, his disturbance of consciousness improved. Simultaneously, he was able to respond to verbal stimuli and partially follow movements. Over the next few days, his cerebrospinal fluid drainage gradually decreased to about 200 ml per day.

Abbreviations: IH, intracranial hypotension; CSF, cerebrospinal fluid; SE, status epilepticus; ECG, electrocardiograph; PH, pondus hydrogenii; PCO_2, partial pressure of carbon dioxide; MRI, magnetic resonance imaging; MR, magnetic resonance; ICU, intensive care unit; CT, computerized tomography; ICP, intracranial pressure; PRES, posterior reversible encephalopathy syndrome.

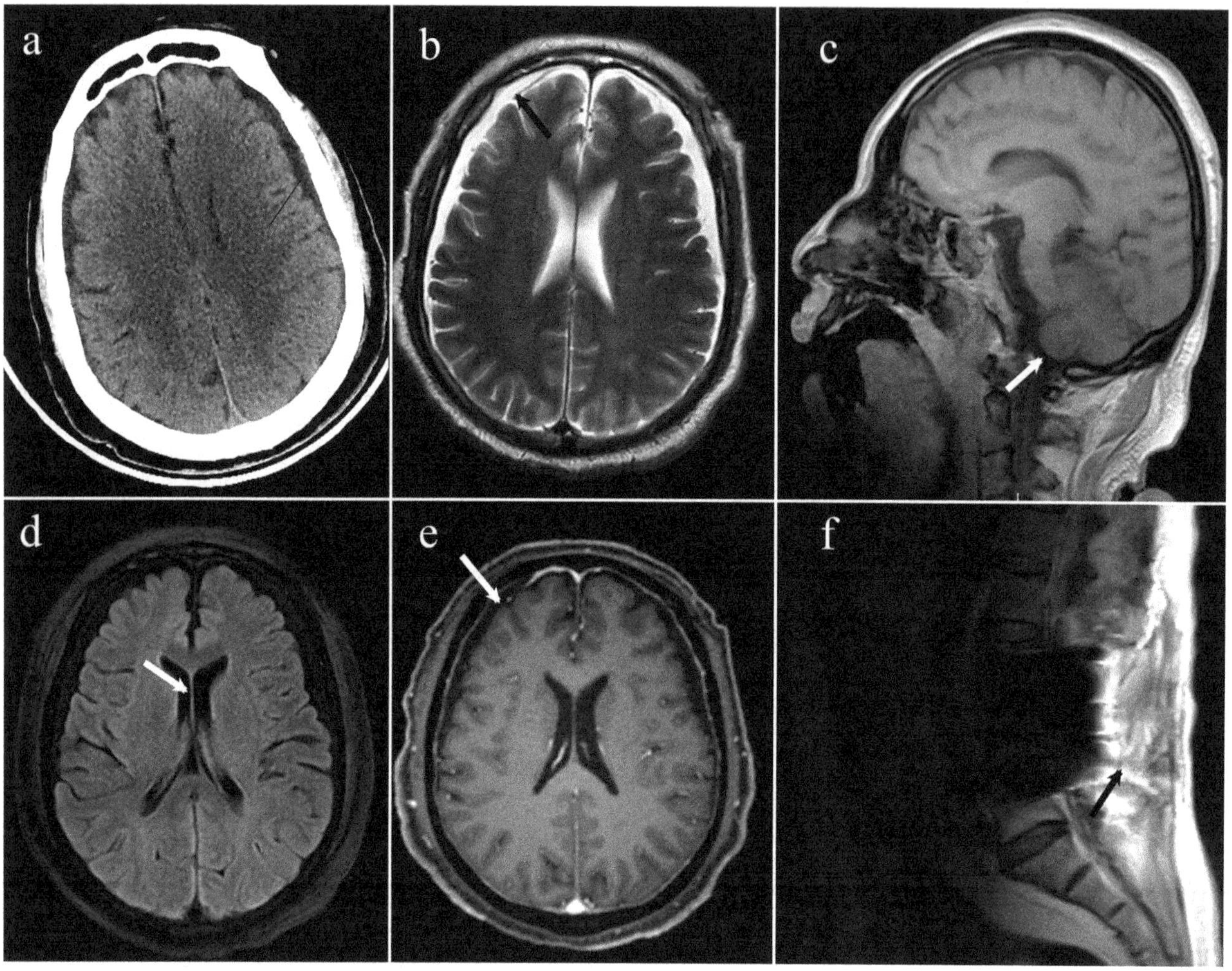

FIGURE 1 | (a) The emergency CT suggested that the space under the inner plate of the skull was widened on both sides, which was considered a subdural effusion; **(b)** axial T2 weighted MRI demonstrates bilateral subdural effusions (arrows); **(c)** sagittal T1-weighted MRI demonstrates sagging of the brain; **(d)** axial T1 weighted MRI demonstrates bilateral ventricles narrowing; **(e)** axial T1 post-gadolinium showing diffuse, mild pachymeningeal thickening, and enhancement (arrow); **(f)** MRI spine sagittal T2 sequence demonstrates a fluid collection within the posterior paraspinal soft tissue.

On day 10, the patient was successfully removed from the ventilator, so he underwent MRI and enhanced MRI of his brain and spinal cord, revealing evidence of bilateral subdural effusion and mild inferior hernia of the bilateral cerebellar tonsil, bilateral ventricles narrowing, pachymeningeal enhancement, which is consistent with intracranial hypotension. Several tiny hemorrhagic foci were also in the left cerebellar hemisphere and right temporal lobe. Spinal MRI demonstrated postoperative changes of the lumbar spine, lumbosacral fascia edema, and fluid collection between the intrathecal site and the soft tissue; however it did not identify the site of cerebrospinal fluid (CSF) leakage (**Figure 2**). These changes in the brain were indicative of typical intracranial hypotension, such as subdural effusion, mild inferior hernia of the bilateral cerebellar tonsil, ventricular narrowing, and pachymeningeal enhancement which could be caused by cerebrospinal fluid leakage.

Taking all the evidence together, we strongly suspected that he had a cerebrospinal fluid leak. Therefore, we contacted an orthopedic surgeon for dural repair and wound debridement and a drainage tube was placed in the operation area. During the operation, CSF leakage was proved to be present. Thus, intracranial hypotension due to cerebrospinal fluid leakage secondary to intraoperative dural tear was diagnosed.

After surgery, we still kept the Trendelenburg position. On the other hand, a neuro-rehabilitation doctor was brought in for muscle massage and acupuncture. Over the next few days, he gradually regained consciousness and was able to follow instructions better, accompanied by a gradual reduction of clear to bloody spinal drainage fluid. At the same time, his upper body strength was gradually recovering to level 2. The drainage tube was removed when the drainage fluid was <50 ml for more than 2 days. As the condition gradually improved, the patient's family requested that he be transferred back to the local hospital

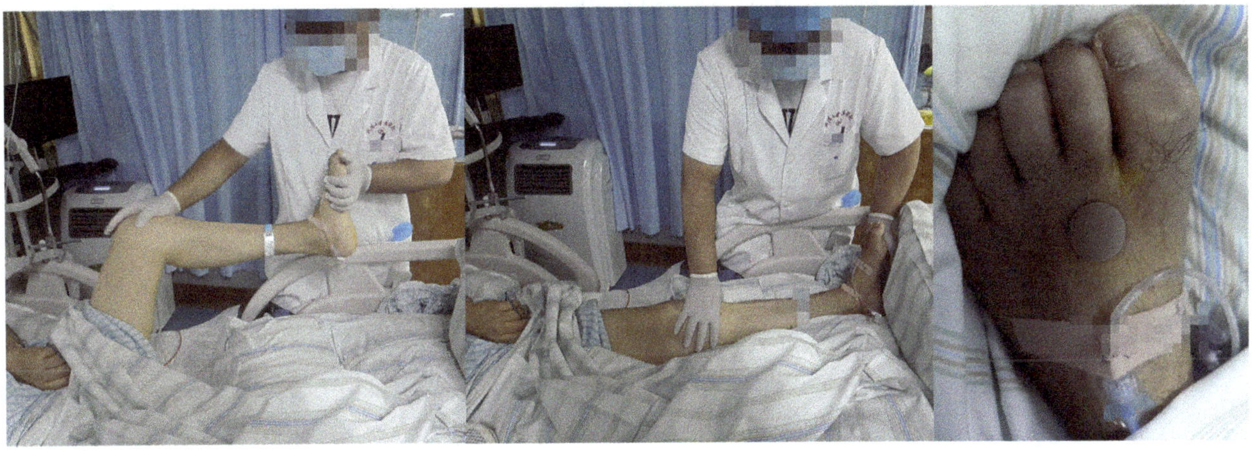

FIGURE 2 | The first two pictures show that the neuro-rehabilitation doctor is giving him muscle massages. The third picture shows the special treatment of Traditional Chinese medicine, acupoint acupuncture.

for further rehabilitation. We followed him up for 3 months. A month after discharge, with his independent diet and defecation, we learned that he had complete sensation in his limbs and level 3 strength in his lower extremities and that his trachea incision had been fully healed and closed. The only problem was the gastrointestinal disturbance, with bloating and constipation, which may be related to the neurotic disorder caused by the operation. Three months after discharge, his gastrointestinal function recovered well and he could walk about 50 m on a flat ground alone.

DISCUSSION

The syndrome of intracranial hypotension (IH) is caused by the leakage of CSF (cerebrospinal fluid) from the thecal sac within or along the spinal canal (3, 4). It is typically manifested by orthostatic headaches that may be associated with one or more of several other symptoms, including pain or stiffness of the neck, nausea, emesis, horizontal diplopia, dizziness, changes in hearing, visual blurring or visual field cuts, photophobia, interscapular pain, and occasionally face numbness or weakness or radicular upper-limb symptoms (5). Seizures caused by IH have also been observed in some rare clinical cases (6, 7). If the leakage can be arrested, it is potentially curable (3, 4, 8).

The most characteristic features of IH on intracranial MR (magnetic resonance) imaging include diffuse pachymeningeal enhancement and "brain sag" (9, 10). Sagging of the brain can cause a subdural hematoma or hygroma, kinking of the midbrain and pons toward the clivus, lessening of the distance (e.g.,) from the optic chiasm to the pituitary gland, and tension on the cranial nerves (3). Other features include dural contrast enhancement and enlargement of the pituitary gland. Homogenous contrast enhancement of the dura mater is the most sensitive sign (3).

Intracranial hypotension is usually treated with a progressive approach. Typically, headaches can be resolved with conservative management, which includes hydration and strict bed rest, allowing for relief of CSF pressure at the site of leakage and thus healing the underlying defect. Caffeine administered intravenously or orally is also effective for post-lumbar puncture IH. If a conservative approach is not effective, epidural blood patches, epidural saline infusion, and surgical correction should be considered (3, 4, 11). However, blood patches are more controversial when used for surgery-related dural leaks, although suggested to be safe in a case series because they can cause seizures and respiratory distress, or other related complications (12). Although the specific mechanism by which IH may cause seizure development and convulsive SE has not been fully elucidated, it has been proposed that IH may cause meningeal irritation or traction on cortical structures of the brain, and finally, result in seizures (6, 13). In addition, the alterations of intracranial pressure (ICP) may result in acute changes in cerebral blood flow, leading to seizure generation (14).

Intracranial hypotension presents in a variety of ways; however, reports of seizures secondary to IH are rare. We summarize the cases of IH presenting as seizures in recent years, including its clinical characteristics and effective treatment (**Table 1**). Gilmour et al. (7) describe a 71-year-old woman with chronic back pain who developed convulsive status epilepticus immediately after scoliosis surgery. MRI was consistent with IH, there was no cortical vein thrombosis, presumably due to an intraoperative dural tear causing status epilepticus, and the seizure terminated after bed rest. Lin et al. (13) describe an individual who had multiple seizures after a thoracic laminectomy and had imaging findings consistent with IH. A thoracic laminotomy was performed on this patient and a dural tear was found and repaired. Chaudhary et al. (6) describe cases of spontaneous intracranial hypotension causing focal onset seizures and impairment of awareness. Other two reports describe patients with hydrocephalus and ventriculoperitoneal shunts who had intractable epilepsy caused by overdrainage (14, 15). Delgado-López et al. (16) present a case of posterior reversible encephalopathy syndrome (PRES) following laminectomy and fixation for L4-5 lumbar stenosis and spondylolisthesis, characterized by status epilepticus, which

TABLE 1 | Summary of some reported cases of seizures secondary to intracranial hypotension (IH).

Article	Patient presentation	Seizure description	The cause of IH	Treatment
Gilmour et al. (7)	A 71-year-old woman with chronic back pain developed convulsive status epilepticus immediately after scoliosis surgery	It was characterized by bilateral clonic movements of her upper and lower extremities, with eyes open and a vertical upward tonic gaze deviation	An intraoperative dural tear secondary to elective redo-scoliosis surgery	Keep on strict bed rest
Lin et al. (13)	A 37-yr-old man with acute spinal cord compression at T9-10 because of pseudoarthritis developed generalized seizure after surgery	30 min postoperative generalized seizures lasting 15 s occurring every 10–15 min	Dural tear after laminectomy	Treated with midazolam, phenytoin, and dural tear repair
Chaudhary et al. (6)	A 60-year-old man who presented with a decreased level of consciousness developed a complex partial seizure involving left-sided facial twitching after the presentation	Focal motor-impaired awareness seizure with left-sided facial twitching	Small bilateral subdural hygromas	Treatment with a 20 cc blood patch in the lumbar spine
	A 37-year-old man who presented with a right-sided acute on chronic SDH which reaccumulated despite burr hole drainage, presenting with decreased level of consciousness	Focal impaired awareness and complex partial seizures	Chiropractic neck manipulation and trivial head trauma, potentially resulting in thoracic dural tear	A 20 cc autologous epidural blood patch was placed at the T12-L1 level
Delgado-López et al. (16)	An 82-year-old woman presented with a generalized tonic-clonic seizure after L4-5 laminectomy and decompression of the dural sac and origin of roots bilaterally	She developed transient hypotension for <1 min presented with a generalized tonic-clonic seizure that lasted 5 days	An unnoticed cerebrospinal fluid leakage secondary to surgery	Antiepileptic drugs, ventilators and other symptomatic support treatment
Pugliese et al. (17)	A 41-year-old woman presented a worsening of the headache and tonico-clonic seizures 7 days after epidural analgesia for a cesarean section	A worsening of the headache which had a gradual onset, was bilateral, pressure-like, with a postural component and tonico-clonic seizures with the left motor syndrome, mild right anisocoria, and rapid deterioration of the mental status	Inadvertent dural puncture during the epidural anesthesia	Treatment with support therapy followed by blood patch
Our report	A 72-year-old Chinese male patient developed seizures, disorder of consciousness, and quadriplegia when he finished spinal surgery	He developed itchy skin and generalized clonic seizures, characterized by bilateral clonic movements in the upper and lower limbs	Cerebrospinal fluid leakage secondary to the spinal surgery of L3/4/5 posterior decompression, interbody fusion, and internal fixation, plus L2/3 left lamina decompression	Treatment with support therapy, trendelenburg position, dural repair surgery, and traditional Chinese acupuncture and massage therapy

IH, intracranial hypotension; SDH, subdural hematomas.

is hypothesized by vasoconstriction, brain hypoperfusion, and cerebrospinal fluid. Pugliese et al. (17) report a case of a woman presenting headache and tonico-clonic seizures 7 days after epidural analgesia for a cesarean section. MRI showed alterations suggestive of the presence of intracranial hypotension (IH), as well as evidence of posterior reversible encephalopathy syndrome (PRES). They suggest that venous stagnation and hydrostatic edema, secondary to intracranial hypotension, probably played a crucial role in the pathogenesis of PRES. In our case, the patient developed seizures after spinal surgery, with imaging revealed bilateral subdural hygromas, which were thought to be related to intracranial hypotension syndrome. It is speculated that the existence of subdural hygromas may lead to the formation of hemorrhagic foci in brain, which felt to be acute, because of the pulling on the brain tissue. This may have caused the seizure due to the highly epileptogenic effect of blood. In addition, during the perioperative period, patients were given a large number of sedative drugs, such as midazolam, and whether these drugs are involved in the seizure is also a thought-provoking question.

Meanwhile, the patient did not develop typical postural headache symptoms but instead presented with a convulsive status epilepticus characterized by impaired limb movement and sensory function as well as impaired consciousness, which was also rare in previous reports. We adopted the Trendelenburg position treatment and a dural repair surgery, which proved to be very therapeutic. Gastrointestinal dysfunction occurred during the patient's subsequent recovery, and it is reasonable to speculate that this may be related to autonomic nervous dysfunction caused by the persistent epileptic state.

CONCLUSION

Unexplained seizures and disorder of consciousness after spinal surgery may be associated with cerebrospinal fluid leakage associated with intracranial hypotension syndrome. Trendelenburg position and dural repair surgery are effective ways to relieve intracranial hypotension and associated symptoms. Better awareness of the association between IH and seizures may help us improve early recognition of the syndrome.

AUTHOR CONTRIBUTIONS

YL wrote the manuscript. HX revised the manuscript. All authors contributed to the article and approved the submitted version.

REFERENCES

1. Gordon N. Spontaneous intracranial hypotension. *Dev Med Child Neurol.* (2009) 51:932–5. doi: 10.1111/j.1469-8749.2009.03514.x
2. Upadhyaya P, Ailani J. A review of spontaneous intracranial hypotension. *Curr Neurol Neurosci Rep.* (2019) 19:22. doi: 10.1007/s11910-019-0938-7
3. Chan SM, Chodakiewitz YG, Maya MM, Schievink WI, Moser FG. Intracranial hypotension and cerebrospinal fluid leak. *Neuroimaging Clin N Am.* (2019) 29:213–26. doi: 10.1016/j.nic.2019.01.002
4. Farb RI, Nicholson PJ, Peng PW, Massicotte EM, Lay C, Krings T, et al. Spontaneous intracranial hypotension: a systematic imaging approach for CSF leak localization and management based on MRI and digital subtraction myelography. *Am J Neuroradiol.* (2019) 40:745–53. doi: 10.3174/ajnr.A6016
5. Mokri B. Spontaneous intracranial hypotension. *Curr Neurol Neurosci Rep.* (2001) 1:109–17. doi: 10.1007/s11910-001-0005-y
6. Chaudhary N, Cooper P, Lownie SP, Ng W, Duggal N. Spontaneous intracranial hypotension: case series of rare clinical presentations. *Can J Neurol Sci.* (2011) 38:54–8. doi: 10.1017/S0317167100011070
7. Gilmour GS, Scott J, Couillard P. Leaking the diagnosis: a case of convulsive status epilepticus due to intracranial hypotension. *Neurocrit Care.* (2019) 31:562–6. doi: 10.1007/s12028-019-00788-3
8. Kranz PG, Malinzak MD, Amrhein TJ, Gray L. Update on the diagnosis and treatment of spontaneous intracranial hypotension. *Curr Pain Headache Rep.* (2017) 21:37. doi: 10.1007/s11916-017-0639-3
9. Bond KM, Benson JC, Cutsforth-Gregory JK, Kim DK, Diehn FE, Carr CM. Spontaneous intracranial hypotension: atypical radiologic appearances, imaging mimickers, and clinical look-alikes. *Am J Neuroradiol.* (2020) 41:1339–47. doi: 10.3174/ajnr.A6637
10. Rahman M, Bidari SS, Quisling RG, Friedman WA. Spontaneous intracranial hypotension: dilemmas in diagnosis. *Neurosurgery.* (2011) 69:4–14; discussion. doi: 10.1227/NEU.0b013e3182134399
11. Paldino M, Mogilner AY, Tenner MS. Intracranial hypotension syndrome: a comprehensive review. *Neurosurg Focus.* (2003) 15:Ecp2. doi: 10.3171/foc.2003.15.6.8
12. Seemiller J, Challagundla S, Taylor T, Zand R. Intrathecal blood injection: a case report of a rare complication of an epidural blood patch. *BMC Neurol.* (2020) 20:187. doi: 10.1186/s12883-020-01763-8
13. Lin SM, Tsou MY, Chan KH, Yin YC, Hsin ST, Liao WW, et al. Myoclonic seizure in the postanesthesia care unit after thoracic laminectomy. *Anesth Analg.* (2002) 95:777–9, table of contents. doi: 10.1213/00000539-200209000-00046
14. Uchida D, Fujimoto A, Yamazoe T, Yamamoto T, Enoki H. Seizure frequency can be reduced by changing intracranial pressure: a case report in drug-resistant epilepsy. *Epilepsy Behav Case Rep.* (2018) 10:14–7. doi: 10.1016/j.ebcr.2017.12.005
15. Agrawal D, Durity FA. Seizure as a manifestation of intracranial hypotension in a shunted patient. *Pediatr Neurosurg.* (2006) 42:165–7. doi: 10.1159/000091860
16. Delgado-López PD, Garcés-Pérez G, García-Carrasco J, Alonso-García E, Gómez-Menéndez AI, Martín-Alonso J. Posterior reversible encephalopathy syndrome with status epilepticus following surgery for lumbar stenosis and spondylolisthesis. *World Neurosurg.* (2018) 116:309–15. doi: 10.1016/j.wneu.2018.05.174
17. Pugliese S, Finocchi V, Borgia ML, Nania C, Della Vella B, Pierallini A, et al. Intracranial hypotension and PRES: case report. *J Headache Pain.* (2010) 11:437–40. doi: 10.1007/s10194-010-0226-z

8

Newly Diagnosed Hepatic Encephalopathy Presenting as Non-convulsive Status Epilepticus: A Case Report and Literature Review

Marco Olivero [1], Delia Gagliardi [1,2], Gianluca Costamagna [1], Daniele Velardo [2], Francesca Magri [3], Fabio Triulzi [4], Giorgio Conte [4], Giacomo P. Comi [1,3], Stefania Corti [1,2] and Megi Meneri [1,2]*

[1] Neuroscience Section, Dino Ferrari Centre, Department of Pathophysiology and Transplantation (DEPT), University of Milan, Milan, Italy, [2] Neurology Unit, Foundation IRCCS Ca' Granda Ospedale Maggiore Policlinico, Milan, Italy, [3] Neuromuscular and Rare Diseases Unit, Department of Neuroscience, Fondazione IRCCS Ca' Granda Ospedale Maggiore Policlinico, Milan, Italy, [4] Neuroradiology Unit, Fondazione IRCCS Ca' Granda Ospedale Maggiore Policlinico, Department of Pathophysiology and Transplantation, Università degli Studi Milano, Milan, Italy

***Correspondence:**
Stefania Corti
stefania.corti@unimi.it*

Background: Hepatic encephalopathy is characterized by psychiatric and neurological abnormalities, including epileptic seizure and non-convulsive and convulsive status epilepticus. Conventional brain magnetic resonance imaging is useful in supporting diagnosis since it can reveal specific radiological findings. In the literature, there is no description of hepatic encephalopathy onset as non-convulsive status epilepticus; we provide the first report.

Case Summary: We report a case of a 67-year-old woman, without history of cirrhosis, presenting altered mental state, normal brain computed tomography imaging, and electroencephalography suggestive of epileptic activity. We suspected non-convulsive status epilepticus, and we administered diazepam and levetiracetam with clinical improvement. Thus, we made a diagnosis of non-convulsive status epilepticus. A radiological study with brain magnetic resonance imaging showed bilateral hyperintensity on T1-weighted sequences of globus pallidus and hyperintensity of both corticospinal tracts on T2-weighted fluid-attenuated inversion recovery sequences. Blood tests revealed hyperammonemia, mild abnormality of liver function indices, and chronic Hepatitis B and D virus coinfection. Hepatic elastosonography suggested liver cirrhosis. The patient started antiviral therapy with entecavir and prevention of hepatic encephalopathy with rifaximin and lactulose; she was discharged with a normal mental state.

Conclusions: Hepatic encephalopathy can present as an initial manifestation with non-convulsive status epilepticus. Electroencephalography is useful for differentiating non-convulsive status epilepticus from an episode of hepatic encephalopathy, and neuroimaging aids the diagnostic process.

Keywords: hepatic encephalopathy, non-convulsive status epilepticus, brain magnetic resonance imaging, case report, corticospinal tract, globus pallidus

INTRODUCTION

Hepatic encephalopathy (HE) is defined as brain dysfunction caused by liver failure or portal systemic shunting, without considering the etiology (1). The clinical picture comprises neurological or psychiatric abnormalities, ranging from subclinical alterations to coma (1). It is one of the most important complications of liver cirrhosis, contributing to both morbidity and mortality (1). From the pathophysiological perspective, ammonia is, probably, the central player in the pathogenesis of HE (1). Considered a metabolic disorder, it is usually reversible by liver transplantation (1). Although rare, HE can present as epileptic seizure; manifestations vary widely, encompassing tonic-clonic seizure, convulsive (CSE), and non-convulsive status epilepticus (NCSE) (2–6). HE can show typical features on brain magnetic resonance imaging (MRI), namely, the bilateral and symmetric hyperintensity of the globus pallidus on T1-weighted (T1W) sequences, and hyperintensity in cerebral white matter, involving corticospinal tract and subcortical hemispheric white matter on T2 weighted (T2W)—"fluid attenuated inversion recovery" (FLAIR) MRI sequences (7). Herein, we report a case of newly diagnosed HE presented as NCSE, in which conventional brain MRI shows some findings associated with this disease, such as the hyperintensity in the globus pallidus on T1 and the hyperintensity along the corticospinal tract on T2-FLAIR.

CASE PRESENTATION

A 67-year-old woman from Romania presented to our Emergency Department for confusion and subacute ideomotor decline in the previous 5 days. Insomnia, nocturnal awakenings, urinary incontinence, and amnesia for recent events were reported in the last month. The patient had a past medical history of paroxysmal atrial fibrillation, previously treated with amiodarone and apixaban, which were self-suspended 1 year ago, obesity, hypertension, and rectal carcinoma which was surgically treated with an enterostomy. The patient had no

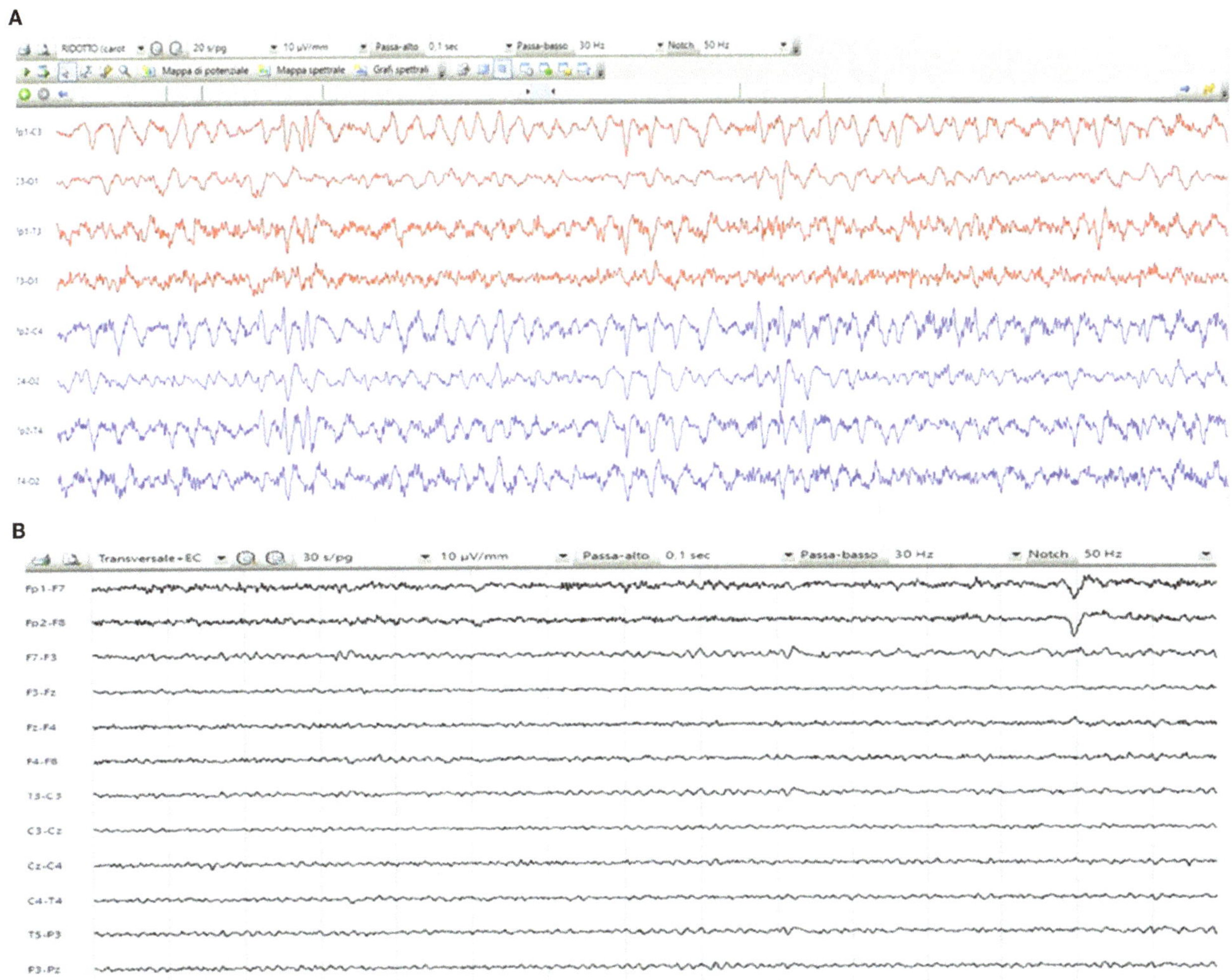

FIGURE 1 | EEG showing status epilepticus **(A)** and resolution after antiepileptic therapy **(B)**.

known history of seizures or other neurological diseases, recent illness, brain trauma, or recent surgical procedures. The chronic therapy encompassed olmesartan, bisoprolol, indapamide, furosemide, amlodipine, acetylsalicylic acid, and ranitidine. The vital parameters were normal, and the Glasgow Coma Scale (GCS) score was 15. The general physical examination did not show pathological items, nor signs of trauma. The chest X-ray was normal, while the electrocardiogram was suggestive of atrial fibrillation. From a neurological point of view, the patient was disoriented in space and time and unable to denominate objects of common use. The pupils were isochoric and reactive to light. The posture was normal and there were no signs of meningism. The cranial nerve examination was normal, except for dubious absence of the menace reflex on the left, not confirmed by a subsequent evaluation. The global strength of the limbs was preserved, as well as tactile sensitivity and coordination. The osteotendinous reflexes were valid, symmetrical in the upper limbs, with a mild prevalence on the right, and weak and symmetrical in the lower limbs. Cutaneous plantar response was mute bilaterally. A stroke was initially suspected, and a neuroimaging study was performed with brain computed tomography (CT), CT angiography, and CT perfusion, which were unremarkable. Because of the persistence of the altered mental state, electroencephalography (EEG) was performed. EEG showed a broadly slowed trace, with a background theta rhythm, which was more expressed on the right. Fast paroxysmal bilateral activity of the type sharp wave was superimposed and more represented on the right and mainly frontotemporal (**Figure 1A**) areas. Herein, NCSE was suspected and 10 mg of diazepam was administered intravenously, with regression of the paroxysmal activity on the synchronous recording of the EEG. Furthermore, antiepileptic therapy with 4,000 mg of intravenous levetiracetam was started, and the mental state progressively improved. The next day, the EEG was repeated, and epileptiform activity did not reappear (**Figure 1B**); levetiracetam was switched to an oral dosage of 2,000 mg daily. The patient was admitted to our Neurology Department with the presumptive diagnosis of NCSE, and a 3 Tesla brain MRI with gadolinium was performed. Bilateral hyperintensity of the lenticular nucleus was detected on T1W sequences (**Figure 2A**), while bilateral hyperintensity of the corticospinal tract signal was displayed on FLAIR (**Figure 2B**). Neuroimaging ruled out an ischemic event and an expansive lesion, with findings suggestive of chronic HE. As a completion, a lumbar puncture with examination of cerebral spinal fluid was performed. It did not show any noteworthy findings, including the real-time polymerase chain reaction for an infectious agent or dosage of autoantibodies associated with autoimmune and paraneoplastic encephalitis. The patient was obese (body mass index = 38.3 kg/m^2) but had no past history of alcoholic abuse. There were no signs of ascites and declining edema. She presented no signs of asterixis. Blood tests performed a few days later revealed: chronic coinfection of Hepatitis B (HBV) and D (HDV) virus, negative Hepatitis C virus (HCV) infection, ammonium 141 umol/L (11.2–48.2 umol/L), albumin 2.7 mg/dl (3.4–4.8), total bilirubin 1.33 (0.12–1.1 mg/dl), INR 1.25 (0.8–1.2), proteins 5.6 g/dl (6.4–8 g/dl), cobalamin 1,121 pg/ml (191–663 pg/ml), and normal levels of folate, transferrin,

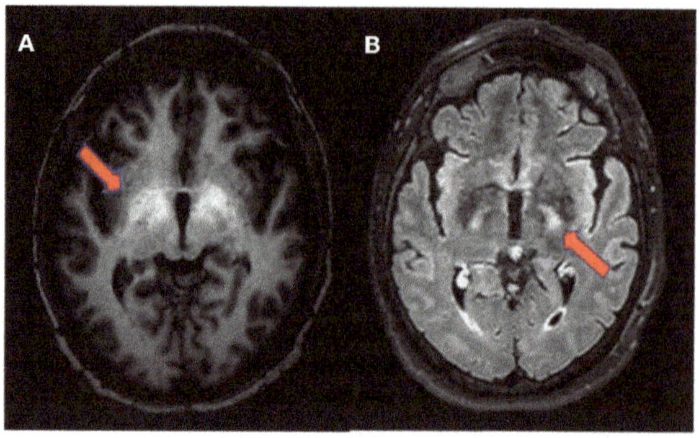

FIGURE 2 | Brain MRI, axial section. T1-weighted imaging showing bilateral symmetrical hyperintensity in the globus pallidus and upper mesencephalon [**(A)**, arrow]. T2-weighted FLAIR imaging depicting hyperintensity of the corticospinal tracts [**(B)**, arrow].

sideremia, and ferritin. Hepatic elastography recorded values compatible with cirrhosis. Hepatic cirrhosis from mixed etiology, chronic HBV-HDV co-infection, and metabolic syndrome was diagnosed. The clinical picture was considered to be an episode of HE, presenting as NCSE. Anti-HBV therapy with entecavir (0.5 mg daily orally) was started, as well as secondary prevention of HE with lactulose (10 g two times daily orally) and rifaximin (400 mg three times daily orally). On the day of discharge, her mental state was normal, and the patient noted improvement in her general health condition (**Figure 3**). Afterwards, she continued to receive levetiracetam for epilepsy, besides lactulose and rifaximine for secondary prevention of HE; relatives reported no other episodes of mental confusion. Three months later, a brain MRI was repeated, and radiological findings were stable.

DISCUSSION

HE is one of the main complications of liver cirrhosis, along with variceal bleeding, hepatorenal syndrome, hepatopulmonary syndrome, and ascites (8). Historically, it has been classified into "overt hepatic encephalopathy" (OHE, clinically manifested neurological and psychiatric abnormalities) and "covert hepatic encephalopathy" (CHE, abnormalities on neuro-psychological and electrophysiological tests without or mild clinically detectable neurological-psychiatric abnormalities) (9). According to the recent "International Society for Hepatic Encephalopathy and Nitrogen Metabolism" (ISHEN) consensus, the onset of disorientation and/or asterixis confirms OHE (10). In cirrhotic patients, OHE develops in 30–40% at some time during their clinical course, while minimal hepatic encephalopathy (MHE) and CHE are seen in 20–80% (11). As HE is a manifestation of serious liver impairment, its outcome depends on the severity of underlying liver disease, its clinical course, and its treatment (1). The serum level of ammonia plays a central role in the pathophysiology of HE, helping physicians in ruling out the diagnosis and defining the

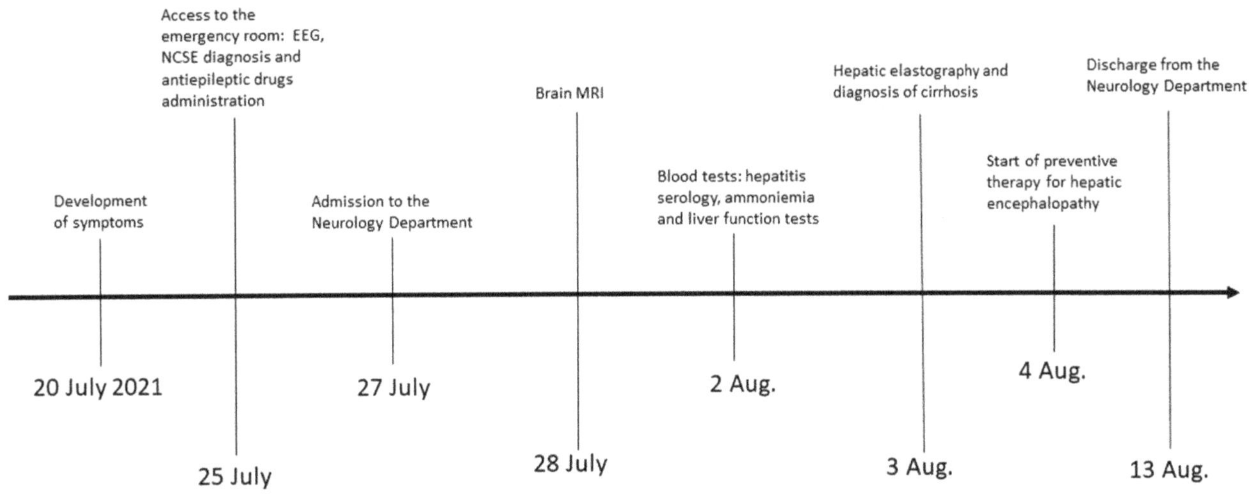

FIGURE 3 | The timeline of the case report.

prognosis; lowering serum ammonia is the main therapeutic goal (1, 9). Apart from hyperammonemia, other pathogenetic factors are implied, such as systemic inflammation, increased blood manganese, circulating bile acids, and lactate (1, 9). Their generation is influenced by common precipitant factors of HE, like malnutrition, infections, electrolyte imbalance, constipation, gastrointestinal bleeding, dehydration, and use of diuretics (1, 9). These pathogenetic factors influence the blood-brain barrier (BBB) by increasing its permeability (1, 9). Anyway, independent of blood-brain barrier status, ammonia passes freely into the brain, which is exclusively removed by astrocytes *via* glutamine synthetase (1, 9). The generation of glutamine renders the astrocyte hypertonic, resulting in swelling, impaired function, and, finally, brain edema (1, 9). Astrocyte swelling causes neuronal dysfunction and clinical manifestations of HE (1, 9). However, as in our case, there may be no clear precipitant factor underlying an episode of OHE (1, 9).

On a neurological point of view, clinical elements are plethoric, encompassing, mostly, the higher cortical functions and the motor system (12). Cognitive findings in patients with chronic HE vary from subtle deficits, not apparent without psychometric and electrophysiological testing (CHE), to clearer findings during periods of decompensation related to higher ammonia levels, such as impairments in attention span, reaction time, and working memory (OHE) (12). Disturbances in the sleep-wake pattern are common initial manifestations of HE and may precede mental state changes or neuromuscular symptoms (13). As HE progresses, patients may develop mood and personality changes, disorientation in time and space, inappropriate behavior, somnolence, confusion, and, finally, the so-called "coma hepaticus" (14). Seizures and status epilepticus are very rarely reported in HE (2). Generally, HE is associated with different EEG patterns, such as delta activity and the more typical triphasic waves (9). In particular, the description of NCSE in HE is anecdotal, probably because cognitive disturbances are shared in the two conditions, and an EEG is not always performed. To the best of our knowledge, just four case reports were previously described, and none of them reported NCSE as the first manifestation of HE (3–6). In our case, NCSE was diagnosed according to Salzburg criteria, since we found epileptiform discharge on the EEG that ceased after antiepileptic drugs administration, associated with a mental state improvement (15). The pathophysiology underlying the development of seizures in the setting of HE remains unknown, although hyperammonemia is likely the most important factor (16). In our case, the patient developed, within a few days, cognitive symptoms of episodical OHE but more likely caused by NCSE secondary to hyperammonemia. Neuroimaging excluded structural causes of seizures, while blood tests showed no other noteworthy metabolic alterations.

Brain MRI is the most useful imaging technique to support the diagnosis of HE in uncertain cases (17). Neuroradiological signs depend on the severity and velocity of development of liver failure, namely, a chronic or acute HE (18). In this case, we observed findings on conventional brain MRI compatible with a chronic form of HE, probably long neglected, not associated with any neurological signs. The bilateral and symmetric T1 hyperintensity involving the globus pallidus and substantia nigra reticulata is characteristic, reported in almost 90% of patients with cirrhosis and likely due to manganese accumulation; it may be associated with Parkinsonism (7, 17). Sometimes, other areas are involved, namely, the subthalamic nucleus, tectal plate, hypothalamus, adenohypophysis, limbic system, and white matter (7, 17, 18). Less commonly, the hyperintensity of both corticospinal tracts is described on T2-FLAIR sequences; it is caused by vasogenic brain edema due to glutamine increase in astrocytes, resulting in loss of organic osmolytes, such as myo-inositol, that accumulate in the extracellular compartment (17). This finding may be associated with subclinical alterations, detectable in electrophysiological studies with motor-evoked potentials, not performed in the case of our patient (19). Similar abnormalities may also be seen in periventricular white matter, the thalamus, posterior limb of internal capsule, and cortex (18). However, hyperintensity along both the corticospinal tracts may be seen in healthy adults and should be interpreted with caution, especially in 3 Tesla MRI (17, 20). These changes are similar to the signal abnormalities observed in patients with other diseases, such as amyotrophic lateral sclerosis, X-linked Charcot-Marie-Tooth, optic neuromyelitis, metabolic disorders (Krabbe disease and X-linked adrenoleukodystrophy), infectious diseases (*Borrelia* spp. and Human T-cell lymphotropic Virus 1), and primary central nervous system lymphoma (21–28). Other neuroradiological findings include an increase of mean diffusivity of hemispheric brain matter on diffusion weighted imaging (DWI); laminar hyperintensities involving the cortical deep layers; white matter focal lesions; and a low magnetization transfer ratio (MTR) in various white matter regions (17, 29). These radiological findings have been shown to be reversible after liver transplantation (30, 31).

CONCLUSIONS

We reported the first description of NCSE as an initial manifestation of HE. Specific brain MRI findings, namely, bilateral hyperintensity on T1 of the globus pallidus and hyperintensity of both corticospinal tracts on T2-FLAIR, were able to suggest the diagnosis of HE. From a general point of view, NCSE is easily underdiagnosed for lack of clear and univocal clinical signs. It is important to understand the possibility of NCSE in patients presenting an altered mental state; EEG is helpful in ruling it out. Hyperammonemia is a possible pathogenetic factor of NCSE, especially in patients with cirrhosis. The problem arises in differentiating acute alteration of the mental state due to an episode of HE from a real NCSE. Again, the EEG is useful for resolving diagnostic doubt, especially in the case of presumed HE that does not respond to empirical treatment.

AUTHOR CONTRIBUTIONS

MO: drafted the manuscript for intellectual content and collected and analyzed the data. DG, GCos, DV, and MM: collected and analyzed the data and revised the manuscript for intellectual content. FM, FT, GCon, GPC, and SC: revised the manuscript for intellectual content. All authors contributed to the article and approved the submitted version.

ACKNOWLEDGMENTS

This work was supported by Italian Ministry of Health ricerca corrente 2022 to GPC.

REFERENCES

1. Rose CF, Amodio P, Bajaj JS, Dhiman RK, Montagnese S, Taylor-Robinson SD et al. Hepatic encephalopathy: novel insights into classification, pathophysiology and therapy. *J Hepatol.* (2020) 73:1526–47. doi: 10.1016/j.jhep.2020.07.013
2. Rudler M, Marois C, Weiss N, Thabut D, Navarro V. Brain-Liver Pitié-Salpêtrière Study Group (BLIPS). Status epilepticus in patients with cirrhosis: How to avoid misdiagnosis in patients with hepatic encephalopathy. *Seizure.* (2017) 45:192–7. doi: 10.1016/j.seizure.2016.12.011
3. Jhun P, Kim H. Nonconvulsive status epilepticus in hepatic encephalopathy. *West J Emerg Med.* (2011) 12:372–4. doi: 10.5811/westjem.2011.1.2125
4. Badshah MB, Riaz H, Aslam S, Badshah MB, Korsten MA, Munir MB. Complex partial nonconvulsive status epilepticus masquerading as hepatic encephalopathy: a case report. *J Med Case Rep.* (2012) 6:422. doi: 10.1186/1752-1947-6-422
5. Jo YM, Lee SW, Han SY, Baek YH, Ahn JH, Choi WJ et al. Nonconvulsive status epilepticus disguising as hepatic encephalopathy. *World J Gastroenterol.* (2015) 21:5105–9. doi: 10.3748/wjgv21.i16.515
6. Hor S, Chen CY, Tsai ST. Propofol pump controls nonconvulsive status epilepticus in a hepatic encephalopathy patient: a case report. *World J Clin Cases.* (2019) 7:2831–7. doi: 10.12998/wjcc.v7.i18.2831
7. Rovira A, Alonso J, Córdoba J, MR. imaging findings in hepatic encephalopathy. *AJNR Am J Neuroradiol.* (2008) 29:1612–21. doi: 10.3174/ajnr.A1139
8. Tsochatzis EA, Bosch J, Burroughs AK. Liver cirrhosis. *Lancet.* (2014) 383:1749–61. doi: 10.1016/S0140-6736(14)60121-5
9. Wijdicks EF. Hepatic encephalopathy. *N Engl J Med.* (2016) 375:1660–70. doi: 10.1056/NEJMra1600561
10. Bajaj JS, Wade JB, Sanyal AJ. Spectrum of neurocognitive impairment in cirrhosis: Implications for the assessment of hepatic encephalopathy. *Hepatology.* (2009) 50:2014–21. doi: 10.1002/hep.23216
11. Vilstrup H, Amodio P, Bajaj J, Cordoba J, Ferenci P, Mullen KD et al. Hepatic encephalopathy in chronic liver disease: 2014 Practice Guideline by the American Association for the Study of Liver Diseases and the European Association for the Study of the Liver. *Hepatology.* (2014) 60:715–35. doi: 10.1002/hep.27210
12. Dellatore P, Cheung M, Mahpour NY, Tawadros A, Rustgi VK. Clinical manifestations of hepatic encephalopathy. *Clin Liver Dis.* (2020) 24:189–96. doi: 10.1016/j.cld.2020.01.010
13. Córdoba J, Cabrera J, Lataif L, Penev P, Zee P, Blei AT. High prevalence of sleep disturbance in cirrhosis. *Hepatology.* (1998) 27:339–45. doi: 10.1002/hep.510270204
14. Weissenborn K. Diagnosis of encephalopathy. *Digestion.* (1998) 59 Suppl 2:22–4. doi: 10.1159/000051415
15. Leitinger M, Beniczky S, Rohracher A, Gardella E, Kalss G, Qerama E et al. Salzburg consensus criteria for non-convulsive status epilepticus—approach to clinical application. *Epilepsy Behav.* (2015) 49:158–63. doi: 10.1016/j.yebeh.2015.05.007
16. Ficker DM, Westmoreland BF, Sharbrough FW. Epileptiform abnormalities in hepatic encephalopathy. *J Clin Neurophysiol.* (1997) 14:230–4. doi: 10.1097/00004691-19970500000008
17. Alonso J, Córdoba J, Rovira A. Brain magnetic resonance in hepatic encephalopathy. *Semin Ultrasound CT MR.* (2014) 35:136–52. doi: 10.1053/j.sult.2013.09.008
18. Bathla G, Hegde AN, MRI. and CT appearances in metabolic encephalopathies due to systemic diseases in adults. *Clin Radiol.* (2013) 68:545–54. doi: 10.1016/j.crad.2012.05.021
19. Córdoba J, Raguer N, Flavià M, Vargas V, Jacas C, Alonso J et al. T2 hyperintensity along the cortico-spinal tract in cirrhosis relates to functional abnormalities. *Hepatology.* (2003) 38:1026–33. doi: 10.1053/jhep.2003.50406
20. Neema M, Guss ZD, Stankiewicz JM, Arora A, Healy BC, Bakshi R. Normal findings on brain fluid-attenuated inversion recovery MR images at 3T. *AJNR Am J Neuroradiol.* (2009) 30:911–6. doi: 10.3174/ajnr.A1514
21. Kono Y, Sengoku R, Mitsumura H, Bono K, Sakuta K, Yamasaki M et al. Clinical characteristics associated with corticospinal tract hyperintensity on magnetic resonance imaging in patients with amyotrophic lateral sclerosis. *ClinNeurolNeurosurg.* (2014) 127:1–4. doi: 10.1016/j.clineuro.2014.09.011

22. Kassubek J, Bretschneider V, Sperfeld AD. Corticospinal tract MRI hyperintensity in X-linked Charcot-Marie-Tooth Disease. *J ClinNeurosci.* (2005) 12:588–9. doi: 10.1016/j.jocn.2004.07.020
23. Zhu R, Liu X, He Z. Widely spread corticospinal tracts lesions in a case of neuromyelitisoptica. *Clin Neurol Neurosurg.* (2017) 161:56–8. doi: 10.1016/j.clineuro.2017.08.010
24. Demaerel P, Wilms G, Verdru P, Carton H, Baert AL, MR. findings in globoid cell leucodystrophy. *Neuroradiology.* (1990) 32:520–2. doi: 10.1007/BF02426470
25. Loes DJ, Fatemi A, Melhem ER, Gupte N, Bezman L, Moser HW et al. Analysis of MRI patterns aids prediction of progression in X-linked adrenoleukodystrophy. *Neurology.* (2003) 61:369–74. doi: 10.1212/01.wnl.0000079050.91337.83
26. Pruvost-Robieux E, Yeung J, Sudacevschi V, Cordoliani Y, De Malherbe M, Pico F. Reversible corticospinal tract hyperintensities in neurologic Lyme disease. *Neurology.* (2016) 87:548–9. doi: 10.1212/WNL.0000000000002913
27. Konagaya M, Iida M. A case of HTLV-1 associated myelopathy with diffuse white matter lesion of the frontal lobe and continuous lesion of the pyramidal tract on cranial MRI. *Rinsho Shinkeigaku.* (1991) 31:875–7.
28. Shi K, Shen J, Yue X. Primary central nervous system lymphoma with symmetrical pyramidal tract hyperintensity. *JAMA Neurol.* (2021) 78:876–7. doi: 10.1001/jamaneurol.2021.1165
29. Matsusue E, Kinoshita T, Ohama E, Ogawa T. Cerebral cortical and white matter lesions in chronic hepatic encephalopathy: MR-pathologic correlations. *AJNR Am J Neuroradiol.* (2005) 26:347–51.
30. Pujol A, Pujol J, Graus F, Rimola A, Peri J, Mercader JM, et al. Hyperintenseglobus pallidus on T1-weighted MRI in cirrhotic patients is associated with severity of liver failure. *Neurology.* (1993) 43:65–9. doi: 10.1212/wnl.43.1_part_1.65
31. Rovira A, Córdoba J, Sanpedro F, Grivé E, Rovira-Gols A, Alonso J. Normalization of T2 signal abnormalities in hemispheric white matter with liver transplant. *Neurology.* (2002) 59:335–41. doi: 10.1212/wnl.59.3.335

Case Report: Not All Neurological Symptoms Respond Well to Penicillin in Patients with Neurosyphilis

Xiaoli Wang [1†], *Pengying Mu* [1,2†], *Wenjuan Zhang* [1] *and Yonghong Liu* [1*]

[1] *Department of Neurology, Xijing Hospital, Fourth Military Medical University, Xi'an, China,* [2] *Department of Neurology, Xing Yuan hospital of Yulin, Shaanxi, China*

***Correspondence:**
Yonghong Liu
liuyhong@fmmu.edu.cn

†These authors have contributed equally to this work

Patients with neurosyphilis present with a wide range of neurological symptoms, the response of which to penicillin is not well known. In this paper, we analyzed the clinical video-electroencephalogram (EEG) features of neurosyphilis in a 54-year-old man who exhibited with rhythmic orofacial involuntary movements, Argyll Robertson pupil, frequent paroxysmal oral-automatism seizures, periodic lateralized discharges (PLEDs) with triphasic waves, behavioral changes, and memory decline. After treatment with penicillin, PLED and seizures disappeared and behavioral changes and memory decline were significantly improved, but rhythmic orofacial involuntary movements and Argyll Robertson pupil persisted, which indicates an irreversible characteristic of late stage neurosyphilis syndromes.

Keywords: neurosyphilis, penicillin, oral-automatism seizures, rhythmic orofacial involuntary movements, periodic lateralized epileptiform discharges, Argyll Robertson pupil

BACKGROUND

Neurosyphilis shows a wide range of clinical symptoms, including seizures, poor vision, stroke, confusion, and personality changes (1). If untreated, the infections may involve the brain parenchyma, and the conditions would be worsened with the appearance of general paresis, tabes dorsalis, and Argyll–Robertson pupil (2). Until now, the response of different clinical symptoms to penicillin is little known. We hereby describe a case of neurosyphilis who presented with severe orofacial involuntary movements, Argyll Robertson pupil, and frequent oral automatism seizures. Meanwhile, his electroencephalogram (EEG) revealed periodic lateralized discharges (PLEDs) consisting of triphasic waves over the right temporal region. After treatment with penicillin, PLED disappeared and seizures diminished, but rhythmic orofacial involuntary movements and Argyll Robertson pupil seem to be unresponsive to treatment and still persisted during wakefulness.

CASE REPORT

A 54-year-old man presented to our hospital with frequent epileptic seizures. The medical history consisted of a 4- to 5-year behavioral change and memory decline, 3 years of involuntary movements of the face and mouth along with sharp clicking sound, and occasional paroxysmal vertigo and tinnitus. By admission, he has taken on valproate at the dose of 50 mg, twice a day for several months but got no obvious benefit. General physical examination was normal. No cerebellar and sensory deficits were detected, and his gait was quite natural. All the cranial nerves were normal on examination except the Argyll Robertson pupil which showed no reaction to the light

(**Supplementary Video 1**). Brain MRI revealed right temporal lobe atrophy. Serologic tests and CSF analysis were both positive for syphilis and so were the serum rapid plasma regain (titer 1:2) and treponema pallidum particle agglutination (TPPA) assay. The serum toludine red unheated serum test (TRUST) titer was 1:2. Cerebrospinal fluid (CSF) TPPA and fluorescent treponemal antibody absorption (TA-Abs) analysis unveiled similar indication. The WBC count and immunoglobulin G in CSF were 20 $\times 10^6$/L and 51.6 mg/L, respectively, higher than normal. The protein (36 mg/dl) and glucose (3.28 mmol/L) levels were in regular range.

EEG Findings at Admission

Video-EEG monitoring showed PLEDs consisting of triphasic waves over the right temporal region (**Figure 1A**). In total, 8 times seizures were recorded, which presented as oral and manual automatism and only lasting about 1 min and occurring during non-rapid eye movement (NREM) sleep (**Supplementary Video 2**). The ictal EEG confirmed a right temporal-frontal region onset theta wave evolution. Meanwhile, rhythmic orofacial involuntary movements arose in wakefulness and disappeared during sleep (**Supplementary Video 3**), indicating an uncontrolled contraction of masticatory muscles.

Treatment and Course

The patient was treated with penicillin (24 MU of intravenous aqueous penicillin G daily, divided every 4 h) for 14 days as a course. After two courses of treatment with penicillin plus valproate 50 mg orally two times/day, significant improvement was observed with his seizures and behavioral symptoms. The patient refused to get CSF test at the time of his second visit, only EEG and Mini-Mental State Examination (MMSE) were performed, and the EEG performed three months after the treatment found no PLEDs and only slow waves over the right temporal region. The MMSE of the patient was 22/30 (with the diploma of primary school), implying a normal range of cognition. However, Argyll Robertson pupil and rhythmic orofacial involuntary movements persisted after the treatment even at 7-month follow-up (**Figure 1B**).

DISCUSSION

In this study, we reported a case of confirmed neurosyphilis presented with PLEDs in EEG and manifested by frequent seizures, Argyll Robertson pupil, and rhythmic orofacial involuntary movements. After the treatment with penicillin, PLED disappeared and seizures diminished, but rhythmic orofacial involuntary movements and Argyll Robertson pupil still persisted.

Periodic lateralized discharges (PLEDs) are often seen with acute stroke, brain tumors, and inflammatory and infectious diseases (3). Whether PLEDs represent an ictal or interictal phenomena remains highly controversial (4). However, lateralized periodic discharges are considered ictal when related to apparent clinical symptoms (4, 5). The higher WBC count in CSF indicated an inflammatory reaction. The PLEDs in neurosyphilis might be a reflection of enhanced neuronal excitability, which is a treatable condition (6, 7). Moreover, PLEDs in this patient was temporally associated with frequent epileptic seizures and behavioral symptoms. In addition, after treatment with penicillin and anti- seizure medicines, PLEDs disappeared and, similarly, the seizures and behavioral disorders were improved. Therefore, our finding stresses the importance of performing syphilis testing for patients with frequent seizures. We postulated that syphilis induces a subacute state of epileptogenicity as the possible pathology, and the PLEDs may represent the peri-ictal pattern (6, 7).

In our case, the video-EEG captured 8 times of automatism seizures, and the ictal EEG confirmed a right temporal-frontal originated theta wave evolution. This finding agrees with previous demonstrations that the oral automatism seizures are typical focal seizure for medial temporal lobe epilepsy (8), and ictal EEG confirmed right temporal-frontal region onset theta wave evolution. Orofacial involuntary movements are well described in neurosyphilis and have been termed as "the candy sign," which is considered the clue to the diagnosis of neurosyphilis (9). Although these two kinds of events manifest similarly, involving the facial and masticatory muscles in a stereotyped manner, there are clear differences in electrophysiological feature. First, oral automatism seizures are associated with ictal epileptic discharges, only lasting about 1 min, and occurring during NREM sleep. However, rhythmic orofacial involuntary movements were continuous and persisted during wakefulness without epileptic discharges. Furthermore, after treatment with penicillin, PLED disappeared and seizures diminished, but rhythmic orofacial involuntary movements were unresponsive to treatment and still persisted during wakefulness. Therefore, the neural pathogenesis underlying these two kinds of events would be different.

Patients with frequent seizures may experience psychiatric symptoms during the period around the ictus (10). However, cognitive decline associated with frequent seizures always indicated a potentially reversible condition (10, 11). Memory is probably affected by focal seizures arising from temporal lobe, which is treatable (12). In line with previous findings, there was notable improvement after two courses of treatment with penicillin in our patient (6, 7). The MMSE scored: 22/30 comparable to the diploma of primary school skill. Meanwhile, seizures, PLEDs, and behavioral symptoms were significantly improved by penicillin treatment.

The late stage neurosyphilis with general paresis is characterized by progressive dementia, psychiatric syndromes, personality change, manic delusions, tremor, and dysarthria (1). Pathologically, there is atrophy of the frontal and temporal lobe. The "Lissauer" form of the disease may also affect the cerebellum and basal ganglia (13). Common neurological signs include pupillary abnormalities (Argyll–Robertson pupils), dysarthria, tremors of facial, lingual, and hand muscles (1, 13). Argyll Robertson pupil is pathognomonic of neurosyphilis, particularly, the pathologic lesion is suspected to be in the midbrain that interrupts the pupillary light reflex pathway (14). The mechanism underlying the rhythmic orofacial involuntary movements in neurosyphilis remains unknown, but a wealth of data implicates the basal ganglia may be involved (15–17). Orofacial involuntary

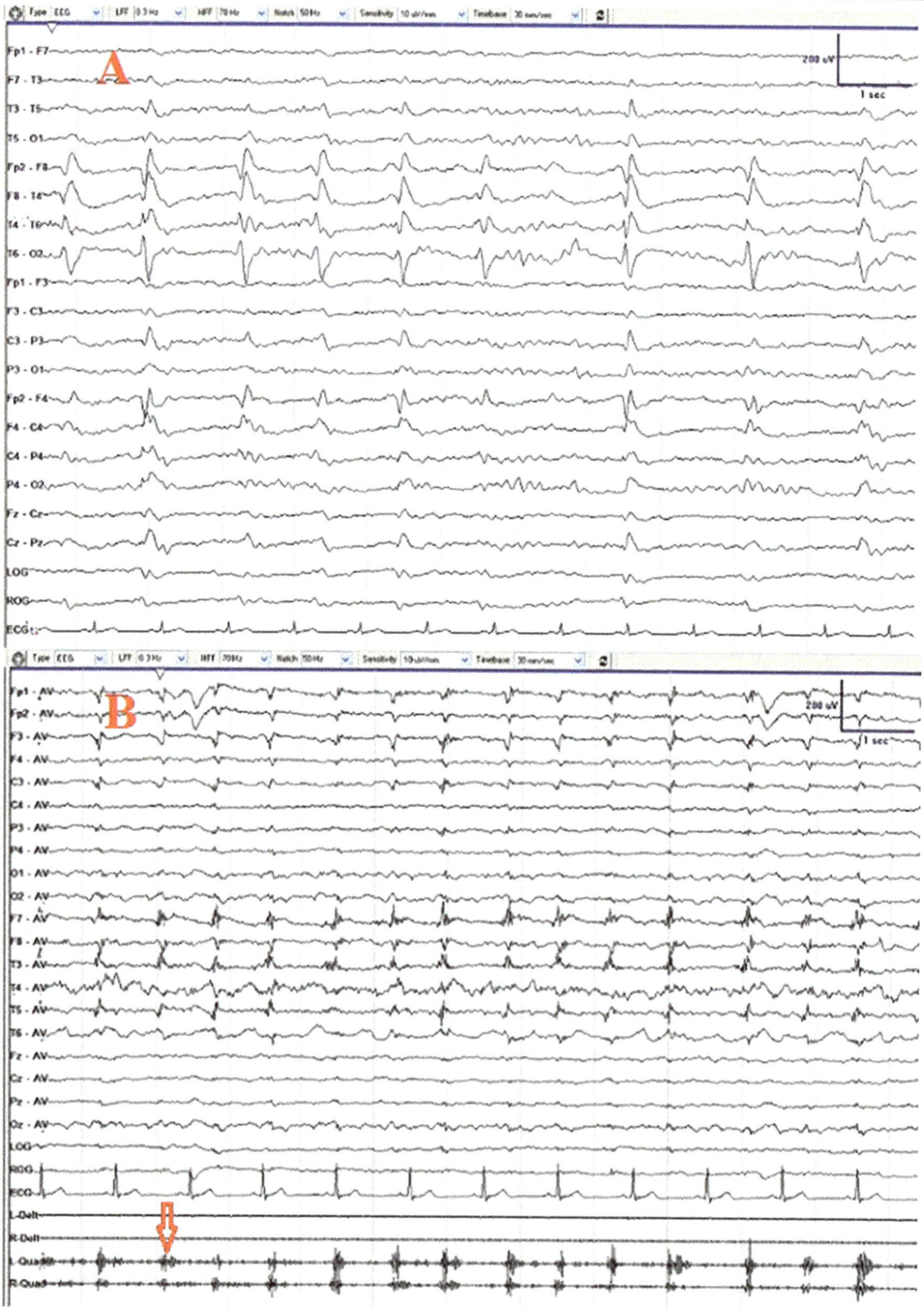

FIGURE 1 | Initial electroencephalogram (EEG) **(A)** showing periodic lateralized discharge (PLED) consisting of triphasic waves over the right temporal region. After treatment with penicillin for 2 courses, PLED disappeared and repeated EEG **(B)** showed only slowing waves and muscle artifacts produced by persisted rhythmic orofacial involuntary movements (red arrow).

movements exhibit with tardive syndromes which presents as vacuous chewing movements accounted by dopamine super sensitivity theory as high expression of D2 receptors has been identified (18). There is some evidence to support the theory. Particularly, an increased number of D2 receptors have been found to correlate with vacuous chewing movement (18). Therefore, the defective dopaminergic pathway in basal ganglia region may also induce the orofacial involuntary movements.

Although neurosyphilis is a treatable condition, the reversibility is dependent on the severity and duration of the disease. Hence, penicillin probably does not improve late neurosyphilitic syndromes (13). Like in our case, Argyll Robertson pupils and rhythmic orofacial involuntary movements did not react to the medical intervention (17).

CONCLUSION

Overall, neurosyphilis related neurologic disorders are diverse. The response of which to penicillin varied according to the severity and duration of the disease. Hence, penicillin probably has little effect on late neurosyphilitic syndromes.

ETHICS STATEMENT

The studies involving human participants were reviewed and approved by Xijing Hospital Research Ethics Committee. The patients/participants provided their written informed consent to participate in this study. Written informed consent was obtained from the individual(s) for the publication of any potentially identifiable images or data included in this article.

AUTHOR CONTRIBUTIONS

XW and PM conducted the clinical assessment. WZ conducted the video recording. XW, PM, and YL assisted in the video editing, initial draft, and revisions of manuscript. XW and YL assisted in the interpretation of clinical data and the revision of the manuscript.

ACKNOWLEDGMENTS

We are grateful to the patient for his cooperation in the work.

SUPPLEMENTARY MATERIAL

Supplementary Video 1 | The pupils constricted poorly to light stimulus. There is no apparent change in pupil size.

Supplementary Video 2 | The pre-ictal electroencephalogram (EEG) shows a focal abnormal triphasic waves and slow waves over the right temporal region during non-rapid eye movement (NREM) sleep, followed by the ictal EEG, revealing a seizure. Ictal EEG presented with attenuation of background, along with movement artifact and then followed by 3–5 Hz slow waves evolution during the seizure. The ictal semiology was characterized by sudden awakening from sleep with movement artifact, and then followed by oral automatism seizures.

Supplementary Video 3 | The rhythmic orofacial involuntary movements detected in the patient is mild, continuous, and repetitive, involving the lower facial and masticatory muscles in a stereotyped manner and producing sharp clicking sound.

REFERENCES

1. Ropper AH. Neurosyphilis. *New England J Med.* (2019) 381:1358–63. doi: 10.1056/NEJMra1906228
2. Drago F, Merlo G, Ciccarese G, Agnoletti AF, Cozzani E, Rebora A, et al. Changes in neurosyphilis presentation: a survey on 286 patients. *JEADV.* (2016) 30:1886–900. doi: 10.1111/jdv.13753
3. Fitzpatrick W, Lowry N. PLEDs: clinical correlates. *Canad J Neurol Sci.* (2007) 34:443–50. doi: 10.1017/S0317167100007332
4. Gelisse P, Crespel A, Genton P, Jallon P, Kaplan PW. Lateralized Periodic Discharges: Which patterns are interictal, ictal, or peri-ictal? *Clin Neurophysiol.* (2021) 132:1593–603. doi: 10.1016/j.clinph.2021.04.003
5. Sen-Gupta I, Schuele SU, Macken MP, Kwasny MJ, Gerard EE. "Ictal" lateralized periodic discharges. *Epilepsy Behav.* (2014) 36:165–70. doi: 10.1016/j.yebeh.2014.05.014
6. Noone ML, Sinha S, Taly AB, Chandrika S. Periodic lateralized epileptiform discharges in neurosyphilis. *Epilepsia.* (2007) 48:390–3. doi: 10.1111/j.1528-1167.2007.00921.x
7. Takagaki K, Morales MK, Vitantonio D, Berkowitz F, Bell WL, Kumar PN, et al. Periodic lateralized epileptiform discharges (PLEDs) in patients with neurosyphilis and HIV infection. *Clin EEG Neurosci.* (2016) 47:247–50. doi: 10.1177/1550059414552704
8. Wang Y, Wang X, Mo JJ, Sang L, Zhao BT, Zhang C, et al. Symptomatogenic zone and network of oroalimentary automatisms in mesial temporal lobe epilepsy. *Epilepsia.* (2019) 60:1150–59. doi: 10.1111/epi.15457
9. Marto JP, Borbinha C, Lampreia T, Alves L, Viana-Baptista M. Teaching video neuroimages: candy sign: the clue to the diagnosis of neurosyphilis. *Neurology.* (2017) 88:e35. doi: 10.1212/WNL.0000000000003544
10. Vijayaraghavan L, Natarajan S, Krishnamoorthy ES. Peri-ictal and ictal cognitive dysfunction in epilepsy. *Behav Neurol.* (2011) 24:27–34. doi: 10.1155/2011/378649
11. González Mingot C, Gil Villar MP, Calvo Medel D, Corbalán Sevilla T, Martínez Martínez L, Iñiguez Martínez C, et al. Epileptic peri-ictal psychosis, a reversible cause of psychosis. *Neurologia.* (2013) 28:81–7. doi: 10.1016/j.nrleng.2012.03.010
12. Baker J, Savage S, Milton F, Butler C, Kapur N, Hodges J, et al. The syndrome of transient epileptic amnesia: a combined series of 115 cases and literature review. *Brain Communic.* (2021) 3:fcab038. doi: 10.1093/braincomms/fcab038
13. Ghanem KG. REVIEW: Neurosyphilis: A historical perspective and review. *CNS Neurosci Ther.* (2010) 16:e157–68. doi: 10.1111/j.1755-5949.2010.00183.x
14. Thompson HS, Kardon RH. The Argyll Robertson pupil. *J Neuro-Ophthalmol.* (2006) 26:134–8. doi: 10.1097/01.wno.0000222971.09745.91
15. Jones AL, Bouchier IA, A. patient with neurosyphilis presenting as chorea. *Scott Med J.* (1993) 38:82–4. doi: 10.1177/003693309303800309
16. Ozben S, Erol C, Ozer F, Tiras R. Chorea as the presenting feature of neurosyphilis. *Neurol India.* (2009) 57:347–9. doi: 10.4103/0028-3886.53277
17. Shah BB, Lang AE. Acquired neurosyphilis presenting as movement disorders. *Movement Disord.* (2012) 27:690–5. doi: 10.1002/mds.24950
18. Teo JT, Edwards MJ, Bhatia K. Tardive dyskinesia is caused by maladaptive synaptic plasticity: a hypothesis. *Movement Disord.* (2012) 27:1205–15. doi: 10.1002/mds.25107

10

Case Report: Triphasic Waves in a 9-Year-Old Girl with Anti-NMDAR Encephalitis

*Ke Zhang, Shuang Xu, Yalan Zhou and Tangfeng Su**

Department of Pediatrics, Tongji Hospital, Tongji Medical College, Huazhong University of Science and Technology, Wuhan, China

***Correspondence:**
Tangfeng Su
stf@tjh.tjmu.edu.cn
orcid.org/0000-0002-1925-5519

Background: Triphasic waves (TWs) are mainly described in association with metabolic encephalopathy, especially hepatic encephalopathy. Now, as different conditions including non-metabolic and structural abnormalities have been reported to be associated with TWs, the presence of TWs becomes a non-specific finding for metabolic encephalopathy.

Case Presentation: We report the first case of anti-NMDAR encephalitis in a 9-year-old girl presenting with TWs on EEG. The TWs background EEG lasted for about 12 h on the 40th day of the disease course. No epileptic wave was found during a series of EEG examinations. The child was discharged from the hospital and no neurological sequelae remained after a six-month follow-up.

Conclusions: TWs are not specific to metabolic encephalopathy, but can also occur in children with autoimmune encephalitis. This case achieved a good prognosis after the early initiation of immunotherapy.

Keywords: triphasic waves, EEG, anti-NMDAR encephalitis, pediatric, metabolic encephalopathy, case report

INTRODUCTION

Background EEG patterns (non-convulsive status epilepticus (NCSE), non-convulsive seizures (NCS), periodic discharges, and triphasic waves) play an important role in the diagnosis and management of patients presenting with encephalopathy in the intensive care unit. Encephalopathy may be secondary to infectious, metabolic and autoimmune etiologies. EEG should be considered as a good tool to assess the functional status of the brain in patients with encephalopathy, especially for prognostic purposes.

Triphasic waves (TWs) are abnormal EEG waveforms, first described as "blunted spike and wave" in patients with hepatic encephalopathy by Foley in 1950 (1). Later, Bickford and Butt proposed the term "triphasic waves" according to the characteristic shape of the waves in 1955 (2). Now, TWs refer to generalized periodic discharges (GPDs) with triphasic morphology for brevity in the American Clinical Neurophysiology Society (ACNS) classification and the revised glossary and updated proposal for EEG terms (3). The typical TWs are composed of three phases: a high-amplitude positive wave preceded and followed by a slow negative deflection, usually occurring periodically in the frequency range of 1.5 to 2 HZ, predominantly in the frontal and central regions. A fronto-occipital lag ranged from 25 to 140 milliseconds can be observed (4). A wide variety of pathological conditions have been reported to be associated with TWs, including hepatic, renal, hypoxia, structural, toxic and metabolic abnormalities (5).

It is worth noting that TWs are not common in people under the age of 30, especially rarely recorded in children (6). Here, we report the first case of anti-NMDAR encephalitis in a young child presenting with TWs on EEG.

CASE PRESENTATION

A 9-year-old girl with uncontrollable twisting of lower limbs was admitted to the pediatric intensive care unit due to a depressed level of consciousness. One month ago, the child developed frequent twitching of the left lower extremities for 1–2 h, with no change in her level of consciousness during those attacks. Except for the abnormal limb movements, her parents complained the child recently had mental disorders, manifesting as low frustration threshold, worse memory, and bouts of involuntary laughter. She was then diagnosed with mental illness by a local hospital after the exclusion of conceivable organic medical conditions and was treated with aripiprazole, lorazepam, magnesium valproate and sertraline hydrochloride. However, involuntary muscle twitches were not alleviated but became more frequent and extended to other body regions.

At admission, the patient exhibited a stuporous mental state, with a Glasgow Coma Scale score of 11 (E3M3V5). Neurological examination revealed no nuchal rigidity, Brudzinski's sign or Kernig's sign. Laboratory tests, including complete blood cell counts, liver and renal functions, serum electrolyte, ammonia, and blood glucose, were all within normal limits. Cranial MRI also revealed no specific abnormality. A subsequent lumbar puncture demonstrated a pressure of 221 mmH2O (80-180 mmH2O), while the routine and biochemical CSF tests showed normal results. Results of the study for microbiological investigations on CSF were negative, including CSF microscopy, CSF culture, CSF serology (herpes simplex virus [HSV] IgG/IgM, cytomegalovirus [CMV] IgG/IgM, varicella-zoster virus [VZV] IgM, measles IgM, Epstein-Barr's virus [EBV] IgM) and polymerase chain reaction (PCR) analysis for neurotropic viruses. EEG on day 2 showed diffuse slow waves without epileptiform discharges (**Figure 1A**). These results suggested a low probability of infectious causes. Besides, the child underwent examination of ultrasound and CT scans, which showed no teratoma or other tumors.

Based on the typical clinical features (rapid onset, psychiatric symptoms, movement disorder, decreased consciousness and abnormal EEG), autoimmune encephalitis was highly suspected, which was later confirmed by positive anti-NMDAR antibodies in serum and CSF. Empirical therapy was immediately administered with intravenous methylprednisolone (500 mg/d) and gamma globulin (12.5 g/d). A 24-h video EEG on day 8 revealed generalized TWs more prominent anteriorly lasting for about 12 h (**Figure 1B** and timeline in **Figure 2**). In addition, the child's frequent involuntary jerking movements were confirmed as non-epileptic seizures by the long-term video EEG monitor. No signs of metabolic dysfunction were displayed. Although long-term video EEG recordings showed a disappearance of TWs the next day, the child's mental status still did not improve. Assessment of the child's consciousness revealed partial recovery on day 17, while simultaneous EEG showed diffuse slow waves. The patient finally recovered and was discharged from hospital on day 37 without any evidence of neurological sequelae. Six months later, a routine EEG follow-up just showed mild slow background activity (**Figure 1C**).

DISCUSSION

Autoimmune encephalitis (AE) is an inflammatory disease of the central nervous system mediated by autoimmune disorders. The main clinical manifestations usually include abnormal mental behavior or cognitive impairments, decreased levels of consciousness, speech dysfunction, dyskinesia, seizures, autonomic nervous dysfunction and central hypoventilation. Anti-NMDAR encephalitis is the most common type of AE, accounting for 4% of all encephalitis (7).

EEG plays an important role in patients with AE, not only for detecting seizures, assessing prognosis, but also for diagnosis in some cases. Almost all patients with AE are found with abnormal EEG findings, which usually showing non-specific diffuse slowing of the background, focal slowing and sometimes accompanied by variable epileptiform activity. Moise et al. described the continuous EEG findings of 64 patients with AE, with generalized rhythmic delta activity more commonly seen in anti-NMDAR encephalitis. They also identified extreme delta brush (EDB) as a signature EEG pattern in anti-NMDAR encephalitis (8). Zhang et al. conducted a study that addressed the EEG features of 34 children with anti-NMDAR encephalitis. EEG characteristics before immunotherapy included generalized slowing (73.5%), focal slowing (5.9%), normal background activity (20.6%) and interictal epileptic paroxysms (47.1%). EDB were recorded in 2 patients (9). EDB, characterized by beta bursts overriding on delta waves in EEG analysis, has been currently considered to be pathognomonic in 5–33% of patients with anti-NMDAR encephalitis, most in more severe cases and with poor prognosis (10). Although a variety of EEG abnormalities associated with anti-NMDAR encephalitis have been reported, to the best of our knowledge, this is the first case report of anti-NMDAR encephalitis presenting with TWs on EEG in a child.

TWs are usually described in association with metabolic encephalopathy, especially hepatic encephalopathy. However, a growing body of case reports indicate that TWs may also occur secondary to other etiologies, such as uremia, hypernatremia, hyponatremia, hypercalcemia, hypoglycemia, hyperthyroidism, hypothyroidism, drug-induced and anoxic encephalopathy. Other causes linked with TWs include stroke, tumors, Creutzfeldt-Jakob disease and dementia (6, 11). Among inflammatory and infectious encephalopathies, TWs are reported in encephalopathy of sepsis, Mollaret's meningitis, herpes simplex encephalitis, Borrelia burgdorferi meningoencephalitis, tuberculous meningitis, carcinomatous meningitis and Hashimoto's encephalopathy (12–14). To our knowledge, only one study reported a case of EEG with TWs in an AE adult case (15).

Although common in adults, TWs are relatively rare in children. Janati et al. reported two cases of TWs in drowning

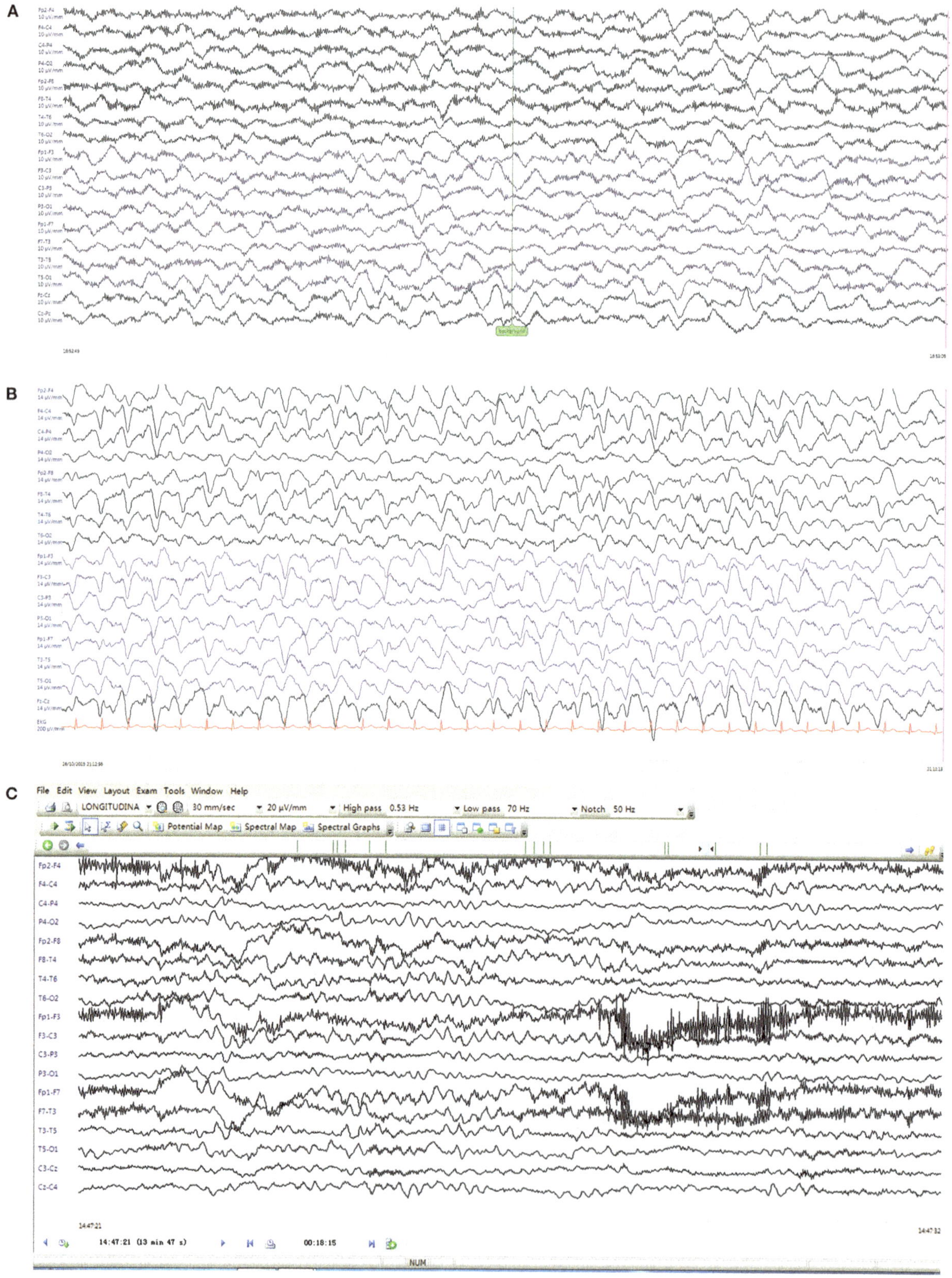

FIGURE 1 | EEG on day 2 **(A)**, day 8 **(B)** after PICU admission, and six months after inpatient discharge **(C)**. **(A)** Day 2, EEG revealed diffuse irregular slow waves. **(B)** Day 8, EEG showed generalized triphasic waves predominantly in frontal regions. **(C)** Six months later, EEG demonstrated mild slow background.

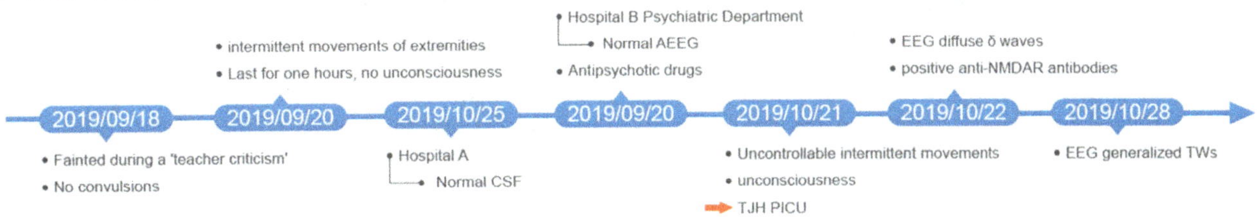

FIGURE 2 | Timeline of the clinical course.

children (16). Hosain et al. analyzed EEGs in 178 children with coma and found that TWs appeared in only 6 children (17). Laan et al. described TWs over the frontal regions on EEG in children with Angelman syndrome, a rare genetic disorder (18). In our case, a 9-year-old girl presented with TWs during the course of anti NMDAR encephalitis.

In view of the numerous causes of TWs, metabolic encephalopathies should be considered first. In our case, the blood ammonia, glucose and electrolyte were at normal levels, so that metabolic encephalopathy could be basically excluded. In addition, TWs have also been described in toxic encephalopathy induced by valproic acid, cefepime, cefoperazone, ceftriaxone, lithium, and pregabalin (19–21). Vulliemoz et al. also reported TWs in a patient with chronic renal failure after administration of levetiracetam (22). Our patient had initially taken valproic acid on admission, but soon changed to levetiracetam. In addition to normal hepatorenal function and no history of the above medicines, the possibility of toxic factors was small. Furthermore, seizure is a common clinical manifestation in children with anti NMDAR encephalitis, and in some cases, NCSE could be present. Dilaver et al. described 15 cases aged 66 ± 8 years with NCSE whose EEGs presented with atypical triphasic waves (23). Sometimes, it is difficult to attribute the presence of TWs to NCSE or encephalopathy. Benzodiazepines (BZPs) or non-sedating anti-seizure drugs (NSAEDs) are commonly administered to differentiate them (24). However, there is debate over the utility of the trials, as the administration of BZPs or NSAEDs may also diminish TWs in metabolic/toxic encephalopathies (25). Nevertheless, patients' mental status should be specially paid attention to after the therapy of BZPs or NSAEDs. In NCSE, both epileptiform discharges and consciousness can be improved or normalized with the medicines, whereas the mental state is not improved in metabolic/toxic encephalopathies (26). Owing to dyskinesia, midazolam was administered to the girl with continuous infusion upon admission, even during the EEG monitor, which signified this EEG pattern occurred in spite of the use of BZPs. Of note, TWs background in this patient was monotonous and did not show highly changing and time-dynamic spatiotemporal evolution. Besides, after TWs disappeared, the child remained comatose. We tend to believe that the TWs on the EEG were indeed due to anti-NMDAR encephalitis.

The mechanism of TWs is still unclear. Bickford et al. considered TWs as a positive traveling wave along the cortex, caused by subcortical disturbance at the thalamocortical level (2). Gloor P et al. suggested that the abnormal oscillatory discharges between cortical and thalamic neurons may be responsible for this EEG pattern (27). Now, it is supposed that TWs may result from metabolic or structural abnormalities at the thalamocortical level, especially in the thalamocortical relay neurons. Abnormal glutamate metabolism is probably one of the mechanisms.

There are different arguments about the prognosis of TWs. Bahamon-Dussan J. E. et al. studied 30 patients with TWs, all of whom had different degrees of altered mental status. After 22 months of follow-up, the overall mortality was 77%. Only three of the seven survivors had normal nervous systems. They concluded that TWs indicated a dismal prognosis (28). Sutter et al. analyzed the EEGs of 154 patients with encephalopathy and found TWs implied higher mortality (29). Whereas, Kaplan et al. believed that the prognosis often depended on the underlying causes. If TWs occurred in the setting of reversible toxic metabolic dysfunction, the outcome could be better. If in the cases of closed head injury or hypoxia, the prognosis could be poor (30). Sutter et al. later followed up 105 patients with TWs. They suggested that the unresponsiveness of EEG, rather than the underlying etiology, could be an independent factor associated with high case fatality rate (31). In our case, the primary disease of the girl was anti-NMDAR encephalitis, having a recovery rate of ~80% (32). Besides, her EEG showed good reactivity. Both the primary disease and EEG reactivity predicted a favorable outcome.

CONCLUSION

Our case report further confirms that TWs are not specific to metabolic encephalopathy, but can also occur in children with autoimmune encephalitis. More importantly, the possibility of metabolic or drug-induced encephalopathy should be first ruled out when TWs appear. To our knowledge, this is the first report of TWs observed in a child with anti-NMDAR encephalitis.

ETHICS STATEMENT

The studies involving human participants were reviewed and approved by the Ethics Committee of Tongji Hospital, Tongji Medical College, Huazhong University of Science and Technology. Written informed consent to participate in this study was provided by the participants' legal guardian/next of kin. Written informed consent was obtained from the individual(s), and minor(s)' legal guardian/next of kin, for the publication of any potentially identifiable images or data included in this article.

AUTHOR CONTRIBUTIONS

KZ prepared the original draft. SX and YZ revised the manuscript. TS reviewed and edited the final manuscript. All authors contributed to drafting or revising the article, gave final approval of the version to be published, and agree to be accountable for this work.

ACKNOWLEDGMENTS

The authors would like to thank all family members for their consent to this publication. We also thank Ms. Xinyi Hu from the University of Geneva in Switzerland for English language editing.

REFERENCES

1. Foley JM, Watson CW, Adams RD. Significance of the electroencephalographic changes in hepatic coma. *Trans Am Neurol Assoc.* (1950) 51:161–5.
2. Bickford RG, Butt HR. Hepatic coma: the electroencephalographic pattern. *J Clin Invest.* (1955) 34:790–9. doi: 10.1172/JCI103134
3. Fernandez-Torre JL, Kaplan PW. Triphasic waves: historical overview of an unresolved mystery. *J Clin Neurophysiol.* (2021) 21:809. doi: 10.1097/WNP.0000000000000809
4. Palanca BJA, Wildes TS, Ju YS, Ching S, Avidan MS. Electroencephalography and delirium in the postoperative period. *Br J Anaesth.* (2017) 119:294–307. doi: 10.1093/bja/aew475
5. Kaplan PW, Sutter R. Affair with triphasic waves-their striking presence, mysterious significance, and cryptic origins: what are they? *J Clin Neurophysiol.* (2015) 32:401–5. doi: 10.1097/WNP.0000000000000151
6. Brigo F, Storti M. Triphasic waves. *Am J Electroneurodiagnostic Technol.* (2011) 51:16–25. doi: 10.1080/1086508X.2011.11079796
7. Gardoni F, Stanic J, Scheggia D, Benussi A, Borroni B, Di Luca M. NMDA and AMPA receptor autoantibodies in brain disorders: from molecular mechanisms to clinical features. *Cells.* (2021) 10:1. doi: 10.3390/cells10010077
8. Moise AM, Karakis I, Herlopian A, Dhakar M, Hirsch LJ, Cotsonis G, et al. Continuous EEG findings in autoimmune encephalitis. *J Clin Neurophysiol.* (2021) 38:124–9. doi: 10.1097/WNP.0000000000000654
9. Zhang M, Li W, Zhou S, Zhou Y, Yang H, Yu L, et al. Clinical features, treatment, and outcomes among Chinese children with anti-methyl-d-aspartate receptor. (Anti-NMDAR) Encephalitis. *Front Neurol.* (2019). 10:596. doi: 10.3389/fneur.2019.00596
10. Liang Z, Yang S, Sun X, Li B, Li W, Liu Z, et al. Teratoma-associated anti-NMDAR encephalitis: Two cases report and literature review. *Medicine.* (2017) 96:e9177. doi: 10.1097/MD.0000000000009177
11. Kaplan PW. The EEG in metabolic encephalopathy and coma. *J Clin Neurophysiol.* (2004) 21:307–318. doi: 10.1097/01.WNP.0000145004.22230.D5
12. Konno S, Sugimoto H, Nemoto H, Kitazono H, Murata M, Toda T, et al. Triphasic waves in a patient with tuberculous meningitis. *J Neurol Sci.* (2010) 291:114–7. doi: 10.1016/j.jns.2009.12.027
13. Eriksson B, Wictor L. EEG with triphasic waves in Borrelia burgdorferi meningoencephalitis. *Acta Neurol Scand.* (2007) 116:133–6. doi: 10.1111/j.1600-0404.2007.00858.x
14. Henchey R, Cibula J, Helveston W, Malone J, Gilmore RL. Electroencephalographic findings in Hashimoto's encephalopathy. *Neurology.* (1995) 45:977–81. doi: 10.1212/WNL.45.5.977
15. Sutter R, Kaplan PW, Cervenka MC, Thakur KT, Asemota AO, Venkatesan A, et al. Electroencephalography for diagnosis and prognosis of acute encephalitis. *Clin Neurophysiol.* (2015) 126:1524–31. doi: 10.1016/j.clinph.2014.11.006
16. Janati A, Erba G. Electroencephalographic correlates of near-drowning encephalopathy in children. *Electroencephalogr Clin Neurophysiol.* (1982) 53:182–91. doi: 10.1016/0013-4694(82)90022-0
17. Hosain SA, Solomon GE, Kobylarz EJ. Electroencephalographic patterns in unresponsive pediatric patients. *Pediatr Neurol.* (2005) 32:162–5. doi: 10.1016/j.pediatrneurol.2004.09.008
18. Laan LA, Brouwer OF, Begeer CH, Zwinderman AH, van Dijk JG. The diagnostic value of the EEG in Angelman and Rett syndrome at a young age. *Electroencephalogr Clin Neurophysiol.* (1998) 106:404–8. doi: 10.1016/S0013-4694(98)00007-8
19. Segura-Bruna N, Rodriguez-Campello A, Puente V, Roquer J. Valproate-induced hyperammonemic encephalopathy. *Acta Neurol Scand.* (2006) 114:1–7. doi: 10.1111/j.1600-0404.2006.00655.x
20. Payne LE, Gagnon DJ, Riker RR, Seder DB, Glisic EK, Morris JG, et al. Cefepime-induced neurotoxicity: a systematic review. *Crit Care.* (2017) 21:276. doi: 10.1186/s13054-017-1856-1
21. Suzuki S, Naito S, Numasawa Y, Asada M, Shoji N, Zeniya M, et al. Encephalopathy induced by high plasma and cerebrospinal fluid ceftriaxone concentrations in a hemodialysis patient. *Intern Med.* (2019) 58:1775–9. doi: 10.2169/internalmedicine.1785-18
22. Vulliemoz S, Iwanowski P, Landis T, Jallon P. Levetiracetam accumulation in renal failure causing myoclonic encephalopathy with triphasic waves. *Seizure.* (2009) 18:376–8. doi: 10.1016/j.seizure.2009.01.006
23. Kaya D, Bingol CA. Significance of atypical triphasic waves for diagnosing nonconvulsive status epilepticus. *Epilepsy Behav.* (2007) 11:567–77. doi: 10.1016/j.yebeh.2007.07.014
24. van Rijckevorsel K, Boon P, Hauman H, Legros B, Ossemann M, Sadzot B, et al. Standards of care for non-convulsive status epilepticus: Belgian consensus recommendations. *Acta Neurol Belg.* (2006) 106:117–24.
25. O'Rourke D, Chen PM, Gaspard N, Foreman B, McClain L, Karakis I, et al. Response rates to anticonvulsant trials in patients with triphasic-wave eeg patterns of uncertain significance. *Neurocrit Care.* (2016) 24:233–9. doi: 10.1007/s12028-015-0151-8
26. Kaplan PW, Gelisse P, Sutter R. An electroencephalographic voyage in search of TWs-the sirens and corsairs on the encephalopathy/EEG horizon: a survey of TWs. *J Clin Neurophysiol.* (2021) 21:725. doi: 10.1097/WNP.0000000000000725
27. Gloor P, Fariello RG. Generalized epilepsy: some of its cellular mechanisms differ from those of focal epilepsy. *Trends Neurosci.* (1988) 11:63–8. doi: 10.1016/0166-2236(88)90166-X
28. Bahamon-Dussan JE, Celesia GG, Grigg-Damberger MM. Prognostic significance of EEG triphasic waves in patients with altered state of consciousness. *J Clin Neurophysiol.* (1989) 6:313–9. doi: 10.1097/00004691-198910000-00002
29. Sutter R, Stevens RD, Kaplan PW. Clinical and imaging correlates of EEG patterns in hospitalized patients with encephalopathy. *J Neurol.* (2013) 260:1087–98. doi: 10.1007/s00415-012-6766-1
30. Kaplan PW. EEG monitoring in the intensive care unit. *Am J Electroneurodiagnostic Technol.* (2006) 46:81–97. doi: 10.1080/1086508X.2006.11079564
31. Sutter R, Stevens RD, Kaplan PW. Significance of triphasic waves in patients with acute encephalopathy: a nine-year cohort study. *Clin Neurophysiol.* (2013) 124:1952–8. doi: 10.1016/j.clinph.2013.03.031
32. Armangue T, Petit-Pedrol M, Dalmau J. Autoimmune encephalitis in children. *J Child Neurol.* (2012) 27:1460–9. doi: 10.1177/0883073812448838

11

Case Report: Ictal Central Apnea as First and Overlooked Symptom in Temporal Lobe Seizures

Elisa Micalizzi[1], *Anna Elisabetta Vaudano*[2], *Giada Giovannini*[2,3,4], *Giulia Turchi*[2], *Leandra Giunta*[2] *and Stefano Meletti*[2,3*]

[1] Department of Brain and Behavioral Sciences, University of Pavia, Pavia, Italy, [2] Neurology Unit, Ospedale Civile di Baggiovara (OCB) Hospital, Azienda Ospedaliera-Universitaria, Modena, Italy, [3] Department of Biomedical, Metabolic and Neural Science, University of Modena and Reggio Emilia, Modena, Italy, [4] PhD Program in Clinical and Experimental Medicine, University of Modena and Reggio Emilia, Modena, Italy

***Correspondence:**
Stefano Meletti
stefano.meletti@unimore.it

Ictal respiratory changes have been mainly described following generalized tonic-clonic seizures and recently considered to be a biomarker to assess the risk of sudden unexplained death in epilepsy (SUDEP). Nonetheless, modification of respiratory pattern can be related also to focal seizures, especially arising from the temporal lobe. Changes in cardiac function such as tachycardia or bradycardia could be often associated. We report a short case series of four patients with temporal lobe epilepsy admitted to our Epilepsy Monitoring Unit (EMU) presenting with an ictal central apnea as the first clinical manifestation of their seizures. None of these patients was aware of the occurrence of respiratory arrest. Age at onset ranged from 15 to 29 years. One patient had seizures with prolonged central apnea accompanied by a significant decrease in oxygen saturation. Neuroimaging in two patients showed alterations of mesial temporal lobe structures, including the amygdala. Recent neurophysiological studies supported the existence of a cortical network involving the limbic system that modulates downstream brainstem respiratory centers. Monitoring for respiratory changes and oxygen saturation in focal seizures is warranted for their potential value in identifying the epileptogenic zone and for a better understanding of ictal respiratory changes that could potentially define a subgroup of patients with high risk of seizure-related autonomic changes.

Keywords: amygdala, temporal lobe epilepsy, seizures, SUDEP, ictal apnea

INTRODUCTION

Peri-ictal autonomic changes might occur in epileptic seizures and are a potential biomarker for the risk of sudden unexplained death in epilepsy (SUDEP), which is the most common direct cause of death in patients with epilepsy (1). Both cardiac and respiratory dysfunction have been implicated as possible precipitating causes in SUDEP (2). Respiratory changes during epileptic seizures have been described in the literature (3, 4). Peri ictal respiratory changes are commonly related to bilateral tonic-clonic seizures (4) but can also be observed in focal seizures originating from the mesial structures of the temporal lobe. Desaturations and ictal central apnea (ICA) occurred most frequently in seizures arising from the temporal lobe (1, 2), and the longer the duration of the seizure, the higher the degree of desaturation. We report four cases of ICA as the first ictal clinical manifestation of seizures originating from the temporal lobe recorded in our epilepsy monitoring unit by means of a 10-20 EEG system integrated with EKG, SpO2, and thoracoabdominal bands for respiratory inductance plethysmography. According to published criteria, we considered as apnea a respiratory arrest of 5 or more seconds on the pneumographic channel; a desaturation was defined as a drop of SpO2 value below 95% (mild 90–94%, moderate 75–89%, severe <75%) (1, 5).

CASES DESCRIPTION

Case 1

The patient is a right-handed 31-year-old female with no relevant past medical history and no family history of epilepsy. At the age of 25, she presented with two possible motor episodes during sleep and was started on antiseizure medication (ASM) with lamotrigine at a low dosage (50 mg/day). Around that time, she referred the occurrence of stereotyped subjective brief episodes characterized by forced thought, intense déjà-vu, anxious feeling associated with an ascending epigastric sensation. She would always be able to recall the events that tended to recur in brief clusters during the menstrual period. After 4 years of treatment, considering the persistence of these subjective episodes and the negative findings on interictal awake/sleep EEG recordings, as well as on 1.5 tesla brain MRI, lamotrigine was stopped in the hypothesis of non-epileptic seizures. A year later, she was admitted to our epilepsy monitoring unit where she underwent a long-term video-EEG monitoring (LTM) during wake and sleep. Routine laboratory findings as well as physical and neurological examinations were normal. A 3T brain MRI showed a slight hyperintensity of the anteromedial structures of the left temporal lobe. FDG-PET imaging was unremarkable. The interictal EEG showed sharp waves on left temporal region only during NREM and REM sleep. During LTM, we recorded three electroclinical seizures, two of them arising from sleep and one during wakefulness, characterized by ICA for around 17 s before any other clinical manifestation (**Figure 1**). In addition, the patient had impairment of awareness with disruption of contact, face pallor, and late oroalimentary automatisms. In each of the three recorded seizures, the respiratory disruption lasted for the entire ictal phase accompanied by drop of oxygen saturation (from 95% to a minimum of 75%) and mean delay between desaturation and clear EEG changes was of 22 s (**Table 1**). On the EEG, a left temporal ictal onset was observed. The patient was not aware of the apnea and did not present any respiratory distress. Lamotrigine was started again (50 mg/day) with complete control of seizures at a 5-month follow-up.

Case 2

The patient is a left-handed 31-year-old male with a past medical history of puberal growth delay treated with GH hormone and negative family history for epilepsy. Since the age of 23, he manifested episodes characterized by sudden appearance of intrusive thoughts and epigastric discomfort followed by staring, unresponsiveness, and oroalimentary automatisms, occurring monthly in short clusters. Hence, in the hypothesis of epileptic seizures, lacosamide was started (up to 200 mg/day) with little or no benefit. In 2018, brain MRI showed a T2 FLAIR cortico-subcortical hyperintensity and T1 hypointensity of the right mesial temporal lobe (amygdala and uncus) without contrast enhancement (**Figure 2A**), interpreted as possible dysplasia or low-grade neuroglial lesion, that remained unvaried on subsequent follow-up. FDG-PET imaging showed right temporal lobe hypometabolism, especially of the temporal pole and of mesial structures (**Figure 2A**). The EEGs performed since the beginning of seizures were characterized by interictal slow abnormalities, spikes, and sharp waves over both left and right temporal derivations, occurring independently. In 2020, neuropsychological tests highlighted deficits of visuo-spatial memory and executive functions. He was admitted to our epilepsy monitoring unit in March 2021. Routine laboratory findings and physical and neurological examinations were unremarkable. He tested negative for anti-CNS antibodies on both serum and CSF. The interictal EEG confirmed spikes and sharp waves on left and right anterior temporal channels during wakefulness and sleep. A total of nine electroclinical seizures were recorded (2/9 during NREM sleep, 7/9 during wakefulness) arising from right anterior temporal channels. In 5/9 artifact-free seizures, ICA, lasting from 7 to 15 s, was recorded, as the first ictal clinical sign, followed by disruption of contact, staring, dystonic posturing of the left hand, oroalimentary automatisms, and eventually nose wiping with the right hand. He was unaware of the occurrence of these seizures and of the apnea. In this patient, no reduction of SpO2 was noticed. A time between 3 and 13 s from ICA onset elapsed before any observable EEG change, longer for the seizures occurring during NREM sleep. Tachycardia was present in all recorded seizures despite of the occurrence of respiratory arrest. He underwent right anterior temporal lobectomy with pathology showing aspecific gliosis. No seizures were reported at a 7-month follow-up.

Case 3

A woman of 25 years, right-handed, reported the occurrence of two episodes of loss of consciousness with motor features during sleep at the age of 15. A first brain MRI was normal. Relying on clinical features, epilepsy was suspected and levetiracetam was started (up to 1,500 mg/day) with consistent efficacy. At the age of 16, during wakefulness, she manifested rare episodes characterized by impairment of awareness, staring, language disturbances, and hypersalivation followed by spontaneous recovery after 1 or 2 min. Right after, she was able to speak properly but not to recall the event. Then, lamotrigine was started (up to 300 mg/day) in association with levetiracetam with slight reduction in frequency of these episodes. After 4 years of seizure freedom, brief but frequent stereotyped episodes with the same features as described above recurred. Lacosamide was added in polytherapy (200 mg/day) without seizures' remission. A second brain MRI (3T) and the FDG-PET were unremarkable. The EEGs performed during the years showed frequent interictal spikes and slow waves over the left temporal lobe derivations. General and neurological examinations were normal. She was admitted to our monitoring unit where we recorded one seizure arising from the left temporal lobe characterized by ICA lasting 23 s, preceding by one second the EEG ictal onset with subsequent moderate

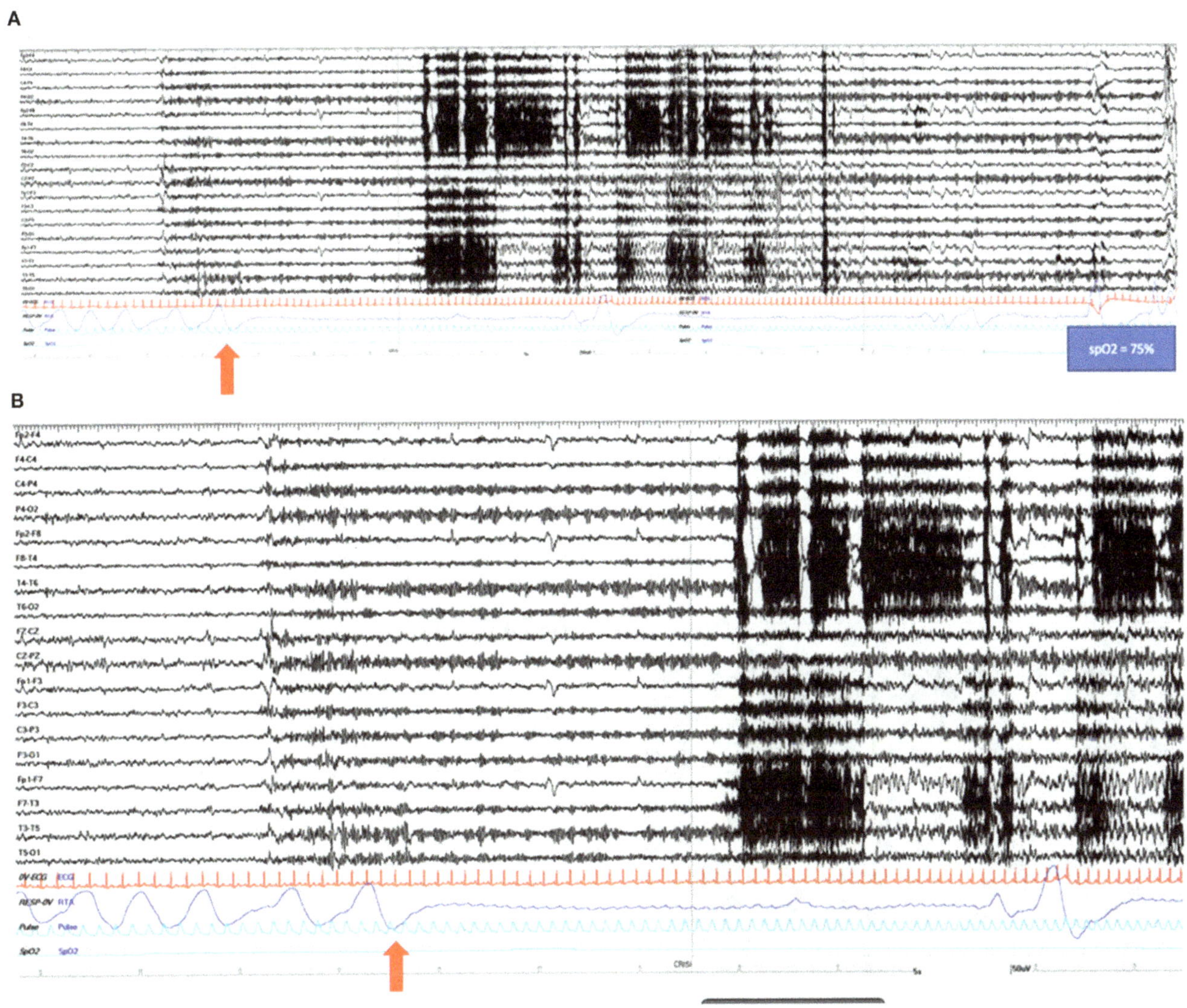

FIGURE 1 | (A) A 2-min view of the EEG pattern with polygraphy of a left temporal lobe seizure characterized by rhythmic theta and delta activity on left fronto-temporal regions in patient 1. This long-lasting apnea induces a severe oxygen desaturation (SpO2 75%). **(B)** A more detailed view of the onset of apnea preceding EEG changes and EMG movement-related artifacts by 20 s. **(A,B)** Red arrows highlight the onset of the apnea. Note the ictal marked increase in heart rate. Red channel: ECG; blue channel: thoracoabdominal respirogram.

desaturation to SpO2 89% and psychomotor arrest (**Table 1**). The patient was unaware for the occurrence of ictal modification of breathing and showed no respiratory distress.

Case 4

This patient is a 31-year-old male, left-handed, with no relevant past medical history except for the recurrence of stereotyped episodes characterized by brief déjà-vu sensations along with a mild headache in the last 2 years. He was admitted to our monitoring unit after a bilateral tonic-clonic seizure. Neurological and general examinations were unremarkable. Laboratory findings were normal. The 1.5 T MRI showed a right mesial temporal cortico-subcortical lesion (amygdala, temporal uncus, hippocampal head, and part of the hippocampal body) with gadolinium enhancement (**Figure 2B**). He underwent video-EEG LTM that showed rare spikes and sharp waves over the fronto-temporal regions during NREM sleep. We recorded four seizures arising from the right temporal regions during wakefulness, with occurrence of central apnea (lasting from 15 to 40 s) preceding the first EEG changes by 6–27 s (**Figure 3**). A mild ictal desaturation (SpO2 nadir 92%) was noted in all seizures. Clinically, the patient did not warn and manifested psychomotor and respiratory arrest, late oroalimentary, and some motor automatisms; when asked, he reported a mental picture which he could not recall but that seemed to be familiar to him. Ictal increase of heart rate was always observed. He was unaware of the occurrence of the apnea and did not report dyspnea. Lacosamide was started (until 200 mg/day); subsequently, the patient was

TABLE 1 | Summary of apnea related findings in the described patients.

Patient	Mean apnea duration (seconds)	Latency of apnea to first EEG changes (seconds)	Max desaturation	Awareness of apnea	Awareness impairment	Heart rate changes	Other ictal manifestations
1	71.7	22	75%	No	Yes	Tachycardia	Psychomotor arrest, staring, oroalimentary automatisms
2	9.8	7.4	No desaturation	No	Yes	Tachycardia	Psychomotor arrest, staring, oromandibular automatisms, contralateral hand dystonia
3	16	1	89%	No	Not known	Tachycardia	Psychomotor arrest
4	19.5	9.5	92%	No	Yes	Tachycardia	Psychomotor arrest, late oromandibular automatisms

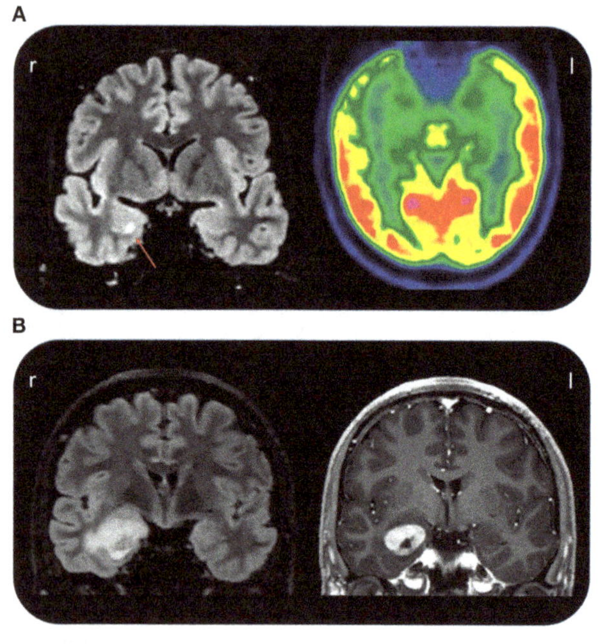

FIGURE 2 | **(A)** Coronal FLAIR MRI of patient 2 (left) showing a hyperintense right amygdala with red arrow pointing to an area of increased signal intensity (red arrow). On the right, the FDG-PET image of the same patient showing right temporal hypometabolism involving the temporal pole and mesial regions. **(B)** Coronal FLAIR MRI of patient 4 (on the left) showing a temporo-mesial lesion that on T1 imaging (on the right) present a clear gadolinium enhancement suggesting a tumoral origin.

addressed to surgery to perform an anterior temporal lobectomy. Pathology revealed a ganglioglioma, a grade I neuronal-glial tumor according to the 2016 CNS WHO classification. The patient appeared seizure-free at a 12-month follow-up.

DISCUSSION

Here, we reported four patients with TLE whose seizures were characterized by an ictal central apnea of variable duration that preceded, or was concomitant, with the scalp-EEG recorded seizures (see **Table 1**). The first description of a respiratory disruption in a patient experiencing focal seizure belongs to Jackson (6). A systematic review and meta-analysis of 21 studies (4) found an incidence of ictal hypoxemia around one third of seizures, with higher estimates found for adult patients presenting with tonic-clonic seizures. Severe peri-ictal desaturation (below 75% of SpO2) were associated to higher risk of SUDEP, considering that respiratory dysfunctions are correlated with increased risk of fatal cardiac rhythm abnormalities (7, 8). While data on peri-postictal apnea in tonic-clonic seizures are well-known, little attention has been paid until recent years toward ictal apnea in focal non-motor/non convulsive seizures. Here, we described four very similar cases in whom ICA was the first ictal symptoms in seizures involving temporo-limbic networks.

Data suggesting a functional connection between the amygdala and neural networks in the brainstem that control the involuntary respiratory drive derive from studies conducted on animals, such as cats (9), rabbits (10), and primates (11). As regards this functional connection between amygdala and brainstem in humans, the only data available come from clinical evidence, especially from invasive neurophysiological and neurosurgical studies. In 1952, Kaada and Jasper reported that intraoperative stimulation of different targets in the temporolimbic cortex-provoked apnea in their subjects (12). In 1954, Penfield and Jasper demonstrated that intraoperative stimulation of the cingulate cortex, rolandic cortex, and uncal regions could also generate brief apneic responses (13). Afterwards, in 1972, Bonvallet and Bobo noted that intraoperative stimulation of the amygdala was associated with

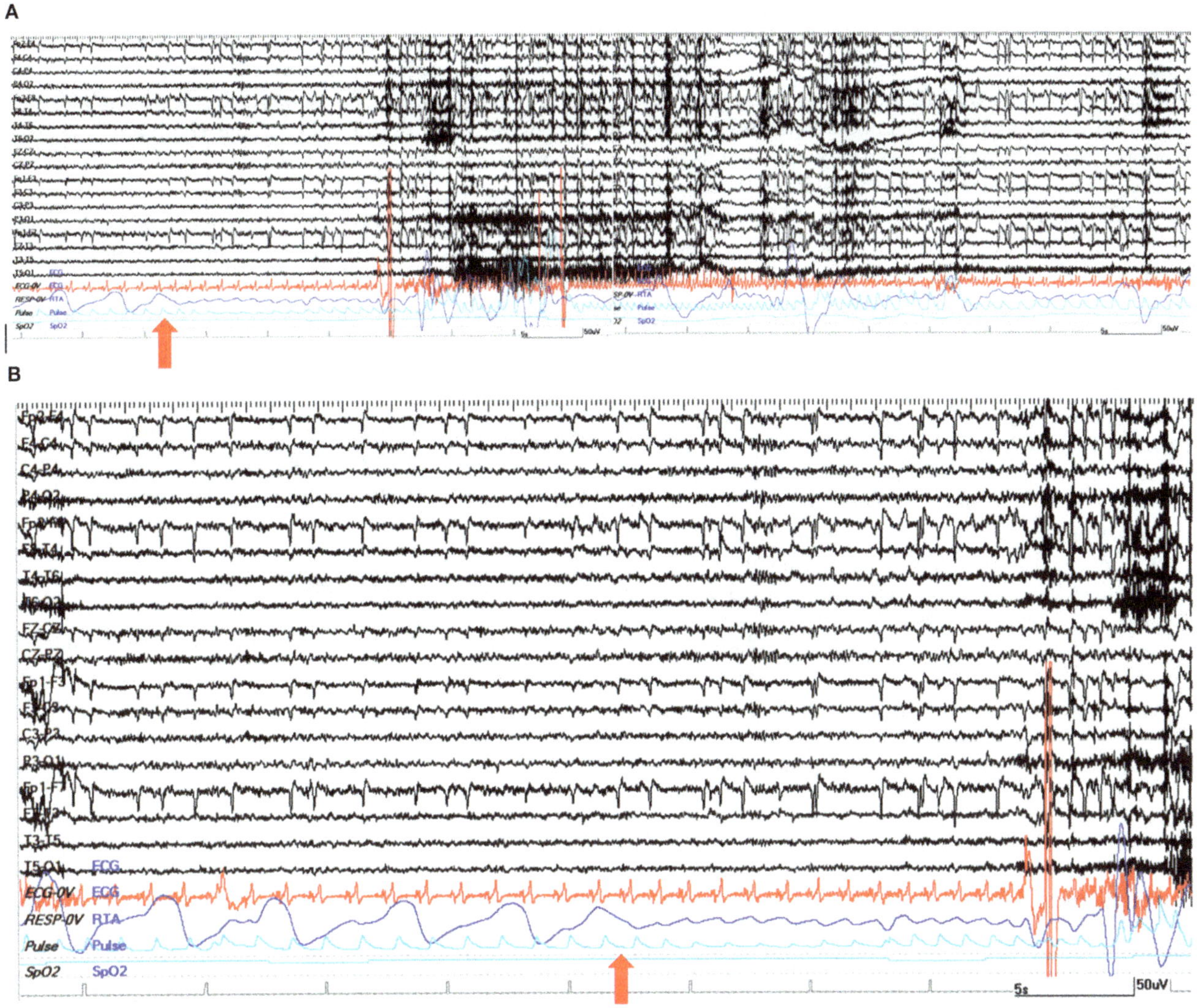

FIGURE 3 | (A) A 120-s view of a right temporal lobe seizure of patient 4. The apnea was the first ictal sign. The ictal EEG is characterized by a slow rhythmic theta activity on right temporal regions. **(B)** Apnea started 15 s before first EEG changes. **(A,B)** Red arrows point at the beginning of apnea on thoraco-abdominal polygraphic channel. Note the ictal marked increase in heart rate. Red channel: ECG; blue channel: respirogram.

apnea and bradycardia (9). Dlouhy et al. (14) documented with intracranial electrodes in one patient that apnea conditioning desaturation could be elicited by seizure spread to basolateral and lateral amygdala (left side) and in three patients upon direct stimulation of these nuclei (both left and right). As it occurred in our patients, none of them was aware of ictal respiratory modification nor appeared distressed. They observed a reduction in heart rate, differently from our four patients who presented tachycardia. They also assessed that unilateral amygdala stimulation is sufficient to cause apnea. More recently, Lacuey et al. (15) reported an incidence of ICA of 68.7% in their patients with mesial temporal lobe seizures, suggesting that this can be a common feature of temporal lobe epilepsy (TLE). They also noted that ICA is often the first clinical sign and sometimes the only clinical manifestation in medial TLE, suggesting its relevance in the anatomo-electro-clinical localization of the seizure onset zone. In another study, Lacuey et al. (15) investigated nineteen consecutive adult patients undergoing stereotactic EEG recordings and elicited a central apnea in 13/19 patients by electrical stimulation of the amygdala, hippocampus head and body, anterior parahippocampal gyrus, and antero-mesial fusiform gyrus. Therefore, they concluded that might exist a limbic and paralimbic network involved in the respiratory regulation of brainstem respiratory centers. Notably, amygdala stimulation might induce functional deafferentation of brainstem structures impairing involuntary breathing controlled by brainstem connections.

The apnea agnosia observed in our patients could be the reason why ICA in focal seizures is often unrecognized by clinicians. Different physiopathological mechanisms underlying this phenomenon have been proposed (14): (i) amygdala stimulation is thought to inhibit forebrain structures (insula or cingulate cortex) that are implicated in the conscious perception of dyspnea (16); (ii) amygdala stimulation can inhibit CO2/pH-sensitive serotoninergic neurons in the midbrain that mediate CO2-evoked arousal (17, 18); (iii) the absence of apnea awareness could be related to the effect of ictal activity on midbrain structures implicated in maintaining arousal/vigilance levels.

Regardless of the pathophysiologic mechanisms underlying ICA, the lack of awareness of apnea could lead to increased risk of SUDEP, especially while sleeping in prone position when self-defense response to respiratory distress could be fundamental (14). ICA is usually a self-limited event but, in some cases, can be prolonged and might be responsible of unobserved death in patients with epilepsy (1). Of course, at present, no data can link ICA to an increased risk of SUDEP; however, ICA could define a subgroup of patients with high-risk of seizure-related autonomic changes that warrant to be studied in more detail. Another interesting finding in our small case series is that apnea precede the scalp-EEG ictal changes by many seconds (up to 20 s in patient 1), suggesting that seizure activity can remain very localized for such a time before spreading to other brain regions, as reported in studies that combined scalp and intracranial EEG (15, 19). Hence, in the absence of an adequate polygraphic monitoring, seizures might go unrecognized, especially if the apnea is the only clinical manifestation. For this reason, we advocate recordings of respiratory changes and oxygen saturation in long-term monitoring of epilepsy patients, that in our view should become a "standard of care" in the context of the epilepsy monitoring unit.

Limitations of our findings may be due to the limited number of our patients and the lack of recordings of intracranial EEG activity that could give more precise information about the symptomatogenic zone of the seizure network. However, we would suggest monitoring of respiratory parameters, such as SpO2 and respiratory inductance plethysmography, also in a diagnostic and pre-surgical work up in patients with focal epilepsy. Data obtained from this type of monitoring could be useful to better localize the epileptogenic zone and to assess potential seizure-related biomarkers of increased SUDEP risk.

AUTHOR CONTRIBUTIONS

All authors listed have made a substantial, direct and intellectual contribution to the work, and approved it for publication.

REFERENCES

1. Vilella L, Lacuey N, Hampson JP, Rani MRS, Loparo K, Sainju RK, et al. Incidence, recurrence, and risk factors for peri-ictal central apnea and sudden unexpected death in epilepsy. *Front Neurol.* (2019) 10:166. doi: 10.3389/fneur.2019.00166
2. Bateman LM, Li CS, Seyal M. Ictal hypoxemia in localization-related epilepsy: analysis of incidence, severity and risk factors. *Brain.* (2008) 131:3239–45. doi: 10.1093/brain/awn277
3. Blum AS. Respiratory physiology of seizures. *J Clin Neurophysiol.* (2009) 26:309–15. doi: 10.1097/WNP.0b013e3181b7f14d
4. Bruno E, Maira G, Biondi A, Richardson MP, on behalf of the RADAR-CNS Consortium. Ictal hypoxemia: a systematic review and meta-analysis. *Seizure Eur J Epilepsy.* (2018) 63:7–13. doi: 10.1016/j.seizure.2018.10.011
5. Lacuey N, Zonjy B, Hampson JP, Sandhya Rani MR, Zaremba A, Sainju RK, et al. The incidence and significance of peri-ictal apnea in epileptic seizures. *Epilepsia.* (2018) 59:573–82. doi: 10.1111/epi.14006
6. Jackson JH. On Asphyxia in slight epileptic paroxysms: On the symptomatology of slight epileptic fits supposed to depend on discharge-lesions of the uncinate gyrus. *Lancet.* (1899) 1:79–8.
7. Kiely DG, Cargill RI, Grove A, Struthers AD, Lipworth BJ. Abnormal myocardial repolarization in response to hypoxaemia and fenoterol. *Thorax.* (1995) 50:1062–6. doi: 10.1136/thx.50.10.1062
8. Roche F, Reynaud C, Pichot V, Duverney D. Effect of acute hypoxia on QT rate dependence and corrected QT interval in healthy subjects. *Am J Cardiol.* (2003) 91:916–9. doi: 10.1016/S0002-9149(03)00040-7
9. Bonvallet M, Bobo EG. Changes in phrenic activity and heart rate elicited by localized stimulation of amygdala and adjacent structures. *Electroencephalog Clin Neurophysiol.* (1972) 32:1–16. doi: 10.1016/0013-4694(72)90223-4
10. Applegate CD, Kapp BS, Underwood MD, McNall CL. Autonomic and somatosensory effects of amygdala central N. stimulaton in awake rabbits. *Physiol Nehav.* (1983) 31:353–60. doi: 10.1016/0031-9384(83)90201-9
11. Reis DJ, McHugh PR. Hypoxia as a cause of bradycardia during amygdala stimulation in monkey. *Am J Physiol.* (1968) 214:601–10. doi: 10.1152/ajplegacy.1968.214.3.601
12. Kaada BR, Jasper H. Respiratory responses to stimulation of temporal pole, insula, and hippocampal and limbic gyri in man. *AMA Arch Neurol Psychiatry.* (1952) 68:609–19. doi: 10.1001/archneurpsyc.1952.02320230035004
13. Penfield W, Jasper H. *Epilepsy and the Functional Anatomy of the Human Brain.* Boston: Little, Brown and Company (1954). p. 830–1.
14. Dlouhy BJ, Gehlbach BK, Kreple CJ, Kawasaki H, Oya H, Buzza C, et al. Breathing inhibited when seizures spread to the amygdala and upon amygdala stimulation. *J Neurosci.* (2015) 35:10281–9. doi: 10.1523/JNEUROSCI.0888-15.2015
15. Lacuey N, Hampson JP, Harper RM, Miller JP Lhatoo D. Limbic and paralimbic structures driving ictal central apnea. *Neurology.* (2019) 92:e655–69. doi: 10.1212/WNL.0000000000006920
16. Buchanan GF, Richerson GB. Role of chemoreceptors in mediating dyspnea. *Respir Physiol Neurobiol.* (2009) 167:9–19. doi: 10.1016/j.resp.2008.12.002
17. Buchanan GF, Richerson GB. Central serotonin neurons are required for arousal to CO2. *Proc Natl Acad Sci USA.* (2010) 107:16354–9. doi: 10.1073/pnas.1004587107

18. Severson CA, Wang W, Pieribone VA, Dohle CI, Richerson GB. Midbrain serotonergic neurons are central pH chemoreceptors. *Nat Neurosci.* (2003) 6:1139–1140. doi: 10.1038/nn1130
19. Lacuey N, Hupp NJ, Hampson J, Lhatoo SD. Ictal Central Apnea (ICA) may be a useful semiological sign in invasive epilepsy surgery evaluations. *Epilepsy Res.* (2019) 156:106164. doi: 10.1016/j.eplepsyres.2019.106164

Case Report: Atonic PNES Capture in fMRI

Emmanuelle Hologne [1], Gabriela Hossu [2,3], Luca Fantin [2,4], Marc Braun [2,5], Cyril Husson [6], Louise Tyvaert [7,8†] and Coraline Hingray [6,7†]*

[1] Département de Neurologie, Centre Hospitalier Universitaire de Reims, Reims, France, [2] IADI, U1254, Institut National de la Santé et de la Recherche Médicale et Université de Lorraine, Nancy, France, [3] Centre d'Investigation Clinique-Innovation Technologique, Centre Hospitalier Régional Universitaire de Nancy, Nancy, France, [4] Laboratoire Développement Adaptation Handicap (DevAH) EA 3450, Nancy, France, [5] Département de Neuroradiologie Diagnostique et Thérapeutique, Centre Hospitalier Universitaire de Nancy, Nancy, France, [6] Pôle Hospitalo-Universitaire de Psychiatrie d'Adultes et d'Addictologie du Grand Nancy, Centre Psychothérapique de Nancy, Laxou, France, [7] Département de Neurologie, Centre Hospitalier Universitaire de Nancy, Nancy, France, [8] Centre de Recherche en Automatique de Nancy, U7039, Centre National de la Recherche Scientifique et Université de Lorraine, Nancy, France

***Correspondence:**
Emmanuelle Hologne
ehologne@chu-reims.fr

† These authors have contributed equally to this work and share last authorship

Psychogenic Non-Epileptic Seizures (PNES) are a misunderstood and disabling pathology, characterized by a paroxysmal occurrence of clinical signs without the epileptic activity. Resting-state functional MRI (fMRI) studies in patients with PNES have shown abnormal functional connectivity of the resting-state networks, especially in the limbic and motor systems, and in the precuneus. However, the transient nature of PNES episodes prevents us from elucidating the underlying mechanisms of seizures. Here, we report the case of a patient who presented an atonic episode of PNES during a 3T fMRI session. The patient is a 23-year-old woman, suffering from post-traumatic stress disorder, with no neurological comorbidities. The preprocessing of the fMRI images involved realignment, co-registration, segmentation, normalization, denoising (PhysIO toolbox), and smoothing. The time boundary of the seizure was defined according to the patient's reports, and the seizure period was contrasted with the resting state period before the seizure. A whole-brain analysis showed significant activations (left inferior temporal gyrus, left temporo-occipital junction) and deactivations (right precuneus, right superior parietal lobule, right postcentral gyrus, bilateral lingual gyri, inferior occipital gyri, and cerebellar lobules; right insula in a sub-thresholded analysis). Activations and deactivations occurred in four cerebral networks: emotional processing, agency, self-perception, and dissociation. To our knowledge, this report is the first published case of functional MRI during PNES. These results could confirm the emotional and dissociative hypothesis of the physiopathology of PNES and highlight future targets for neuromodulation.

Keywords: functional imaging, functional neurological disorder, case report, conversion disorder, PNES, article types: case report

INTRODUCTION

Psychogenic non-epileptic seizures (PNES) are a frequent and disabling pathology (1) with a substantial societal cost (2). They are characterized by a paroxysmal occurrence of clinical signs without a visible epileptic activity on electroencephalography (EEG) (3). However, although its clinical presentation is wellknown, its physiopathology remains enigmatic. The PNES are probably a dissociative and emotional pathology. Indeed, emotional processing in PNES is probably different from a healthy state, and overwhelming emotions must be suppressed. The PNES would be the result of an excessive suppression or an emotional inhibition of this emotion (4). However, this emotional inhibition could provoke side effects such as dissociation, defined as the disruption and/or discontinuity in the normal integration of consciousness, memory, identity, emotion, perception, body representation, motor control, and behavior (according to the Diagnostic and Statistical Manual of Mental Disorders Fifth Edition).

Because PNES are unpredictable and transient, two types of studies investigating the PNES physiopathology were performed: ictal (during the seizure) and interictal studies (between seizures). Regarding ictal studies, one work has shown a decreased functional connectivity between the anterior insula, hippocampus, amygdala, parietal, and prefrontal cortices during PNES (5). This work used a stereo-electroencephalography in two patients with epilepsy, which is a technology providing high temporal resolution but a low spatial sampling. Thanks to an excellent spatial resolution of the whole brain, functional MRI (fMRI) can supply evidence of brain areas and networks involved in this pathology. Therefore, inter-ictal studies have used neuroimaging to investigate resting-state networks in patients with PNES. The findings of these studies have shown that the precuneus involved in dissociation (6) was rather involved in the default mode network (DMN) in patients with PNES (7), and the insula, known to be involved in the neural network of emotional processing, was more connected to the sensorimotor network (8). These results suggest that the resting network in patients with PNES is different for the healthy ones, with a higher tendency to dissociation and high connection between the emotional process and motor behavior. This provides evidence of the proposed model of PNES physiopathology (4). However, these works have a strong limitation, as they used a resting-state methodology, during which there are neither emotional nor dissociative tasks, nor clinical signs. Therefore, brain mechanisms occurring during seizures remain unknown, preventing the emergence of neuro-modulating targeted treatments.

Here, we report the first case of a patient who presented a spontaneous episode of PNES recorded in 3-Tesla (3T) fMRI. This analysis allows us, at least a little, to unravel the mysteries of PNES.

CASE DESCRIPTION

Patient

The patient is a 23-year-old right-handed woman. She presents a post-traumatic stress disorder with reviviscences linked to physical and emotional abuse during childhood and adolescence. The diagnosis of PNES was clinically established by an experienced epileptologist according to the ILAE report (3). Her PNES began at 16 years old, and she is used to presenting around 4 episodes of PNES per month. Her seizures are atonic (9); she presents a global hypotonia and, sometimes, few clonic movements of limbs. A few moments before the hypotonia, she feels an undefined prodromal sensation that prevents her. Then, she describes a feeling of "blocking" with an absolute impossibility to voluntarily move and without alteration of consciousness. Interictal physical examination was normal. She has no further medical history, specifically no epilepsy or cranial injury, and no other psychiatric comorbidity. She takes no psychiatric or neurological drugs and receives cognitive-behavioral therapy and hypnotherapy at the psychiatric department of the University.

fMRI Acquisition

Whole-brain functional MR images were acquired using a 3T magnet (Magnetom Prisma; Siemens Healthcare GmbH, Germany) with a 64-channel receive-only head coil. High-resolution anatomical images were acquired using a 3D Turbo Flash sequence (TR = 2,200 ms; TE = 2.93 ms; TI = 900 ms; flip angle = 8°; in plane resolution =0.90 × 0.90 mm2; slice thickness = 1 mm). 160 volumes parallel to the anterior–posterior commissural line were acquired, covering the whole brain. Functional images were acquired using a GE-EPI sequence (TR = 2,000 ms; TE = 30 ms; 48 axial slices; slice thickness = 2.5 mm; slices order: interleaved; in plane resolution = 1.97 × 1.97 mm^2; flip angle = 77°).

The patient gave free and informed written consent to participate in the study Emotional Lived in Patients Suffering From Psychogenic Non-epileptic Seizures (EMOCRISES) (NCT02976545). We asked the patient to keep her eyes closed during the resting-state session of 8 min and 40 s, without falling asleep, and to stay still during the acquisition. In the context of EMOCRISES, the patient had an answer box in her right hand to interact during the experimental session. In this case, the patient used the answer box to inform the staff of the beginning and the end of her seizure.

MRI Data Analysis

Images were preprocessed using SPM12 (Statistical Parametric Mapping, Version 12, Revision 7219, Welcome Department of Cognitive Neurology, London, UK, RRID: SCR_007037) on Matlab [version 7.10.0 (R2010a). Natick, Massachusetts: The MathWorks Inc.; 2010, RRID: SCR_001622]. To optimize the movement correction, we applied the first co-registration between each functional image and the anatomical image. We then applied a standard preprocessing (realignment, co-registration, normalization, and smoothing). We used TAPAS PhysIO Toolbox (The PhysIO Toolbox for Modeling Physiological Noise in fMRI Data) (10) to denoise functional volumes of white matter and a cerebrospinal fluid signal.

We defined the control period from the 20 s after the beginning of the resting-state session to 20 s before the beginning of the seizure (total duration: 60 s). We defined the seizure period as the period between the two moments of patient reports. Using an SPM 12, we modeled the GE-EPI time series using a first-level general linear model (11), with regressors representing the expected BOLD fMRI response to seizure and to rest according to a block-paradigm and hemodynamic response function (HRF). Realignment parameters and denoising regressors were added to the regression models. Finally, we used a 128-s-high-pass filter to remove the non-physiological slow signal shifts.

The T-maps were calculated between rest and seizure. Results were visualized using the BSPMVIEW toolbox for SPM (10.5281/zenodo.168074).

Statistical Analysis

We performed statistical analyses in the whole brain and in regions of interest (ROI) (using Neuromorphometrics atlas). We explored both activations and deactivations. The T-maps were thresholded to obtain an uncorrected $p < 0.001$, and we applied a spatial extent threshold on the activated clusters to obtain $p < 0.05$, corrected for the multiple comparisons (the FWE method) (11). We also performed a sub-thresholded analysis by decreasing T-threshold, to explore other areas eventually involved in PNES mechanisms.

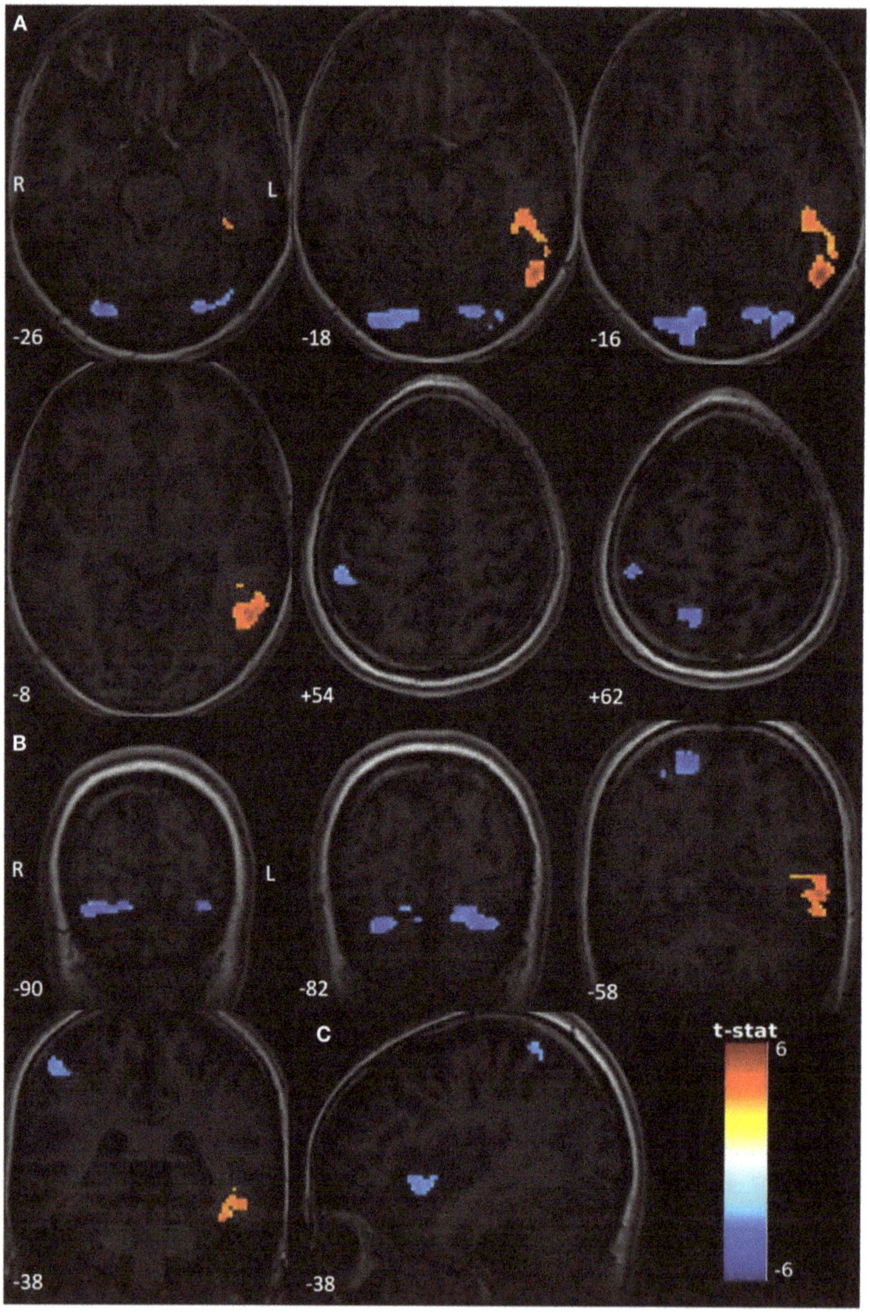

FIGURE 1 | Functional activations and deactivations during contrast PNES > rest (p uncorr < 0.001; cluster-level FWE $p < 0.05$; neuroradiological convention). The numbers on the bottom left correspond to the MNI coordinates [**(A)** Z coordinate, **(B)** Y coordinate, and **(C)** X coordinate]. The letters L and R correspond respectively to the left and right sides. The palette in warm tones corresponds to activations and the one in cold tones to deactivations. The color bar corresponds to T-scores. **(A)** Significant activations and deactivations for $T > 3.1595$, axial slices. **(B)** Significant activations and deactivations for $T > 3.1595$, coronal slices. **(C)** Sub-thresholded deactivations of right insula for $T > 3.1$.

DIAGNOSTIC ASSESSMENT: FMRI RESULTS

Seizure Features

The subject presented one typical PNES event during the fMRI resting-state session. The atonic seizure lasted 220s.

Whole-Brain Analysis

Compared to the rest period, we found significant activations ($T > 3.1595$, $p < 0.001$) in the left inferior temporal gyrus (ITG) and the left temporo-occipital junction (TOJ) during the seizure period. Deactivations involved the right precuneus, the right superior parietal lobule (SPL), and the right postcentral gyrus (PoG), bilateral lingual gyri, bilateral inferior occipital gyri (IOG), and bilateral cerebellar lobule (Crus 1). Interestingly, using a sub-threshold analysis ($T > 3.1$; $p < 0.001$), we observed an additional deactivation in the anterior right insula (**Figure 1**, **Table 1**).

ROI Analysis

Regarding the emotional hypothesis of PNES mechanisms, we defined ROIs as regions involved in emotional processing: the anterior cingular cortex, and both the insula and amygdala bilaterally. No significant deactivations or activations were found.

DISCUSSION

This is, according to our knowledge, the first report of functional MRI of a spontaneous PNES. Significant brain activations (left ITG; left TOJ) and deactivations (right insula, right precuneus, right SPL, right PoG, bilateral lingual gyri, IOG, and cerebellar lobule) were observed during PNES in contrast to a resting period immediately preceding the seizure. Our data had high quality. The recorded seizure was atonic, which gives low-motion artifacts, and, unlike SEEG, fMRI allows for whole-brain analyses. This quality allows us to make assumptions about activations and deactivations during this type of seizure. It seems to involve specific networks: emotional processing, dissociation, self-perception, and sense of agency.

TABLE 1 | Anatomical localization of the significant clusters.

	Area	MNI coordinates			Cluster size	*T*-value
	Positive	**X**	**Y**	**Z**		
Left	Temporoccipitaljunction	−54	−64	−16	573	6,4
	Inferior temporal gyrus	−48	−34	−18		4,95
	Negative					
Left	Crus 1	−26	−82	−24	200	−4,95
	Inferior occipital gyrus	−30	−90	−14		−4,65
	lingual gyrus	−14	−84	−16		−4,26
Right	Crus 1	26	−84	−24	301	−6,6
	lingual gyrus	30	−90	−16		−5,1
	Inferior occipital gyrus	20	−98	−14		−4,42
	Precuneus	16	−58	−64	149	−5,62
	Post central	48	−34	−62	106	−4,68

Emotional Network

We showed a deactivation in the right anterior insula, strongly related to emotional processing (12). The left ITG, involved in the ventral visual pathway, could be also involved in emotional regulation (13), like bilateral lingual gyri (14). Moreover, bilateral Crus 1 is involved in multisensory emotional processing (15).

Dissociation

We found out deactivation in the precuneus, which is involved in dissociation (6), that is to assay a disconnection between the mind and the body. As already described above, patients with PNES had a higher involvement of the precuneus in the DMN than healthy controls. Moreover, this involvement was correlated with dissociation scores (7).

Body Ownership (BO) and Peripersonal Space (PPS)

We showed a deactivation in the right PoG and SPL and an activation in the left TOJ. The BO is the faculty to recognize one's own body as being part of oneself. The PPS is a neuronal network, where each neuron is able to encode multisensory inputs in a receptive field localized close to the body. These two concepts lead to self-construction and self-perception. The right PoG and SPL are involved in these processes (16, 17). The left TOJ is a highly associative region (notably related to vestibular illusions), and it could be involved in BO (16).

Agency

The right PoG, right SPL, and left TOJ could be also involved in the self-agency network. On the one hand, self-agency is the ability to recognize oneself as the agent of one's actions. This network involves the associative motor cortices and the primary and associative sensory cortices like the right PoG and SPL (18). On the other hand, a negative agency is the experience of reduced control of motility, and the left TOJ cluster is spatially close to this network (19).

Our work has limitations. Indeed, we only recorded one "declared" PNES, and we do not know if the activation/deactivation pattern is reproducible. Moreover, it could be surprising to observe that there is no involvement of the motor network, especially, given the atonic type of PNES in this patient. However, our analysis was performed on the global timing of the PNES to increase the signal-to-noise ratio, and we did not analyze the dynamic BOLD signal changes over the duration of the PNES. Motor networks could be involved, but in a time-limited manner, which is a lead that was not explored here. Furthermore, the rest period defined just before PNES may not be fully occupied by rest, as the brain activity could change before the subject's perception of the onset of her seizure. This rest period could also be noisy by voluntary motor action of the use of the press button. Moreover, ROI analyses may not have demonstrated any significant responses due to the weak power of our work based on a single case. Finally, these involved areas are highly associative regions involved in other networks, and our interpretation could be disputable. However, given the PNES pathology and the semiology of our patient, this interpretation seems, to us, to be the more relevant.

To summarize, body scheme, agency, emotional processing, and dissociation appear to be involved in PNES. However, none of these networks have been completely activated or deactivated, as if PNES were not the result of activation or deactivation of one or more welldefined networks but, rather, as an intrinsic imbalance of these networks. This pattern highlights the fundamental role of self-perception and emotional processing during PNES, as it has been suggested for years (4). This work ought to be replicated on larger samples in order to improve our understanding of the physiopathology of PNES, which will lead to precise targets for neuromodulation and more specific treatment.

AUTHOR CONTRIBUTIONS

GH, CHu, CHi, and LT conceived the experiment. GH, CHi, and MB performed the experiment. EH, GH, CHi, and LT analyzed the data. EH wrote the manuscript in concertation with LF, GH, MB, CHu, CHi, and LT. All authors contributed to the article and approved the submitted version.

REFERENCES

1. Asadi-Pooya AA, Sperling MR. Epidemiology of psychogenic non-epileptic seizures. *Epilepsy Behav. 1 mai.* (2015) 46:60-5. doi: 10.1016/j.yebeh.2015.03.015
2. Magee JA, Burke T, Delanty N, Pender N, Fortune GM. The economic cost of non-epileptic attack disorder in Ireland. *Epilepsy Behav EB. avr.* (2014) 33:45–8. doi: 10.1016/j.yebeh.2014.02.010
3. LaFrance WC, Baker GA, Duncan R, Goldstein LH, Reuber M. Minimum requirements for the diagnosis of psychogenic nonepileptic seizures: a staged approach. *Epilepsia.* (2013) 54:2005-18. doi: 10.1111/epi.12356
4. Roberts NA, Reuber M. Alterations of consciousness in psychogenic nonepileptic seizures: Emotion, emotion regulation and dissociation. *Epilepsy Behav. janv.* (2014) 30:43-9. doi: 10.1016/j.yebeh.2013.09.035
5. Madec T, Lagarde S, McGonigal A, Arthuis M, Benar C-G, Bartolomei F. Transient cortico-cortical disconnection during psychogenic nonepileptic seizures (PNES). *Epilepsia.* (2020) 61:e101-6. doi: 10.1111/epi.16623
6. Terpou BA, Densmore M, Théberge J, Frewen P, McKinnon MC, Lanius RA. Resting-state pulvinar-posterior parietal decoupling in PTSD and its dissociative subtype. *Hum Brain Mapp.* (2018) 39:4228-40. doi: 10.1002/hbm.24242
7. van der Kruijs SJM, Jagannathan SR, Bodde NMG, Besseling RMH, Lazeron RHC, Vonck KEJ, et al. Resting-state networks and dissociation in psychogenic non-epileptic seizures. *J Psychiatr Res. 1 juill.* (2014) 54:126-33. doi: 10.1016/j.jpsychires.2014.03.010
8. Li R, Liu K, Ma X, Li Z, Duan X, An D, et al. Altered Functional Connectivity Patterns of the Insular Subregions in Psychogenic Nonepileptic Seizures. *Brain Topogr. 1 juill.* (2015) 28:636-45. doi: 10.1007/s10548-014-0413-3
9. Hubsch C, Baumann C, Hingray C, Gospodaru N, Vignal J-P, Vespignani H, et al. Clinical classification of psychogenic non-epileptic seizures based on video-EEG analysis and automatic clustering. *J Neurol Neurosurg Psychiatry.* (2011) 82:955-60. doi: 10.1136/jnnp.2010.235424
10. Kasper L, Bollmann S, Diaconescu AO, Hutton C, Heinzle J, Iglesias S, et al. The PhysIO Toolbox for Modeling Physiological Noise in fMRI Data. *J Neurosci Methods.* (2017) 276:56-72. doi: 10.1016/j.jneumeth.2016.10.019
11. Friston KJ, Holmes AP, Worsley KJ, Poline J-P, Frith CD, Frackowiak RSJ. Statistical parametric maps in functional imaging: A general linear approach. *Hum Brain Mapp.* (1994) 2:189–210. doi: 10.1002/hbm.460020402
12. Adolfi F, Couto B, Richter F, Decety J, Lopez J, Sigman M, et al. Convergence of interoception, emotion, and social cognition: A twofold fMRI meta-analysis and lesion approach. *Cortex. 1 mars.* (2017) 88:124-42. doi: 10.1016/j.cortex.2016.12.019
13. Pollatos O, Gramann K. Attenuated modulation of brain activity accompanies emotion regulation deficits in alexithymia: Emotion regulation in alexithymia. *Psychophysiology. mai.* (2012) 49:651–8. doi: 10.1111/j.1469-8986.2011.01348.x
14. Rubin-Falcone H, Weber J, Kishon R, Ochsner K, Delaparte L, Doré B, et al. Longitudinal effects of cognitive behavioral therapy for depression on the neural correlates of emotion regulation. *Psychiatry Res.* (2018) 271:82-90. doi: 10.1016/j.pscychresns.2017.11.002
15. Stoodley CJ. The cerebellum and cognition: evidence from functional imaging studies. *The Cerebellum.* (2012) 11:352-65. doi: 10.1007/s12311-011-0260-7
16. Seghezzi S, Giannini G, Zapparoli L. Neurofunctional correlates of body-ownership and sense of agency: A meta-analytical account of self-consciousness. *Cortex.* (2019) 121:169-78. doi: 10.1016/j.cortex.2019.08.018
17. Grivaz P, Blanke O, Serino A. Common and distinct brain regions processing multisensory bodily signals for peripersonal space and body ownership. *NeuroImage.* (2017) 147:602-18. doi: 10.1016/j.neuroimage.2016.12.052
18. Seghezzi S, Zirone E, Paulesu E, Zapparoli L. The brain in (willed) action: a meta-analytical comparison of imaging studies on motor intentionality and sense of agency. *Front Psychol.* (2019) 2:804. doi: 10.3389/fpsyg.2019.00804
19. Zito GA, Wiest R, Aybek S. Neural correlates of sense of agency in motor control: A neuroimaging meta-analysis. *PLoS ONE.* (2020) 15:321. doi: 10.1371/journal.pone.0234321

13

Case Report: Novel Homozygous Likely Pathogenic *SCN1A* Variant with Autosomal Recessive Inheritance and Review of the Literature

Ana Victoria Marco Hernández [1,2], Miguel Tomás Vila [1], Alfonso Caro Llopis [2,3], Sandra Monfort [3] and Francisco Martinez [2,3]*

[1] Neuropediatrics Section, Hospital Universitari i Politècnic La Fe, Valencia, Spain, [2] Genetics Unit, Hospital Universitari i Politècnic La Fe, Valencia, Spain, [3] Genomics Unit, La Fe Health Research Institute, Valencia, Spain

***Correspondence:**
Ana Victoria Marco Hernández
marco_anaher@gva.es

Dominant pathogenic variations in the *SCN1A* gene are associated with several neuro developmental disorders with or without epilepsy, including Dravet syndrome (DS). Conversely, there are few published cases with homozygous or compound heterozygous variations in the *SCN1A* gene. Here, we describe two siblings from a consanguineous pedigree with epilepsy phenotype compatible with genetic epilepsy with febrile seizures plus (GEFS+) associated with the homozygous likely pathogenic variant (NM_001165963.1): c.4513A > C (p.Lys1505Gln). Clinical and genetic data were compared to those of other 10 previously published patients with epilepsy and variants in compound heterozygosity or homozygosity in the *SCN1A* gene. Most patients (11/12) had missense variants. Patients in whom the variants were located at the cytoplasmic or the extracellular domains frequently presented a less severe phenotype than those in whom they are located at the pore-forming domains. Five of the patients (41.7%) meet clinical criteria for Dravet syndrome (DS), one of them associated acute encephalopathy. Other five patients (41.7%) had a phenotype of epilepsy with febrile seizures plus familial origin, while the two remaining (17%) presented focal epileptic seizures. *SCN1A*-related epilepsies present in most cases an autosomal dominant inheritance; however, there is growing evidence that some genetic variants only manifest clinical symptoms when they are present in both alleles, following an autosomal recessive inheritance.

Keywords: *SCN1A*, Dravet syndrome, GEFS+, homozygous, autosomal recessive inheritance

INTRODUCTION

SCN1A gene encodes the alpha 1 subunit of the sodium channel, Nav1.1, an important protein that makes up the voltage-dependent sodium channels. Pathogenic variants cause a reduction in sodium currents in gamma-aminobutyric acid (GABA)-ergic inhibitory interneurons, leading to hyperexcitability of neuronal network and the appearance of seizures (1–3). *SCN1A* is associated with several epilepsy syndromes and a range of other diseases (4, 5). The most common is Dravet syndrome (DS), but it is also associated with generalized epilepsy with febrile seizures plus (GEFS+), familial hemiplegic migraine (FHM), autism spectrum disorder (ASD), Sudden

Unexpected Death Epilepsy (SUDEP), and epilepsy of infancy with migrating focal seizures (EIMFS) and very rarely involved in infantile spasms (4, 6–9). Genetic epilepsy with febrile seizure plus (GEFS+) is a familial epilepsy syndrome in which affected individuals within a family typically have a variety of epilepsy phenotypes, varying from simple febrile seizures and febrile seizures plus with a good outcome to severe epileptic encephalopathies (10).

About 1,871 *SCN1A* pathogenic variants have been identified so far (11), almost all of them under an autosomal-dominant fashion.

An attempt has been made to explain the phenotypic variability associated with *SCN1A* based on the type of mutation or functional alteration; in general, missense mutations are negatively correlated with a severe phenotype, and mutations with severe phenotypes are more frequently located in the pore region (12). Pathogenic variants that lead to a complete loss of function of the channel are virtually always associated with severe phenotypes, whereas milder impairments in channel function usually cause milder phenotypes (5, 12). Mutations that produce gain of function have also been described, as missense p.Thr226Met variant, which associates a severe clinical phenotype of early-onset epileptic encephalopathy, with profound developmental delay and hyperkinetic movement disorder (13, 14). However, in clinical practice, it remains difficult to fully predict the effects of novel variants on channel function. Recently, Jaber et al. have published original research reporting three patients with arthrogryposis multiplex congenita (AMC) in relation to other heterozygous missense variants of *SCN1A* (15).

To date, only 10 patients with *SCN1A*-related epilepsy due to autosomal recessive inheritance have been identified. In 2015, Brunklaus et al. published for the first time two novel homozygous missense mutations of the *SCN1A* gene in four children with infantile epilepsies from two consanguineous pedigrees. In both families, the heterozygous-carrier parents remained unaffected while their homozygous children developed *SCN1A*-related epilepsies, including DS and GEFS + (14). Since then, six more patients have been published (16–20). Here, we report two siblings, sons of a family with high consanguinity, with GEFS+ associated with the homozygous c.4513A > C variant in the SCN1A gene.

MATERIALS AND METHODS

Participants

The study was carried out in patients affected by homozygous *SCN1A* pathogenic or likely pathogenic variants, according to the American College of Medical Genetics and Genomics criteria (21), from Hospital La Fe. One family was recruited for inclusion. Informed consent was obtained from the parents of both participants. A systematic search was carried out in the scientific literature for other patients diagnosed with *SCN1A*-related epilepsy with recessive inheritance. The search terms in Pubmed were "*SCN1A*," "homozygous," and "recessive inheritance."

A brief clinical description of this cohort can be seen in **Table 1**.

This study was approved by the local ethics committee of the Hospital Universitari i Politècnic La Fe (Valencia, Spain).

Genetic Studies

Peripheral blood samples from individuals and their parents were collected by standard methods for the genetic studies. Genomic DNA was isolated using the Qiacube extractor (QIAGEN, Hilden, Germany). DNA purity and concentration were measured using the NanoDrop 8000 spectrophotometer (Thermo Scientific) and a Qubit 2.0 fluorometer (Invitrogen), respectively.

Massive parallel sequencing for exome sequencing was performed by using the SureSelect Clinical Research Exome (Agilent Technologies). The libraries were sequenced on an Illumina NextSeq 500 following the manufacturer's protocol to get a mean reading depth of 100 X. Sequence read alignments, variant calling, and annotation were performed in the *Alissa Interpret* platform (Agilent Technologies). All disease-causing genes related with epilepsy and/or neurodevelopmental disorders described in different databases were analyzed. To evaluate the clinical impact and to assess the pathogenicity of variants in exome sequencing, we applied the previously described criteria (22). All clinically relevant genetic variants detected were confirmed by Sanger sequencing from purified PCR products. Primers for amplification and Sanger sequencing were designed with exon-primer (primers and PCR conditions are available on request).

CASE STUDIES

Patient 1

Patient 1 is a 4-year-old female born to healthy consanguineous parents (see **Figure 1**). During pregnancy, no antenatal problems were detected, neither any problem during delivery. The patient lived in her country of origin (Romania) for up to 12 months. The family reported that, at 4 months of age, she presented the first febrile status epilepticus (SE) (20 min). At 7 months, she presented a 10-min febrile seizure (FS), for which phenobarbital was prescribed. She presented two more FS up to 11 months. At 11 months, she presented first generalized tonic-clonic seizure (GTCS) lasting 5 min without fever. So, treatment with valproic acid was established. At 12 months, she was assessed for the first time in our center. She presented age-appropriate psychomotor development. Brain MRI and electroencephalogram study were normal. In the metabolic study, lactic acid, ammonium, and organic acids were normal. In the acylcarnitine profile, a slight decrease in free carnitine 11.95 μmol/L (12.92–36.88) was detected, probably secondary to treatment with valproate, so it was decided to suspend phenobarbital and valproic acid to start treatment with levetiracetam. Since then, she has presented four more FS in the context of infectious illness, and her psychomotor development and neurological examination are normal. The clinical phenotype of the patient is GEFS+.

TABLE 1 | Clinical information on 12 patients with pathogenic or likely pathogenic *SCN1A* variants with autosomal recessive inheritance NM_001165963.1 (see **Figure 2**).

	Patient 1 **4 y female**	**Patient 2** **35 mo male**	**Patient 3** **9 y male**	**Patient 4** **7 y female**	**Patient 5** **30 y male**	**Patient 6** **19 y female**
Variant	chr2:166852591T>G c.4513A>C (p.Lys1505Gln)		chr2:169915161C>T c.302G>A (p.Arg101Gln) chr2:166850781A>G c.4727T>C (p.Ile1576Thr)		c.2768T>G, p.(Ile923Ser) Homozigous	c.824A >G, p.(Asn275Ser) Homozigous
Medical history	None	None	None	None	None	None
Family background	Consanguineous (**Figure 1**) Mother's sister and first-counsin with S Second paternal uncle with S		Consanguineous Sister died at 2 months from SE Asymptomatic father, mosaic		Consanguineous Sister with similar phenotype, age at seizure onset 10 mo	Consanguineous (first cousins) Brother is patient 11
Age al seizure onset	4 mo	7 mo	3 mo	11 mo	19 mo	3 mo
Seizure type al onset	FS (20 min)	FS (3 min)	GTCS and PS	GTCS and PS		FS
Seizure types	FS, FSE, GTCS	FS, FSE (30 min)	MS, AS	FS, MS, AS	FS, HCS afebrile and febrile	FS, PS, AS, GTCS
Seizure triggers	Fever	Fever			Fever	Fever, LMT, CBZ
Medication trials **Actual medication**	FB, VPA. **LEV**	**LEV**			**LEV, ZNS** (others)	LMT, CBZ, LEV, TPM, CLB, **VPA**
Additional clinical features	None	Sensorineural deafness	Weight and height measurements $p < 3$			ADHD
Intellectual disability	No	No Hypotonia	Yes	Yes	No, learning difficulties, slow reasoning	Borderline,
Type of movement disorder/Neurologic examination	None/Normal	None/Normal			"Clumsy"	
Language disturbance	No	No				
Brain MRI	Normal	Normal	Mild asymmetric widening of the posterior horn of the left ventricle, slight non-specific white matter change in T2 weighted images	Normal	Normal	Normal
EEG	Normal	Normal		Generalized epileptiform activity with no distinctive photosensivity	Normal, minor fronto.temporal abnormalities	Normal, diffuse spike-waves in temporal and frontal
Phenotype	GEFS+	GEFS+	DS	DS	GEFS+	GEFS+
Reference	This work	This work	Tuncer et al. (17)		Moretti et al. (20)	
	Patient 7 14 y female	Patient 8 4.5 y male	Patient 9 17 y male	Patient 10 5 y female	Patient 11 8 y male	Patient 12 3 y male

(Continued)

TABLE 1 | Continued

	Patient 7 **14 y female**	**Patient 8** **4.5 y male**	**Patient 9** **17 y male**	**Patient 10** **5 y female**	**Patient 11** **8 y male**	**Patient 12** **3 y female**
Variant	chr2:166903459T>C c.1198A>G (p.Met400Val)		chr2:166900370G>A c.1852C>T (p.Arg618Cys)		chr2:166856252G>A c.4319C>T (p.Ala1440Val)	chr2:166850711AT>A c.4796delA (p.Tyr1599Phefs*19)
Medical history			None		None	None
Family background	Parents are first-cousins Young brother with bilateral sensorineural hearing loss Maternal first cousin with febrile seizures until age five.		Parents are first-cousins Older sister with sensorineural hearing impairment due to connexin 26 mutation		Non-consanguineous parents	Both parents are heterozygous for this variation
Age al seizure onset	5 mo	15 mo	6 mo	13 mo	6 mo	4 mo
Seizure type al onset	FS 10 min	FS 20 min	Febrile GTCS 5 min	FS 10 min	FS	Afebrile left FMS
Seizure types	FS, Hemiclonic, GTCS, FSE, AA (atypical absences)	FSE, afebrile GTCS.	FS, Short afebrile focal seizures, night-time S frontal semiology	FS, PS with ASC characterized by behavioral arrest followed by head turning and hemi-clonic jerking	FS, GTCS, afebrile HCS, febrile HCS (5–15 min), MS ("head nodding," and "jerking of the legs"), PS, SE (>30 min), multiple types S.	FMS, AAS
Seizure triggers	CBZ, fever	Fever	Fever	Fever	Fever	Fever
Medication trials	CBZ	None	CBZ, LMT, TPM, LEV, STP, VPA, CZ	CBZ, VPA	VPA, LEV, TPM, BZD, FB, P	OXC, FTN, VPA, LEV, FB.
Actual medication						**VPA, TPM, CZ**
Additional clinical features					AE: SE at 2y→F0E0 no eye contact	Hepatomegaly
Intellectual disability	Yes, profound learning disability	No	DMD Severe learning difficulties	5y No	Hyperactive behavior, DMD. After AE: Profound DMD, behavior problems autistic traits	Neuromotor developmental retardation
Type of movement disorder/Neurologic examination	Diskinetic movement disorder characterized by mixed spasticity and dystonia		Balance and motor coordination problems		Ataxia After AE: spastic quadriplegia	Ataxic walking without support. Hand stereotypic movements
Language disturbance					After AE: total loss of speech	Meaningless word repetitions

(Continued)

TABLE 1 | Continued

	Patient 7 14 y female	Patient 8 4.5 y male	Patient 9 17 y male	Patient 10 5 y female	Patient 11 8 y male	Patient 12 3 y female
Brain MRI	20 mo: small corpus callosum with markedly delayed myelination and an AC	15 mo: normal	8 and 12 y: normal	4 y: normal	1 y: normal	Normal
EEG	19 mo: diffusely slow 11 y: awake: slow background of low amplitude.Sleep recurrent bursts of rhythmic sharp w. 14 y: interictal epileptiform activity	15 mo: normal		14 mo: normal 3 y: bilateral bursts of 3–4 Hz spike and wave. No photosensitivity	1 y: normal 21 mo: epileptic activity with slow waves and multifocal spike and spike-wave discharges which tended to increase with photic stimulation	4 mo: normal 3 y: frequent repetitive generalized spike-slow waves and multiple spike-slow wave activities
Phenotype	DS	FS+	FS+ PS	FS+ PS	DS and AE	DS
Reference		Brunklaus et al. (16)			Khanh Van et al. (19)	Aslan et al. (18)

AAS, atypical absence seizure; AC, atrophic cerebellum; AE, Acute encephalopathy; AS, absence seizure; ASC, absence seizure; ASC, altered state of ccnsciousness; CBZ, carbamazepine; CZ, clobazam; DS, Dravet syndrome; FSE, febrile status epilepticus; FB, fenobarbital; FS, febrile seizures; FTN, fenitoina; GEFS+, genetic epilepsy with febrile seizures plus; GTCS, Generalized tonic-clonic seizure; HCS, hemiclonic seizure; LEV, levetiracetam; LMT, lamotrigine; mo, months; MS, myoclonic seizures; OXC, oxcarbazepine; P, propofol; PS, partial seizure; S, seizure; STP, stiripentol; TPM, topiramato; VPA, valproate; Y, year w, waves.

Patient 2

Patient 2 is a 35-month-old male, the brother of Patient 1 (see **Figure 1**). The child was born from uneventful eutocic delivery after a 37-week regular gestation, with a birth weight 3,580 g; Apgar score, 8/9/10. In the screening with otoacoustic emissions carried out at birth, hearing loss was detected, which was confirmed by performing auditory-evoked potentials of the trunk (response, 70 dB in both ears with dysmorphic curves). At 7 months of age, he presented the first FS (3 min). Furthermore, at that age, significant axial hypotonia was detected, without maintaining head support and little visual contact. For this reason, it was decided to perform an MRI study and electromyogram, which were normal. Metabolic study was extended to ammonium, amino acids in serum and cerebrospinal fluid, acylcarnitines, and organic acids, all in the normal range. At 10 months of age, hearing aids were placed, and early stimulation was started with very good evolution. In the following months, the patient presented a total of four more typical FS. At 20 months of life, he presented a febrile SE of 30 min in the context of high fever, so it was decided to start treatment with levetiracetam. Subsequently, he has only presented a more typical FS.

Currently, psychomotor development is at the lower limit of normality, and the neurological examination is normal. The clinical phenotype of the Patient 2 is compatible with GEFS+.

Genetics

Initially, Paticnt 2 was genetically studied due to hearing loss; only the heterozygous variant c.269T > C (p.Leu90Pro) in the *GJB2* gene was considered of relevance. The inheritance pattern of hearing loss due to this gene is autosomal recessive and requires the presence of a second mutation in this gene to confirm the genetic diagnosis of hearing loss. It is possible that there might be a second undetected mutation or that there is another genetic or non-genetic cause of the hearing loss. On the other hand, Patient 2 presents the homozygous variant c.4513A > C in the *SCN1A* gene as the only clinically relevant result. This variant causes the substitution of the highly conserved amino acid lysine by glutamine in position 1,505 of the protein (p.Lys1505Gln), predicted as likely pathogenic by most of the *in silico* predictors (see **Table 2**). This variant has not been previously described. The variant is located between the repeat Domains III and IV at the cytoplasmic domain (see **Figure 2**). According to the ACMG criteria, this variant was classified as likely pathogenic (PP3, PM1, PM2, and PP2).

Familial segregational study by Sanger sequencing confirmed that Patient 1 shares the variant c.4513A > C in *SCN1A* gene in homozygous state, while the healthy parents of the two patients were heterozygous carriers.

DISCUSSION

So far, thousands of patients with heterozygous variants in the *SCN1A* gene have been published. The spectrum of the clinical phenotype associated with variations in the *SCN1A* gene is wide. Numerous studies have attempted to correlate the clinical phenotype according to the genotype (5, 12, 23), and there is evidence that, depending on the type and location of the

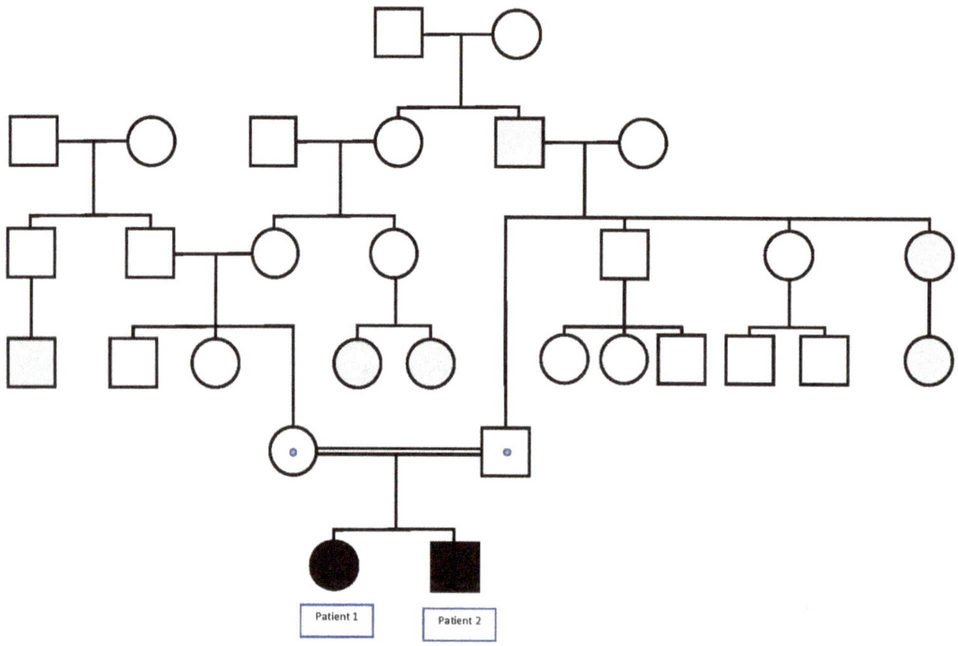

FIGURE 1 | Pedigree of the family in which the p.Lys1505Gln variant in the *SCN1A* gene segregates with GEFS+. Black symbols denote homozygous patients, and dotted symbols denote obligate or confirmed heterozygous healthy carriers. Gray symbols denote patients with FS or FS+.

mutation in the gene, the severity of the clinical picture varies. However, predicting the clinical consequences of novel genetic variants found in routine clinical practice is not an easy task. On the other hand, new phenotypes associated with *SCN1A* are continually being published (13, 15, 24–27).

The majority of published patients with pathogenic variants in *SCN1A* have autosomal dominant inheritance, more frequently by *de novo* mutation, although there are also many inherited cases (28). However, in recent years, several individuals who presented epilepsy in relation to homozygous or compound heterozygous variants in *SCN1A*, that is, with autosomal recessive inheritance, have been published. We have collected all the published cases and added our patients in order to broaden the phenotypic and genotypic spectrum associated with *SCN1A*.

In 2015, Brunklaus et al. published for the first time two novel homozygous missense mutations of the *SCN1A* gene in four children. Then, Tuncer et al. published two brothers with compound heterozygosity in *SCN1A* with symptoms compatible with DS (17). Subsequently, Aslan et al. and Van et al. have published two more cases with homozygous variants in patients with DS (18, 19), and Moretti et al. published two novel homozygous missense variations of the *SCN1A* gene in two individuals from two different families from consanguineous pedigrees. Both of them encompassed with GEFS+ (20) (see **Tables 1, 2**).

Ten of the total 12 patients were children of families with consanguinity. Patient 11, published by Van et al. presented the variant p.Ala1440Val in homozygosity, but the authors verified that it was a *de novo* mutation, since, despite having verified the paternity of the parents, none of them were carriers (19).

Regarding the clinical phenotype, five of the patients (41.7%) are clinically encompassed by Dravet syndrome (DS), one of them associated acute encephalopathy (AE). Five (41.7%) had a phenotype of GEFS+ of familial origin. Two (16.7%) of the patients presented FS+ and focal epileptic seizures (10). In **Table 1**, we have collected the description of all the patients.

Patient 2 presented sensorineural deafness, of unknown etiology, despite having carried out an extensive etiological study. Furthermore, Patients 7 and 8 had a younger brother with sensorineural hearing loss without a specified cause, and Patients 9 and 10 had an older sister with sensorineural hearing impairment due to connexin 26 mutation. Therefore, of the eight families in the series, three of them had individuals with sensorineural deafness. There are no publications linking *SCN1A* variants with sensorineural deafness, despite the large number of published patients with variants in this gene. For this reason, we think that this finding is probably related to consanguinity of the family rather than to *SCN1A* gene. The concurrence in a family of two autosomal recessive inherited diseases is not so uncommon when it comes to consanguineous families (29). Sensorineural deafness of genetic cause is mostly (about 80%) due to genetic variants of autosomal recessive inheritance (30, 31).

In the same way, we think that, possibly, the hepatomegaly that Patient 12 presented is unrelated to the variants in *SCN1A* gene.

Missense variants in *SCN1A* gene have variable effects, depending on the functional regions in which they occur and the nature of amino acid substitutions (11).

Missense mutations leading to disease are more likely to occur in the voltage sensor (S4) and the pore region (S5-S6

TABLE 2 | Genetic information on 12 patients with pathogenic or likely pathogenic *SCN1A* variants with autosomal recessive inheritance NM_001165963.1.

Patient	Patient 1 and 2	Patient 3 and 4	Patient 5	Patient 6	Patient 7 and 8	Patient 9 and 10	Patient 11	Patient 12
Variant	chr2:166852591 T>G c.4513A>C (p.Lys1505Gln)	chr2:166915161 C>T c.302G>A (p.Arg101Gln) chr2:166850781 A>G c.4727T>C (p.Ile1576Thr)	chr2:166894464 A>C c.2768T>G (p.Ile923Ser)	Chr2: 166908369 T>C c.824A>G (p.Asn275Ser)	chr2:166903459 T>C c.1198A>G (p.Met400Val)	chr2:166900370 G>A c.1852C>T (p.Arg618Cys)	chr2:166856252 G>A c.4319C>T (p.Ala1440Val)	chr2:166850711 AT>A c.4796delA (p.Tyr1599Phefs*19)
Classification	Likely pathogenic	Pathogenic Likely pathogenic	Uncertain significance	Likely pathogenic	Pathogenic	Uncertain significance/Likely pathogenic	Likely pathogenic	Pathogenic
Inheritance	Inherited homozygous (from both parents)	Compound heterozygous	Homozygous		Inherited homozygous (from both parents)	Inherited homozygous (from both parents)	Homozygous *de novo*	Inherited homozygous (from both parents)
ACMG criteria	PM1 moderate, PM2 moderate, PP2 supporting, PP3 supporting	PM5 very strong, PM1 moderate, PM2 moderate, PM5 moderate, PP2 supporting, PP3 supporting, PP5 supporting PM1 moderate, PM2 moderate, PP2 supporting, PP3 supporting	PM2 moderate, PP2 supporting, PP3 supporting	PM1 moderate, PM2 moderate, PP2 supporting, PP3 supporting	PM1 strong, PM2 moderate, PM5 moderate, PP2 supporting, PP3 supporting, PP5 supporting	PM2 moderate, PP2 supporting, PP3 supporting	PM1 moderate, PM2 moderate, PP2 supporting, PP3 supporting	PVS1 very strong, PM2 moderate, PP3 supporting
CADD	28.6	29.6/26.9	26.9	23.1	23.7	29.6	33	33
Phenotype	GEFS+ (both)	DS (both)	GEFS+	GEFS+	DS (p7) FS (p8)	FS+ PS (both)	DS and AE	DS
Reference	This work	Tuncer et al. (17)	Moretti et al. (20)		Brunklaus et al. (16)		Khanh et al. (19)	Aslan et al. (18)

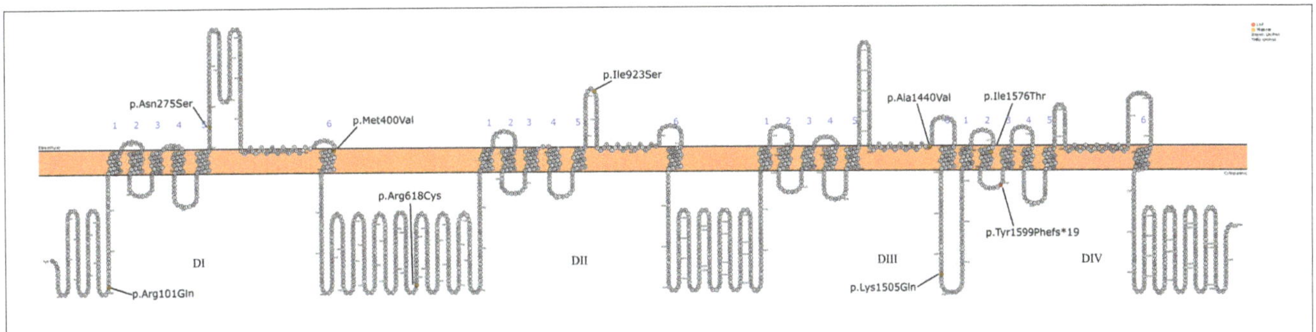

FIGURE 2 | Schematic representation of the *SCN1A* gene mutations detected in the 12 patients.

segments) of the four homologous domains, as in the case of Patients 3, 4, 7, and 11 of this series (32). As an exception, Patient 8 (the brother of Patient 7) presents the variant in the pore and a mild phenotype. In some pairs of siblings, a marked heterogeneity of the phenotype is observed. It has been proposed that variations in other epilepsy genes can modify the clinical phenotype associated with variants in *SCN1A* (33). This phenomenon has also been described in other genetic epilepsies associated with other ion channels, such as *SCN2A* (34). This variability associated with the same variation in *SCN1A* has been described both in individuals from the same family and at the interfamily level. However, further unknown environmental or epigenetic factors have been also proposed to play a significant role in the development and evolution of the epilepsy phenotype (35, 36).

All the variants described in the series are missenses, except for the frames hit variant in Patient 12, who presents a severe DS phenotype even though it is located at the intracytoplasmic level. So, due to the characteristics of the variant, the effect on the protein can be variable. Pathogenic variants that lead to a complete loss of function of the channel are virtually always associated with severe phenotypes.

It is difficult to establish a correlation between the genotype phenotype with such a small series; however, the data suggest that the variants located at the intracytoplasmic or extracellular level (Patients 1, 2, 5, 6, 9, 10, and 12) present a less severe epileptic phenotype. Conversely, those variants found at the pore region (Patients 3, 4, 7, 8, and 11) more frequently present a more severe phenotype, with a phenotype of Dravet syndrome in most patients.

It is worth noting that heterozygous carrier parents or other relatives are asymptomatic. Therefore, the variants described in this work are probably hypomorphic, both due to their location within the gene and because of their intrinsic properties, and they are only capable of altering the function of the Nav1.1 protein when they are in homozygous state. In any case, it is also remarkable that the phenotypic spectrum of the whole series of patients presenting the autosomal recessive phenotype related to SCN1A is quite similar to the phenotypic spectrum of most patients with autosomal dominant inheritance, as well as a similar genotype-phenotype correlation.

CONCLUSIONS

The 12 patients published so far with an autosomal recessive epileptic phenotype associated with *SCN1A* show that not all patients with symptoms associated with this gene have autosomal dominant inheritance. On the other hand, it is worth noting that the resulting phenotypes do not differ from those usually caused by dominant heterozygous variants. Furthermore, the analysis of the variants found in each patient, correlating it with the phenotype he or she presents, allows us to know a little better the correlation of genotype-phenotype associated with *SCN1A*. It is possible that hypomorphic heterozygous variants only manifest when affecting the two alleles of this gene.

ETHICS STATEMENT

The studies involving human participants were reviewed and approved by Comité de ética del Instituto de Investigación Sanitaria La Fe. Written informed consent to participate in this study was provided by the participants' legal guardian/next of kin. Written informed consent was obtained from the minor(s)' legal guardian/next of kin for the publication of any potentially identifiable images or data included in this article.

AUTHOR CONTRIBUTIONS

AM: drafting of the article, clinical examination of the patients, and bibliographic search. AC and SM: substantial contributions to analysis and interpretation of genetic data. MT: revising the article for important intellectual content and contribution to clinical data analysis. FM: analysis and interpretation of genetic data and revising of the article and final approval. All authors contributed to the article and approved the submitted version.

ACKNOWLEDGMENTS

We warmly thank all the patients and their families for their involvement in this study.

REFERENCES

1. Catterall WA, Kalume F, Oakley JC. Nav1.1 channels and epilepsy. *J Physiol.* (2010) 588:1984–59. doi: 10.1113/jphysiol.2010.187484
2. Yu FH, Mantegazza M, Westenbroek RE, Robbins CA, Kalume F, Burton KA, et al. Reduced sodium current in GABAergic interneurons in a mouse model of severe myoclonic epilepsy in infancy. *Nat Neurosci.* (2006) 9:1142–9. doi: 10.1038/nn1754
3. Ogiwara I, Miyamoto H, Morita N, Atapoui N, Mazaki E, Inoue I, et al. Nav1.1 localizes to axons of parvalbumin-positive inhibitory interneurons: a circuit basis for epileptic seizures in mice carrying an *Scn1a* gene mutation. *J Neurosci.* (2007) 27:5903–14. doi: 10.1523/JNEUROSCI.5270-06.2007
4. Scheffer IE, Nabbout R. *SCN1A*-related phenotypes: epilepsy and beyond. *Epilepsia.* (2019) 60:S17–24. doi: 10.1111/epi.16386
5. de Lange IM, Koudijs MJ, van't Slot R, Gunning B, Sonsma ACM, van Gemert LJJM, et al. Mosaicism of *de novo* pathogenic *SCN1A* variants in epilepsy is a frequent phenomenon that correlates with variable phenotypes. *Epilepsia.* (2018) 59:690–703. doi: 10.1111/epi.14021
6. Mei D, Cetica V, Marini C, Gerrini R. Dravet syndrome as part of the clinical and genetic spectrum of sodium cannel epilepsies and encephalopathies. *Epilepsia.* (2019) 60:S2–7. doi: 10.1111/epi.16054
7. Carranza Rojo D, Hamiwka L, McMahon JM, Dibbens LM, Arsov T, Suls A, et al. *De novo SCN1A* mutations in migrating partial seizures of infancy. *Neurology.* (2011) 77:380–3. doi: 10.1212/WNL.0b013e31822 7046d
8. Hirose S, Scheffer IE, Marini C, De Jonghe P, Andermann E, Goldman AM, et al. *SCN1A* testing for epilepsy: application in clinical practice. *Epilepsia.* (2013) 54:946–52. doi: 10.1111/epi.12168
9. Claes L, Del-Favero J, Ceulemans B, Lagae L, Van Broeckhoven C, De Jonghe P. *De Novo* mutations in the sodium-channel gene *SCN1A* cause severe myoclonic epilepsy of infancy. *Am J Hum Genet.* (2001) 68:1327–32. doi: 10.1086/320609
10. Myers KA, Scheffer IE, Berkovic SF, on behalf of the ILAE Genetics Commission. Genetic literacy series: genetic epilepsy with febrile seizures plus. *Epilepstic Disord.* (2018) 20:232–8. doi: 10.1684/epd.2018.0985
11. *SCN1A* mutation database. *Institute of Neurosciences, Guangzhou Medical University.* C2021 – (2021). Available online at: http://scn1a.caae.org.cn (accessed July 8, 2021)
12. Meng H, Xu HQ, Yu L, Lin GW, He N, Su T, et al. The *SCN1A* mutation database: updating information and analysis of the relationships among genotype, functional alteration, and phenotype. *Hum Mutat.* (2015) 36:573–80. doi: 10.1002/humu.22782
13. Sadleir LG, Moutier EI, Gill D, Davis S, Joshi C, DeVile C, et al. Not all *SCN1A* epileptic encephalopathies are Dravet syndrome: early profound Thr226Met phenotype. *Neurology.* (2017) 89:1035–42. doi: 10.1212/WNL.0000000000004331
14. Beck VC, Hull JM, Isom LL. Beyond dravet syndrome: characterization of a novel, more severe *SCN1A*-linked epileptic encephalopathy. *Epilepsy Curr.* (2019) 19:266–8. doi: 10.1177/1535759719858339
15. Jaber D, Gitiaux C, Blesson S, Marguet F, Buard D, Varela Salgado M, et al. *De novo* mutations of *SCN1A* are responsible for arthrogryposis broadening the *SCN1A*-related phenotypes. *J Med Genet.* (2020) 20:1–6. doi: 10.1136/jmedgenet-2020-107166
16. Brunklaus A, Ellis R, Stewart H, Aylett S, Reavey E, Jefferson R, et al. Homozygous mutations in the *SCN1A* gene associated with genetic epilepsy with febrile seizures plus and Dravet syndrome in 2 families. *Eur J Paediatr Neurol.* (2015) 19:484–8. doi: 10.1016/j.ejpn.2015.02.001

17. Tuncer FN, Gormez Z, Calik M, Uzun GA, Sagiroglu MS, Yuceturk B, et al. A clinical variant in *SCN1A* inherited from a mosaic father cosegregates with a novel variant to cause Dravet syndrome in a consanguineous family. *Epilepsy Res.* (2015) 113:5–10. doi: 10.1016/j.eplepsyres.2015.02.020
18. Aslan M, Ozgor B, Kirik S, Gungor S. A novel *SCN1A* mutation: a case report. *J Pediatr Neurosci.* (2020) 15:120–3. doi: 10.4103/jpn.JPN_118_18
19. Khanh Van LT, Hien HTD, Kieu HTT, Hieu NLT, Vinh LS, Hoa G, et al. *De novo* homozygous variant of the *SCN1A* gene in patient with severe Dravet syndrome complicated by acute encephalopathy. *Neurogenet.* (2021) 22:133–6. doi: 10.1007/s10048-021-00636-7
20. Moretti R, Arnaud L, Bouteiller D, Trouillard O, Moreau P, Buratti J, et al. SCN1A-related epilepsy with recessive inheritance: two further families. *Eur J Paediatric Neurol.* (2021) 33:121–4. doi: 10.1016/j.ejpn.2021.05.018
21. Richards S, Aziz N, Bale S, Bick D, Das S, Gastier-Foster J, et al. Standards and guidelines for the interpretation of sequence variants: a joint consensus recommendation of the American college of medical genetics genetics and genomics and the association for molecular pathology. *Genet Med.* (2015) 17:405–24. doi: 10.1038/gim.2015.30
22. Martinez F, Caro-Llopis A, Rosello M, Oltra S, Mayo S, Monfort S, et al. High diagnostic yield of syndromic intellectual disability by targeted next-generation sequencing. *J Med Genet.* (2017) 54:87–92. doi: 10.1136/jmedgenet-2016-103964
23. Brunklaus A, Schorge S, Smith AD, Ghanty I, Stewart K, Gardiner S, et al. *SCN1A* variants from bench to bedside-improved clinical prediction from functional characterization. *Hum Mutat.* (2019) 41:363–74. doi: 10.1002/humu.23943
24. Spagnoli C, Frattini D, Rizzi S, Salerno GG, Fusco C. Early infantile *SCN1A* epileptic encephalopathy: expanding the genotype-phenotype correlations. *Seizure.* (2019) 65:62–4. doi: 10.1016/j.seizure.2019.01.002
25. Berecki G, Bryson A, Terhag J, Maljevic S, Gazina EV, Hill SL, et al. *SCN1A* gain of function in early infantile encephalopathy. *Ann Neurol.* (2019) 85:514–25. doi: 10.1002/ana.25438
26. Ohashi T, Akasaka N, Kobayashi Y, Magra S, Kawashima H, Matsumoto N, et al. Infantile epileptic encephalopathy with a hyperkinetic movement disorder and hand stereotypies associated with a novel *SCN1A* mutation. *Epileptic Disord.* (2014) 16:208–12. doi: 10.1684/epd.2014.0649
27. Ohtsuka Y, Ohmori I, Ogino T, Ouchida M, Shimizu K, Oka E. Paroxysmal movement disorders in severe myoclonic epilepsy in infancy. *Brain Dev.* (2003) 25:401–5. doi: 10.1016/S0387-7604(03)00025-1
28. Scheffer IE, Berkovic S, Capovilla G, Connoly MB, French J, Ghilhoto L, et al. ILAE classification of the epilepsies position paper of the ILAE comission for classification and terminology. *Epilepsia.* (2017) 58:512–21. doi: 10.1111/epi.13709
29. Romdhane L, Mezzi N, Hamdi Y, El-Kamab G, Barakat A, Abdelhak S. Consanguinity and inbreeding in health and disease in North African populations. *Annu Rev Genomics Hum Genet.* (2019) 20:155–79. doi: 10.1146/annurev-genom-083118-014954
30. Yang T, Guo L, Wang L, Yu X. Diagnosis, intervention, and prevention of genetic hearing loss. *Adv Exp Med Biol.* (2019) 1130:73–92. doi: 10.1007/978-981-13-6123-4_5
31. Petersen MB, Willems PJ. Non-syndromic, autosomal-recessive deafness. *Clin Genet.* (2006) 69:371–92. doi: 10.1111/j.1399-0004.2006.00613.x
32. Zuberi SM, Brunklaus A, Birch R, Reavey E, Duncan J, Forbes GH. Genotype-phenotype associations in *SCN1A*-related epilepsies. *Neurology.* (2011) 76:594–600. doi: 10.1212/WNL.0b013e31820c309b
33. De Lange IM, Mulder F, van't Slot R, Sonsma ACM, van Kempen MJA, Nijaman IJ, et al. Modifier genes in *SCN1A*-related epilepsy syndromes. *Mol Genet Genomic Med.* (2020) 8:e1103. doi: 10.1002/mgg3.1103
34. Nieto-Barceló JJ, Gonzalez Montes N, Gonzalo Alonso I, Martínez F, Aparisi MJ, Martínez-Matilla M, et al. Variant in CACNA1G as a posible genetic modifier of neonatal epilepsy in an infant with a De Novo SCN2A mutation. *J J Pediatr Genet.* (2021). doi: 10.1055/s-0041-1723958
35. Suls A, Velizarova R, Yordanova I, Deprez L, Van Dyck T, Wauters J, et al. Four generations of epilepsy caused by an inherited microdelection of the epilepsy caused by an inherited microdeletion of the *SCN1A* gene. *Neurology.* (2010) 75:72–6. doi: 10.1212/WNL.0b013e3181e62088
36. Guerrini R, Cellini E, Mei D, Metitieri T, Petrelli C, Pucatti D, et al. Variable epilepsy phenotypes associated with a familial intragenic deletion of the *SCN1A* gene. *Epilepsia.* (2010) 51:2474–7. doi: 10.1111/j.1528-1167.2010.02790.x

14

Case Report: Late-Onset Lennox-Gastaut Syndrome Treated with Stereotactic Electroencephalography-Guided Radiofrequency Thermocoagulation before Craniotomy

Sixian Li[1]*, Xiaodong Cai*[1]*, Chen Yao*[1]*, Yuanqing Wang*[1]*, Xiaohua Xiao*[1]*, Huafeng Yang*[1]*,*
Yi Yao[2] *and Lei Chen*[3*]

[1] *Department of Neurosurgery, Shenzhen Second People's Hospital, The First Affiliated Hospital of Shenzhen University, Shenzhen, China,* [2] *Department of Functional Neurosurgery, Xiamen Humanity Hospital, Xiamen, China,* [3] *Department of Neurology, West China Hospital in Sichuan University. Chengdu, China*

Correspondence:
Lei Chen
leilei_25@126.com

The onset of Lennox-Gastaut syndrome (LGS), a severe epilepsy syndrome, is typically before 8 years of age. Late-onset LGS (with onset in adolescence and adulthood) is relatively rare clinically and has some differences from classical LGS. Herein, we describe the case of a patient with late-onset LGS and provide a literature review of such cases. The patient had focal epilepsy onset at 8 years of age. After a 9-year evolution, he suffered seizures of different types and had a diagnosis of late-onset LGS. Drug treatment was ineffective. Nothing was found on stereotactic electroencephalography (SEEG) and magnetic resonance imaging (MRI) during the course of the disease. After the second presurgical evaluation, we found a suspicious focus on high-resolution structural MRI which was verified by SEEG at last. After SEEG-guided radiofrequency thermocoagulation (RFTC), his seizures were controlled, and his cognitive function and quality of living clearly improved. However, his seizures recurred 2 years later, and he underwent left occipital resection. Thereafter, his seizures have been controlled until now. This case emphasizes the importance of high-resolution structural MRI in the treatment of LGS. Furthermore, it suggests that late-onset LGS may be caused by focal lesions and evolve from focal epilepsy. Thus, characterizing the clinical symptoms and performing individualized electroencephalographic follow-up are both very important. Additionally, the clinical outcome in this case implies the value and limitations of RFTC in patients with epilepsy and a clear focal lesion. Moreover, this case further supports differences between late-onset and classical LGS in terms of clinical manifestation, cognitive changes, prognosis, and treatment.

Keywords: Case Report, refractory epilepsy, late-onset Lennox-Gastaut syndrome, stereotactic electroencephalography, radiofrequency thermocoagulation

INTRODUCTION

Lennox-Gastaut Syndrome (LGS) is a severe epilepsy syndrome, with onset typically before 8 years of age and comprising a variety of seizure types. LGS is often accompanied by specific changes on electroencephalography (EEG) and cognitive impairment. Herein, we describe a patient with late-onset LGS who had onset after 8 years of age. For a comprehensive analysis, previous cases of late-onset LGS were reviewed and compared to this case.

CASE PRESENTATION

Patient Information

A 19-year-old man first experienced a generalized seizure attack without any cause at 8 years of age. Subsequently, he sometimes complained of bright or colorful flashing lights, blurry vision, and distance changes in both visual fields before seizures, especially on the right side. The visual auras usually lasted several min and sometimes occurred alone. At 17 years of age, he experienced transient nodding attacks, frequently without an aura. At 18 years of age, dropping attacks occurred frequently, with accompanying gripped hands and slight forearm flexion. After the attacks, he could stand by himself without an aura or a memory. The nodding and dropping attacks could occur 2–10 times in 4–5 days and in a series. He was diagnosed with refractory epilepsy and underwent presurgical evaluation at another hospital. Magnetic resonance imaging (MRI) scans were considered negative, and he was monitored by stereotactic electroencephalography (SEEG) focusing on the temporal, parietal, and occipital (TPO) regions, especially on the left side, but without lateralization or localization. Although he underwent vagal nerve stimulation (VNS) using five types of antiepileptic drugs, there was no significant improvement. Thus, he was admitted to our hospital for further treatment.

Clinical Findings

His family, perinatal, and growth history, and physical examination results were normal. Wakeful background on video electroencephalography showed 9–10 Hz alpha rhythm in bilateral occipital regions. Interictal EEG showed generalized 2–2.5 Hz slow spike waves (SSWs) during wakefulness and generalized paroxysmal fast activities (GPFAs) during sleep. There were also multifocal independent spikes, especially in the bilateral occipital and posterior temporal regions where the left side was more predominant than the right. Compared with SSWs and occipital discharges, GPFA was more prominent, followed by occipital discharges. Epileptic spasms, tonic seizures, and atypical absence were recorded, which showed EEG onsets with a little localization value. MRI showed a suspiciously unclear gray-white matter boundary around the left calcarine sulcus (**Figures 1**, **2**), which also showed low metabolism on positron emission tomography (**Figure 1**). Neuropsychological tests showed moderate cognitive impairment. No abnormalities were found on genetic testing and perimetry. Accordingly, the clinic diagnoses were as follows: refractory epilepsy, late-onset LGS, possible onset zone at the left occipital cortex, and postoperative VNS.

Therapeutic Intervention

We analyzed his previous SEEG even though the former hospital considered the SEEG result without lateralization or localization value and performed the VNS, but we found there were rhythmic discharges mainly in the left TPO region, which also had the most obviously electrical evolution during tonic and spasm seizures onset. Combining the imaging finding, we considered the seizure onset was most likely to be on the left TPO region and re-inserted six electrodes in total, of which five were focused on left TPO region and one was focused on the left hippocampus. During the SEEG monitoring, there were plentifully rhythmic interictal discharges in the left occipital region and higher frequency of fast activities during spasm and tonic seizures onset, which verified the left occipital lesion as the epileptogenic zone. Radiofrequency thermocoagulation (RFTC) was performed on this lesion and the surrounding region, with five electrodes and 17 contacts in total.

Follow-Up and Outcomes

Following the treatment with RFTC, he did not experience seizures for more than 1 year, but the right visual hemianopsia remained. There were a few spikes on EEG (only one during a 24-h test), and his cognition improved. However, he again experienced tonic seizures 2 years after the RFTC; thus, he underwent left occipital resection. The pathology indicated micro-malformation of cortical development (mMCD) (1, 2). As yet, he has remained seizure-free for 1 year following the occipitectomy.

DISCUSSION

The onset of LGS is typically before 8 years of age, with a peak at 4–5 years (3). Late-onset LGS, occurring in adolescents or adults (> 8 years old), is relatively rare and accounts for 10–15% of all LGS cases (4, 5). Thus, we collected data on all cases of late-onset LGS that have been reported since 1991; the 42 identified cases are summarized in **Table 1** (6–13). The age of seizure onset ranged from 6 weeks to 28 years, while the age at LGS diagnosis ranged from 8 to 64 years, The lag time between seizure onset and LGS diagnosis is mostly due to ictal semiology and electroclinical findings not having been fulfilled, suggesting that electroclinical changes in LGS follow a gradual evolutionary process, as in this case. It generally takes 1–2 years from seizure onset to a definite diagnosis of LGS (14, 15) because of differences in etiology, clinical characteristics, and disease progression between patients. This emphasizes the importance of individual electroclinical follow-up for early diagnosis of LGS. Additionally, for patients with a definite LGS diagnosis, a retrospective analysis of the characteristics of their electroclinical evolution is necessary and useful for precise treatment.

Among the identified 42 cases of late-onset LGS, 13 showed chromosome variations. Of the 29 remaining cases, 17 showed normal cognition and had a disease course of 5–32 years, while 12 showed cognitive impairment (mild cognitive impairment in two cases) and a course of 5–25 years. This indicates that unlike early-onset LGS, cognitive function, and daily viability are relatively preserved in late-onset LGS; additionally, cognitive function is

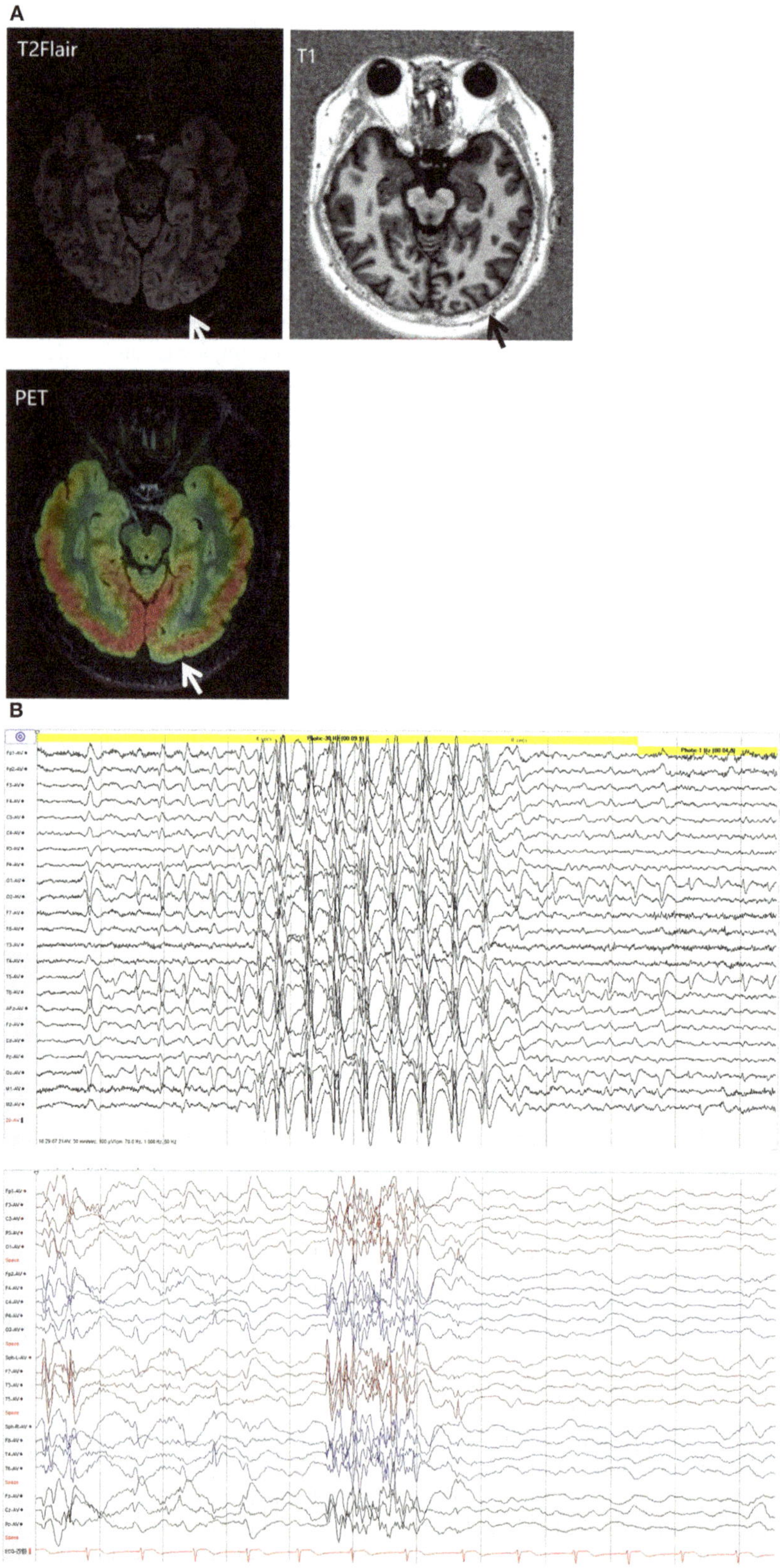

FIGURE 1 | (A) T2 fluid-attenuated inversion recovery (T2-FLAIR) magnetic resonance imaging showing a suspiciously unclear gray-white matter boundary around the left calcarine sulcus (white arrow). T1 magnetic resonance imaging showing a suspiciously unclear gray-white matter boundary around the left calcarine sulcus (black arrow). Positive emission tomography showing low metabolism at the cortex around the left calcarine sulcus (white arrow). **(B)** EEG background: generalized 2-2.5 Hz slow spike waves (SSWs) during wakefulness and generalized paroxysmal fast activity (GPFA) during sleep.

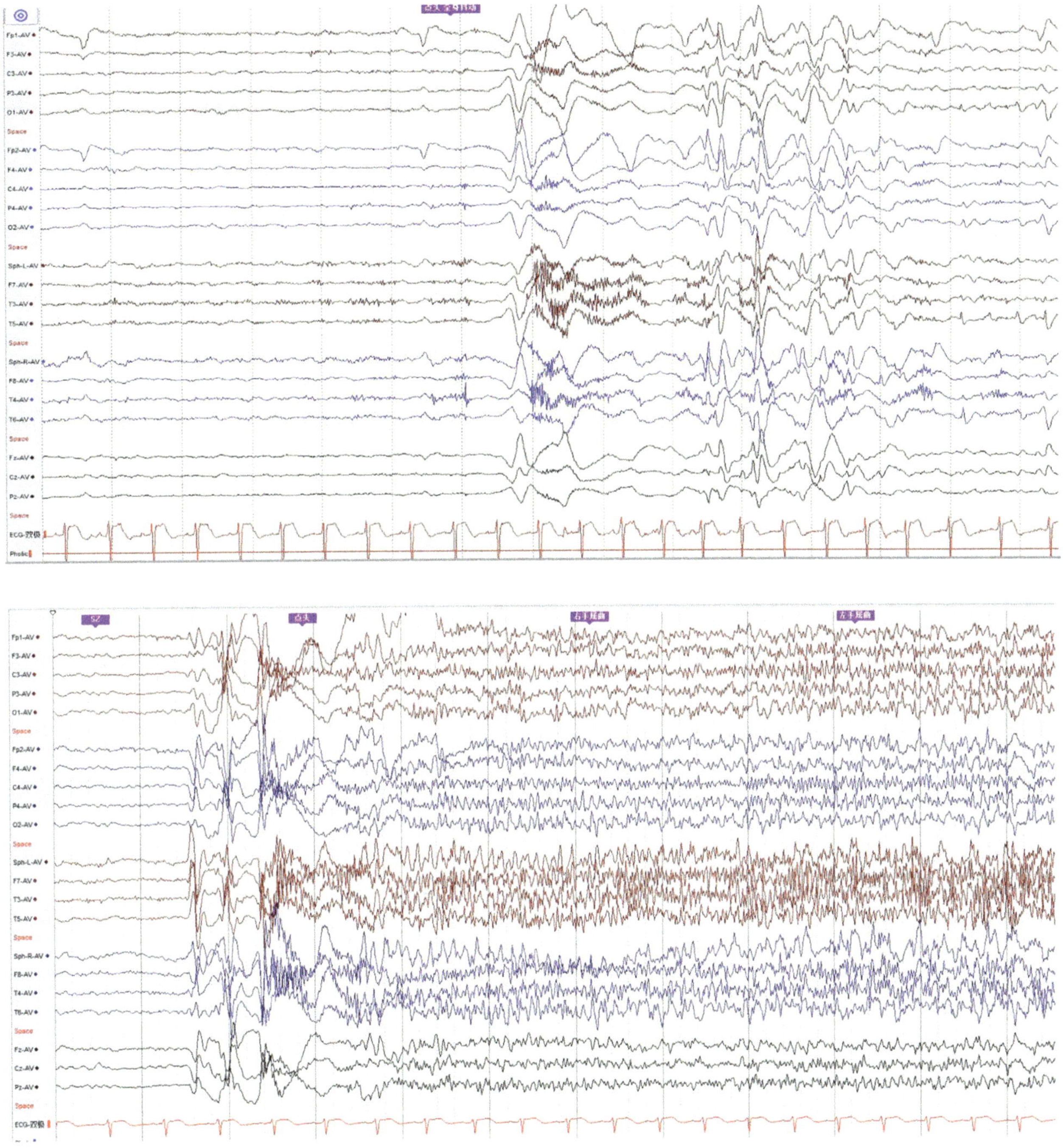

FIGURE 2 | EEG onset: epileptic spasm and tonic seizure involved general EEG onsets with little localization value.

not significantly related to disease course (4, 5, 8). This case had a disease course of 9 years, but the patient's cognitive function had only moderately declined. Furthermore, neurological examination results were mentioned in 38 of the 42 cases, among which four patients had abnormal neurological signs related to intracranial infection, cerebral infarction, perinatal injury, etc. Additionally, the EEG background was mentioned in 16 of the 42 cases, among which 10 showed normal EEG background, and six showed nonspecific slow waves. These findings suggest that late-onset LGS mostly shows no positive neurological signs or special abnormalities in the EEG background, as observed in this case.

Among the 42 cases, MRI findings were negative in 17, nonspecific or subcortical changes were found in 12, local cortical lesions were found in 5, and MRI findings were not mentioned in the remaining 8, suggesting that the cortical

TABLE 1 | Clinical characteristics, EEG and imaging findings, and other case details in 42 cases of late-onset Lennox-Gastaut Syndrome (LGS).

NO.	Sex	Seizure onset (age, y)	Diagnosis (age, y)	Seizure types	Cognition	Living independently	Neurologic exam	EEG background	EEG epileptiform discharges	Imaging	Etiology	AEDS(≥3)	VNS	Prognosis
1	M	14	22	T, AA, GTC	N	N	N	N	GPFA, SSWs	N	/	Y	N	/
2	M	12	17	T, AA, P	N	N	N	N	GPFA, SSWs, MS	N	/	Y	N	/
3	M	17	46	T, P	N	N	N	N	GPFA, SSWs, MS	N	/	Y	N	/
4	M	6w	8	A, AA, T	AB	AB	VI	/	GPFA, SSWs, MS	/	Infection	Y	N	/
5	M	18m	8	A, T	AB	AB	/	/	GPFA, SSWs, MS	/	/	Y	N	Mostly controlled
6	F	9	19	A, GTC	mild	AB	/	Slow	SSWs	/	/	Y	Y	Mostly controlled
7	F	28	28	AA, GTC	mild	AB	LH	Slow	SSWs	Right hemispheric stroke	Stroke	Y	Y	/
8	F	7	32	A, P, SI	AB	AB	/	Slow	SSWs	/	/	Y	Y	/
9	F	13	27	A, T, AA, GTC	N	N	N	N	GPFA, SSWs, GS	N	/	Y	N	/
10	F	12	49	T, AA, A, GTC	N	N	N	N	GPFA, SSWs, GS	N	/	Y	N	/
11	M	17	61	T, AA, M, GTC	N	N	N	N	GPFA, SSWs, GS	N	/	Y	N	/
12	F	12	44	T, AA, A, GTC	N	N	N	N	GPFA, SSWs, GS	N	/	Y	N	/
13	F	16	41	T, A, M, GTC	N	N	N	N	GPFA, SSWs, GS	N	/	Y	N	/
14	M	11	40	T, AA, A, GTC	N	N	N	N	GPFA, SSWs, GS	N	/	Y	N	/
15	F	17	22	T, AA, A, GTC	N	N	N	Slow	GPFA, SSWs, GS	N	/	Y	N	/
16	M	13	26	T, AA, A, GTC	N	N	N	Slow	GPFA, SSWs, GS	N	/	Y	N	/
17	/	20	20	T, AA, A, M, GTC	AB	/	/	/	GPFA, SSWs, MS	N	Brain injury	Y	N	/
18	F	16	16	T, A, GTC	N	/	N	/	GPFA, SSWs, GS	Low-lying cerebellar tonsils just below the foramen magnum level	/	Y	Y	Encephalopathy, DS
19	M	5	32	T, AA, A, GTC	N	/	N	/	GPFA, SSWs, GS	Small probable arachnoid cyst in the left frontal region	/	Y	Y	DS
20	F	9	14	T, AA, A, M, GTC	AB	/	N	/	GPFA, SSWs, GS	Modest ventricular dilatation	ALL with MTX	Y	N	Encephalopathy, DS
21	F	15	26	T, AA, A, M, GTC	N	/	N	/	GPFA, SSWs, GS	N	/	Y	Y	Encephalopathy, DS, SUDEP
22	M	19	19	T, A, GTC	AB	/	N	/	GPFA, SSWs, GS	N	Infection	Y	N	DS
23	F	15	15	T, AA, A, GTC	AB	/	N	/	GPFA, SSWs, GS	Single non-enhancing 6 mm focus in the paramedian inferior left cerebellum	/	Y	Y	VNS partially effective, DS
24	F	11	11	T, AA, A, GTC	N	/	N	/	GPFA, SSWs, GS	Gray matter of heterotopia with transmantle dysplasia	ALL with MTX; MCD	Y	Y	Encephalopathy, DS

(Continued)

TABLE 1 | Continued

NO.	Sex	Seizure onset (age, y)	Diagnosis (age, y)	Seizure types	Cognition	Living independently	Neurologic exam	EEG background	EEG epileptiform discharges	Imaging	Etiology	AEDS(≥3)	VNS	Prognosis
25	F	11	11	T, AA, A, GTC	N	/	N	/	GPFA, SSWs, GS	Cerebellar atrophy	/	Y	Y	Encephalopathy, DS
26	F	11	11	T, A, GTC	AB	/	N	/	GPFA, SSWs, GS	Pachygyria, diffuse bilateral lissencephaly and band heterotopia	MCD	Y	Y	DS
27	F	10	10	T, AA, A, M, GTC	AB	/	N	/	GPFA, SSWs, GS	Mild cerebellar and cortical cerebral atrophy	/	Y	N	DS
28	F	14	64	AA, GTC, A	N	/	N	N	GPFA, SSWs, MS	N	/	Y	N	/
29	F	9	27	T, AA	AB	/	N	/	GPFA, SSWs	Moderate diffuse atrophy	trisomy 21	Y	N	Weekly seizures, SUDEP
30	F	8	12	T, AA, A	AB	/	N	/	GPFA, SSWs	/	trisomy 21	Y	N	DS
31	M	11	14	T, AA, A	AB	/	N	/	GPFA, SSWs	Multiple small subcortical calcification	trisomy 21	Y	N	DS
32	F	12	30	T, AA	AB	/	N	/	GPFA, SSWs	N	trisomy 21	Y	N	Seizures decreased
33	F	8	33	AA, A	AB	/	N	/	GPFA, SSWs	/	trisomy 21	Y	N	Weekly seizures, SUDEP
34	M	5	30	T, GTC	AB	/	LH	/	GPFA, SSWs	/	trisomy 21	Y	N	DS
35	M	12	17	T, AA	AB	/	N	/	GPFA, SSWs	Mild diffuse atrophy	trisomy 21	Y	N	DS
36	M	6	36	T, AA, P, GTC	AB	/	N	/	GPFA, SSWs	/	trisomy 21	Y	N	DS
37	M	16	23	T, AA, GTC	AB	/	N	/	GPFA, SSWs	Moderate diffuse atrophy	trisomy 21	Y	N	DS
38	M	11	12	T, M, P	AB	/	N	/	GPFA, SSWs	Mild diffuse atrophy	trisomy 21	Y	N	DS
39	M	7	11	T, AA, A, GTC	AB	/	N	/	GPFA, SSWs	N	trisomy 21	Y	N	Weekly or monthly seizures
40	M	10	43	T	AB	/	N	/	GPFA, SSWs, MS	Dilation cortical sulci, calcification globus pallidus	trisomy 21	Y	N	DS
41	M	7	34	T, AA	AB	/	N	/	GPFA, SSWs	Mild diffuse atrophy	trisomy 21	Y	N	DS
42	M	9	30	T, AA, GTC	AB	/	slight cerebellar sign	Slow	GPFA, SSWs, MS	Asymmetrical cystic lesions in bilateral parietooccipital regions	Perinatal injury	/	/	/

/, information not available; M, male; F, female; y, year; w, week; m, month; N, normal; AB, abnormal; A, atonic; AA, atypical absence, T, tonic; IS, infantile spasm; GTC, generalized tonic-clonic; P, partial; SI, startle induced; M, myoclonic; VI, visual impairment; LH, left hemiparesis; GPFA, generalized paroxysmal fast activity; SSWs, slow spike waves; MS, multifocal spikes; GS, generalized spike; ALL, acute lymphoblastic leukemia; MTX, methotrexate; MCD, malformations of cortical development; AEDs, antiepileptic drugs; VNS, vagal nerve stimulation; Y, yes, N, none; SUDEP, sudden unexpected death in epilepsy; DS, daily seizures.

structure in late-onset LGS mostly showed no specific changes. However, this substantially differs from previous reports on classical LGS, which indicate that more than 2/3 of patients show cortical structural lesions on MRI (3, 16), including focal, multifocal, and diffuse abnormalities, with static pathological lesions predominating (e.g., focal cortical dysplasia), while progressive or metabolic lesions are relatively rare (17, 18). This may reflect a difference between early- and late-onset LGS, but it may also be related to a case inclusion bias and skill in image reading; thus, this potential distinction needs to be confirmed by accumulating more cases. However, the progression of neuroimaging technology and the quality of MRI scans may also contribute to focal structural lesion identification. In this case, nothing was found in the initial clinical work-up, and the epileptic focus was found during the re-evaluation process by high-resolution structural MRI and later confirmed by SEEG and RFTC, indicating the important role of high-resolution structural MRI in the etiological diagnosis and treatment of late-onset LGS. Routine MRI should include three-dimensional T1, T2 FLAIR, and coronal thin-layer scanning of the long axis of the vertical hippocampus (3).

In the 29 cases without chromosome variations, the prognosis was not mentioned in 6 cases, 11 cases had independent viability, 2 cases had well-controlled seizures, and the remaining 10 cases had a poor prognosis, including frequent seizures, encephalopathy, sudden unexpected death in epilepsy, etc. This indicates that the prognosis of late-onset patients is relatively good. Furthermore, although most of the 42 identified cases had tried more than three antiepileptic drugs, none underwent surgery, which may be related to an unclear etiology. In total, 10 cases had tried VNS, which was clearly mentioned as effective in only 1 case, suggesting that VNS has a poor effect on late-onset LGS, as observed in this case, which showed obvious improvement after surgery, suggesting the effectiveness and necessity of early surgery for patients with late-onset LGS with definite focal lesions (15, 18).

For 1 year after the RFTC, not only were the patient's seizures well controlled, but his cognition improved and the EEG spikes "calmed down" gradually for 2 years. Such changes were first mentioned in 1979 (19). These observations not only suggest that electroclinical changes in late-onset LGS are the result of secondary alterations in brain networks (20), but also confirm the efficacy of RFTC. However, his seizure recurred and he eventually underwent left occipital resection and has been seizure free until now. This indicated the limited efficacy and scope of RFTC compared to craniotomy in lesion damage and pathological network disconnection in some cases with accurate lesion targets, which may be the main reason explaining the low rate of seizure-free cases with RFTC (21). However, the improvement of clinical outcomes after RFTC may further suggest the correct location of epileptic foci and good prognosis after craniotomy, as in this case. Nevertheless, RFTC is superior in some small foci that can be located precisely and destroyed completely but are inaccessible by surgery, and has the advantages of less damage to brain function, fewer complications, and faster postoperative recovery (22, 23).

In summary, LGS, with onset after 8 years of age known as late-onset LGS, may be caused by focal lesions. Individualized follow-up is necessary. Late-onset LGS and classical LGS have some differences in terms of clinical manifestation, cognitive changes, prognosis, and treatment. MRI is important in determining the etiology of late-onset LGS and is useful for early treatment. Comparing to craniotomy, RFTC is limited and less effective in lesion damage. However, clinical improvement after RFTC would support the appropriate identification of seizure onset zone location indicated by SEEG results and therefore help with surgical plan for cortical resection.

PATIENT PERSPECTIVE

We spent a lot of money and time in the treatment of our son's disease before the second evaluation. After the RFTC, our son's seizures were miraculously controlled and he could go to school again. This was beyond our expectations.

AUTHOR CONTRIBUTIONS

All authors listed have made a substantial, direct, and intellectual contribution to the work and approved it for publication.

REFERENCES

1. Piao YS, Lu DH, Chen L, Liu J, Wang W, Liu L, et al. Neuropathological findings in intractable epilepsy: 435 Chinese cases. *Brain Pathol.* (2010) 20:902–8. doi: 10.1111/j.1750-3639.2010.00386.x
2. Blumcke I, Spreafico R, Haaker G, Coras R. Histopathological findings in brain tissue obtained during epilepsy surgery. *N Engl J Med.* (2017) 377:1648–56. doi: 10.1056/NEJMoa1703784
3. Bourgeois BF, Douglass LM, Sankar R. Lennox-Gastaut syndrome: a consensus approach to differential diagnosis. Epilepsia. (2014) 55 (Suppl 4):4–9. doi: 10.1111/epi.12567
4. Goldsmith IL, Zupanc ML, Buchhalter JR. Long-term seizure outcome in 74 patients with Lennox-Gastaut syndrome: effects of incorporating MRI head imaging in defining the cryptogenic subgroup. *Epilepsia.* (2000) 41:395–9. doi: 10.1111/j.1528-1157.2000.tb00179.x
5. Asadi-Pooya AA, Sharifzade M. Lennox-Gastaut syndrome in south Iran: electro-clinical manifestations. *Seizure.* (2012) 21:760–3. doi: 10.1016/j.seizure.2012.08.003
6. Park KM, Hur YJ, Kim SE. Brainstem dysfunction in patients with late-onset Lennox-Gastaut syndrome: voxel-based morphometry and tract-based spatial statistics study. *Ann Indian Acad Neurol.* (2016) 19:518–22. doi: 10.4103/0972-2327.194462
7. Piña-Garza JE, Chung S, Montouris GD, Radtke RA, Resnick T, Wechsler RT. Challenges in identifying Lennox-Gastaut syndrome in adults: a case series illustrating its changing nature. *Epilepsy Behav Case Rep.* (2016) 5:38–43. doi: 10.1016/j.ebcr.2016.01.004
8. Chourasia N, Maheshwari A, Kalamangalam G. Cognitive and functional status in late-onset Lennox-Gastaut syndrome: variation on a classic phenotype. *Epilepsy Behav.* (2020) 102:106660. doi: 10.1016/j.yebeh.2019.106660

9. Trevisol-Bittencourt PC, Sander JW. [Lennox-Gastaut syndrome of late onset? Report of a case] *Arq Neuropsiquiatr.* (1990) 48:520–4. doi: 10.1590/S0004-282X1990000400020
10. Smith KM, Britton JW, Cascino GD. Late-onset Lennox-Gastaut syndrome: diagnostic evaluation and outcome. *Neurol Clin Pract.* (2018) 8:397–402. doi: 10.1212/CPJ.0000000000000527
11. Benbadis SR, Dinner DS. Lennox-Gastaut syndrome in the elderly? *Clin Electroencephalogr.* (1994) 25:142–7. doi: 10.1177/155005949402500406
12. Ferlazzo E, Adjien CK, Guerrini R, Calarese T, Crespel A, Elia M, et al. Lennox-Gastaut syndrome with late-onset and prominent reflex seizures in trisomy 21 patients. *Epilepsia.* (2009) 50:1587–95. doi: 10.1111/j.1528-1167.2008.01944.x
13. Ono T, Ishii T. Multicystic encephalomalacia in an adult case of Lennox-Gastaut syndrome: a case report. *Jpn J Psychiatry Neurol.* (1991) 45:435–6. doi: 10.1111/j.1440-1819.1991.tb02513.x
14. Al-Banji MH, Zahr DK, Jan MM. Lennox-Gastaut syndrome. *BMC Neurosci.* (2015) 20:207–12. doi: 10.17712/nsj.2015.3.20140677
15. Resnick T, Sheth RD. Early diagnosis and treatment of Lennox-Gastaut Syndrome. *J Child Neurol.* (2017) 32:947–55. doi: 10.1177/0883073817714394
16. Panayiotopoulos CP. *The Epilepsies: Seizures, Syndromes and Management* Oxfordshire: Bladon Medical Publishing (2005).
17. Blume WT. Pathogenesis of Lennox-Gastaut syndrome: considerations and hypotheses. *Epileptic Disord.* (2001) 3:183–96.
18. Asadi-Pooya AA. Lennox-Gastaut syndrome: a comprehensive review. *Neurol Sci.* (2018) 39:403–14. doi: 10.1007/s10072-017-3188-y
19. Angelini L, Broggi G, Riva D, Lazzaro Solero C, A case of Lennox-Gastaut syndrome successfully treated by removal of a parietotemporal astrocytoma. *Epilsia.* (1979) 20:665–9. doi: 10.1111/j.1528-1157.1979.tb04850.x
20. Archer JS, Warren AE, Stagnitti MR, Masterton RA, Abbott DF, Jackson GD. Lennox-Gastaut syndrome and phenotype: secondary network epilepsies. *Epilepsia.* (2014) 55:1245–54. doi: 10.1111/epi.12682
21. Bourdillon P, Cucherat M, Isnard J, Ostrowsky-Coste K, Catenoix H, Guénot M, et al. Stereo-electroencephalography-guided radiofrequency thermocoagulation in patients with focal epilepsy: a systematic review and meta-analysis. *Epilepsia.* (2018) 59:2296–304. doi: 10.1111/epi.14584
22. Cossu M, Cardinale F, Casaceli G, Castana L, Consales A, D'Orio P, et al. Stereo-EEG-guided radiofrequency thermocoagulations. *Epilepsia.* (2017) 58 (Suppl 1):66–72. doi: 10.1111/epi.13687
23. Youngerman BE, Khan FA, McKhann GM. Stereoelectroencephalography in epilepsy, cognitive neurophysiology, and psychiatric disease: safety, efficacy, and place in therapy. *Neuropsychiatr Dis Treat.* (2019) 15:1701–16. doi: 10.2147/NDT.S177804

15

Late-Onset Ictal Asystole and Falls Related to Severe Coronary Artery Stenosis: A Case Report

*Francesco Fortunato[1], Angelo Labate[1], Michele Trimboli[1], Carmen Spaccarotella[2], Ciro Indolfi[2] and Antonio Gambardella[1]**

[1] Department of Medical and Surgical Sciences, Institute of Neurology, University Magna Graecia, Catanzaro, Italy,
[2] Cardiology Unit, Department of Medical and Surgical Sciences, University Magna Graecia, Catanzaro, Italy

***Correspondence:**
Antonio Gambardella
a.gambardella@unicz.it

Introduction: Ictal asystole (IA) is a rare, underestimated, and life-threatening cause of transient loss of consciousness and fall. Current treatment options for seizures associated with IA usually include cardiac pacemaker implantation. We report, for the first time, a case of IA that is related to coronary stenosis, which was resolved after coronary angioplasty.

Case Presentation: A 73-year-old man had a 2-year history of focal seizures with impaired awareness. Three months before our observation, he started to have sudden falls resulting in injury on several occasions. General and neurological examinations, as well as brain MRI, were unremarkable. Interictal electroencephalography (EEG) showed bitemporal spiking. Ictal video-polygraphy revealed a diffuse electrodecrement, followed by a buildup of rhythmic 4–6 Hz sharp activity, which was more evident in the left temporal region. After the seizure onset, the ECG showed sinus bradycardia, followed by sinus arrest that was associated with the patient's fall from the standing position. Afterwards, sinus rhythm returned spontaneously. A diagnosis of IA was made. A comprehensive cardiologic evaluation revealed a sub-occlusive stenosis of the left anterior descending artery. Successful coronary angioplasty resolved IA, levetiracetam was added, and no seizure or fall has occurred in the following 20 months. Moreover, he underwent a 7-day Holter ECG monitoring, and no asystole was depicted.

Conclusion: The present case was unique as it shows the potential association between IA and coronary stenosis, also suggesting a possible therapeutic role for coronary angioplasty. It also highlights the importance of carefully investigating epilepsy patients with falls, especially in the elderly, since IA-related falls can be easily misdiagnosed in older age. Thus, if IA is identified, a deeper cardiac evaluation should be considered. As seen in our patient, non-invasive diagnostic examination including routine, prolonged, and exercise ECG, as well as echocardiogram, were readily available and were informative in diagnosing cardiac abnormalities that are amenable to specific treatment.

Keywords: seizure, ictal asystole, SUDEP, ischemic heart, cardiac arrhythmia

INTRODUCTION

Ictal asystole (IA) is a rare, underestimated, and life-threatening cause of transient loss of consciousness, which usually leads to traumatic falls with significant morbidity (1–3). An IA and a non-epileptic syncope may be difficult to distinguish if based solely on clinical grounds due to the similarity of the clinical features, as both are most likely the result of cerebral hypoperfusion (4, 5). Semiologic features supporting an epileptic origin include behavioral arrest and blank stare, preceding falls (4, 5). Also, anamnestic findings of automatisms, visual, olfactory, auditory or gustatory hallucinations, or the déjà vu sensations are indicative of a seizure origin (4, 5), as these symptoms are not observed with reflex faints. On the other hand, post-ictal confusion, a key distinguishing feature of IA, may be misdiagnosed with situational disorientation that occurs in some patients recovering from cardiac syncope (6). Likewise, some patients with focal epilepsy may have seizures presented with isolated syncope that may be challenging to diagnose (7). Moreover, the ECG evolution during an IA is largely indistinguishable from that of a vasovagal faint, with sinus tachycardia being followed by progressive heart rate slowing, which at times progresses to an asystolic pause (5). Consequently, it may be difficult to establish an unequivocal clinical distinction by clinical features or ECG alone (5). Therefore, the diagnosis of IA can be challenging unless the clinician suspects it, or if it is captured on video-polygraphic monitoring with the documentation of asystole, as produced by an ictal electroencephalography (EEG) discharge (1–3).

Most reported cases had late-onset IA on the ground of long-standing drug-resistant focal epilepsy, and IA typically appeared after the onset of epilepsy with delay of many years (1). Nonetheless, it has also been recognized as a new-onset IA group with high prevalence of pre-existing heart conditions (1, 8, 9). IA has been hypothesized as one of the several mechanisms of sudden unexpected death in epilepsy (10), and this risk highlights the need for complete seizure control, cardiac evaluation, and potential cardiac intervention (11). Indeed, current treatment options for seizures associated with IA include anti-seizure medications, epilepsy surgery, and cardiac pacemaker implantation (11), but no treatment guidelines currently exist. We report, for the first time, a case of IA related to coronary artery stenosis that was resolved after coronary angioplasty. We present the following case in accordance with the CARE reporting checklist. The study was approved by the local ethics committee and the patient gave the consent.

CASE PRESENTATION

A 73-year-old man had a 2-year history of occasional episodes of impaired awareness and arrest of behavior, which lasted in <1 min. Three months before our observation, he started to have sudden falls resulting in injury on several occasions. He has never experienced chest pain or other cardiac symptoms.

General and neurological examinations, as well as brain MRI, were unremarkable. Interictal EEG showed sharp waves bilaterally located over the temporal regions (**Figure 1**). Video-polygraphic monitoring captured three typical epileptic seizures. The ictal EEG revealed a diffuse electrodecrement followed by buildup of rhythmic 4–6 Hz sharp activity more evident in the left temporal region (**Figure 2**). After seizure onset, the ECG always showed sinus bradycardia, followed on one occasion by eight-second sinus arrest that was associated with the patient's fall from the standing position (**Figure 2**). No fall occurred during the two ictal events with ictal bradycardia. Sinus rhythm returned spontaneously in all seizures. During the video-polygraphic monitoring, the episodes of asystole, and bradycardia coincided only with the ictal events. A diagnosis of ictal asystole (IA) (1) was made, and he underwent a thorough cardiologic investigation, in accordance to standardized protocol (12).

Electrocardiogram (ECG) recording and echocardiogram were unremarkable; tilt-test and cardiac enzymes were negative, while exercise ECG revealed ST elevation in V1, V2, and V4. Coronary angiogram showed sub-occlusive stenosis of the left anterior descending artery (**Figure 2**). Angioplasty with implantation of three everolimus-eluting stents resolved the coronary stenosis (Figure). In the following month, he continued to have staring spells, but no fall occurred. The Holter ECG monitoring result was normal. Interictal EEG continued to show bi-temporal spiking. During the follow-up video-polygraphic monitoring, three seizures were recorded, but none was associated with bradycardia or IA (Figure). Then, he started levetiracetam (1.0 g/day), and no seizure or fall, which was suspicious for seizure-induced cardiac asystole, has occurred in the following 20 months. Moreover, he underwent a 7-day Holter ECG monitoring, and no asystole was depicted.

DISCUSSION

Ictal asystole (IA) has been considered a rare complication of epileptic seizures, affecting <1% of patients with refractory seizures who underwent video-EEG monitoring (9). The IA seems to be a multifactorial condition and different predisposing factors seem to contribute to the ictal manifestation depending on whether it appears at the beginning of the epilepsy or later (6). In the new-onset IA, female gender and a preexisting heart condition may serve as predispositions in an otherwise mild epilepsy, while in late-onset IA, neuronal network changes in a chronic and therapy-resistant epilepsy may contribute to the ictal manifestation (6). Growing evidence also indicates that IAs are more frequent than was previously recognized and represent an important cause of falling (1, 2, 10). It is also likely that IA may be more common in the elderly, since epilepsy and seizure-induced falls are common in older adults, as well as cardiac and autonomic changes that are more frequently seen in old age (13). In addition, IA-related falling can be easily misdiagnosed in the elderly, since falls occur in more than one-third of the older population. Furthermore, not all seizures in the same patient

Abbreviations: ECG, electrocardiogram; MRI, magnet resonance imaging.

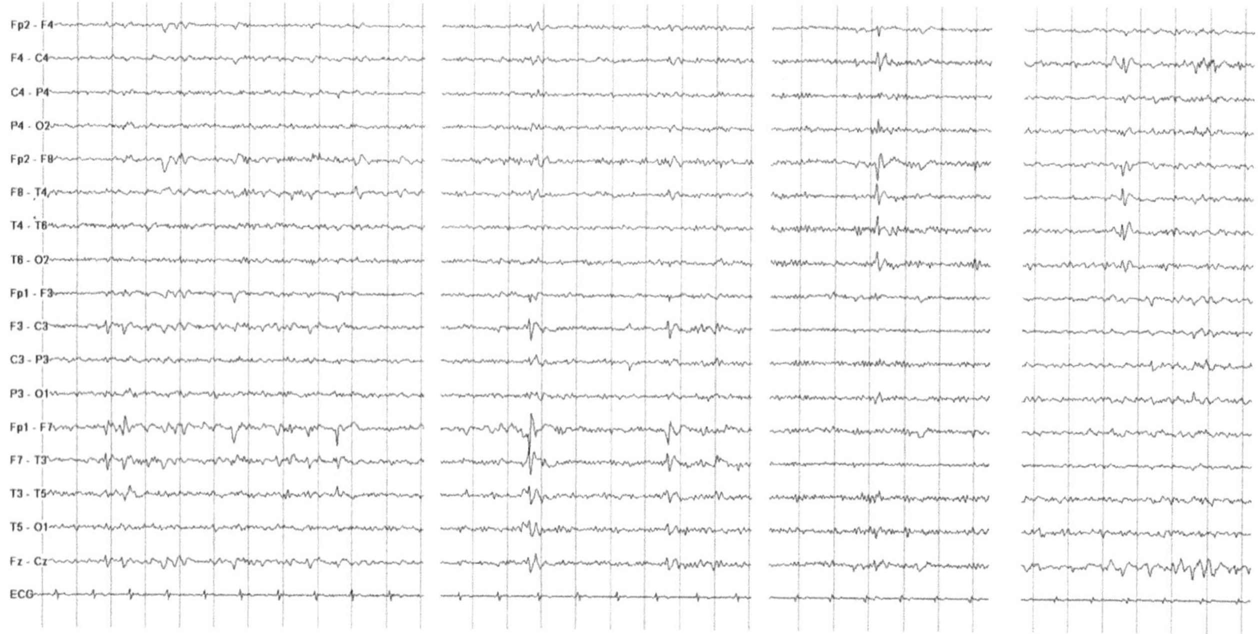

FIGURE 1 | Interictal electroencephalography (EEG) shows spiking activity and slow sharp waves located over the temporal regions bilaterally.

give rise to IA. A systematic review quantified the short-term recurrence risk of IA to about 40%, suggesting also that in case of clinically suspected IA the recording of one or two seizures is not sufficient to rule out IA (14). Moreover, as seen in our patient, those with IA and longer asystole duration were considered "high risk patients," since asystole duration >6 s is strongly associated with ictal syncope and falls (15). Therefore, a correct diagnosis is of paramount importance in such patients, as aggressive seizure control and cardiac pacemaker implantation are advocated to prevent serious injuries from falls related to IA. In this way, the present case was unique as IA and sudden falls were resolved after successful coronary angioplasty. Thus, awareness of this previously unrecognized triggering relationship has important implications for treatment and prognosis.

In our patient, it might be questioned whether coronary artery disease and IA are causally related. We believe that the interaction of the ictal temporal discharge superimposed on a chronic coronary is probably responsible for the genesis of ictal asystole in our patient. There is now a large body of evidence of frequent peri-ictal cardiac dysfunction and stress in association with different seizure types (8, 10, 12, 13). Indeed, a seizure activity may have deleterious impact on the structural integrity of the heart and its vasculature leading to myocardial fibrosis, accelerated atherosclerosis, systolic and diastolic dysfunction, and arrhythmias. Likewise, coronary artery diseases, especially stenosis of left anterior descending artery, are risk factors for almost any kind of arrhythmia, and contribute to ictal heart rate abnormalities, altered autonomic function, and potentially deleterious arrhythmias (16, 17), which may be a pre-requisite for sudden unexpected death in epilepsy (8, 10, 12, 13). During our patient's first video-EEG/ECG monitoring prior to angioplasty, all recorded seizures were always associated with bradyarrhythmia or asystole. Conversely, no change of heart rate occurred during seizures was recorded after coronary angioplasty. Moreover, at longer follow-up, the patient has no further experience of sudden fall, which is suspicious for seizure-induced cardiac asystole, as the 7-day ambulatory ECG monitoring has ruled out any asystole. Thus, it is conceivable that the damaged myocardium related to severe coronary disease greatly contributed to asystole during seizures in our patient. Obviously, further studies with longer follow-up and preferably long-term cardiac monitoring with a loop recorder are warranted to strengthen this relationship between IA and cardiac disease.

It is well-known that ictal epileptic discharges can cause changes in cardiac rhythm: they are more frequently associated with ictal tachycardia, while more rarely connected with ictal bradycardia or IA (18). Both ictal bradyarrhythmia and IA mostly coincide with focal seizures with impaired awareness and are predominantly seen in temporal lobe epilepsy (1, 13, 19, 20). Also, our patient had focal seizures of temporal origin, and video-EEG monitoring was a valuable tool for diagnosing seizure-induced cardiac asystole, as well as for guiding subsequent therapy. Our patient has EEG recordings that demonstrated diagnostic focal changes in the temporal regions at seizure onset, with the characteristic semiologic features of unresponsiveness and of staring, then, after about 15 s, short periods of sinus bradycardia followed in, on occasion by asystole, with a duration of 8 s.

Experimental evidence points to an early involvement of sympathetic and/or parasympathetic discharges in triggering the ictal cardiac changes, but the autonomic alterations in epilepsy are complex, and so are the mechanisms and interactions that support them. The IA is considered as primarily a seizure-driven

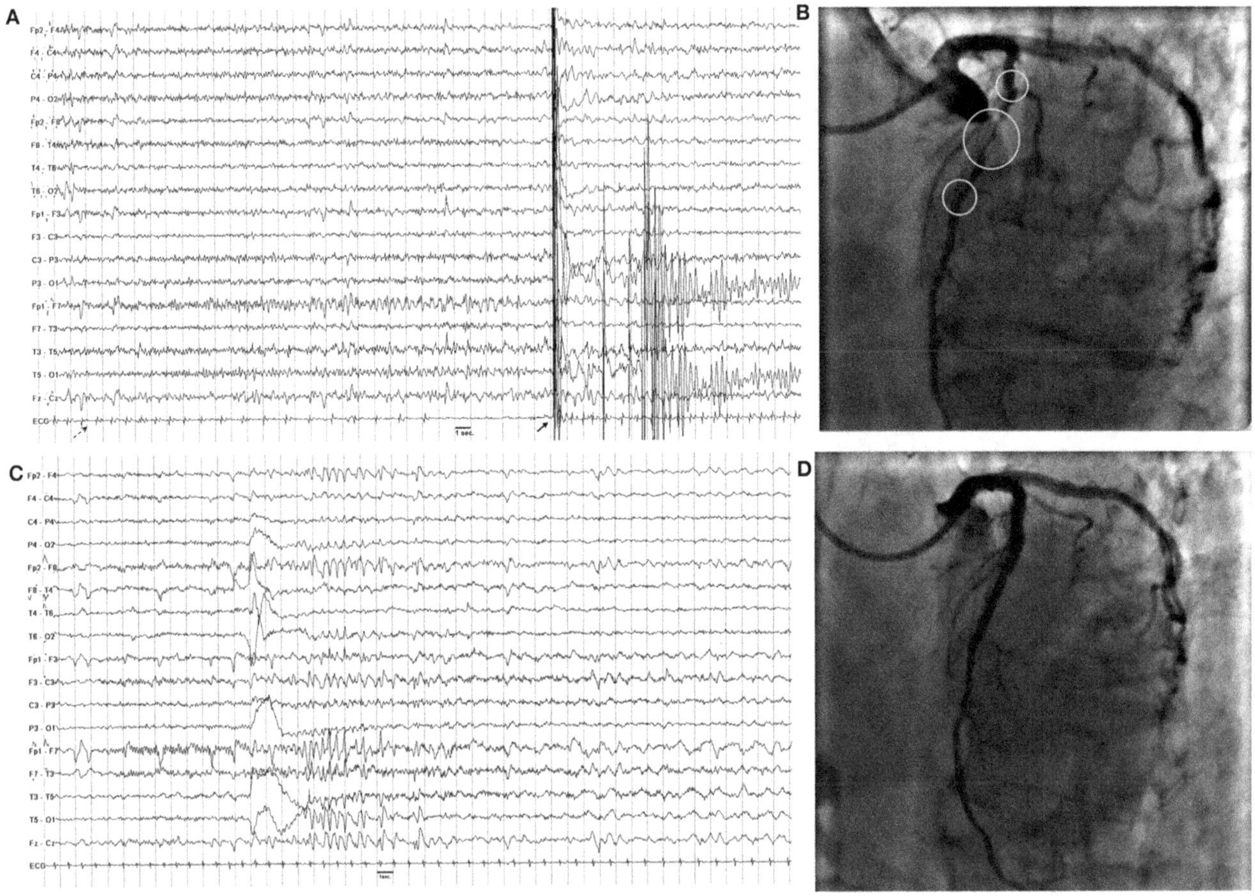

FIGURE 2 | (A) Ictal asystole. On ictal EEG recording note the diffuse electrodecrement followed by buildup of rhythmic 4–6 Hz sharp activity more evident in the left temporal regions. On ECG, there is a progressive slowing of heart followed by asystole of 8 s. The dashed arrow indicates seizure onset, while the full arrow indicates the artifact due to the patient's fall from standing position. **(B)** Coronary angiography shows sub-occlusive stenotic traits (circles) of the left anterior descending coronary. **(C)** Ictal EEG after angioplasty shows a similar pattern with no modification of hearth rate on ECG channel. **(D)** Coronary angiography after angioplasty shows normal flow of the left anterior descending coronary.

phenomenon: cortical centers comprising the central autonomic network thought to be primarily responsible for triggering a "vagal storm" in ictal-induced bradycardia and IA (5). The hypothesis is that IA might be a direct consequence of epileptic activity involving cortical and subcortical structures, especially amygdala nucleus, cingulate gyrus, insula cortex, thalamus, and/or hypothalamus, all linked to the central regulation of cardiovascular functions (17).

Furthermore, many patients manifest both ictal bradycardia or tachycardia at various times in conjunction of their seizures (5). Many intriguing hypotheses have been proposed to explain the "tachycardia-bradycardia dichotomy" in epilepsy (17, 19). Moreover, the background cardiovascular status of patients with epilepsy is expected to influence the cardiac responses during seizures (9, 16). As far as we are aware, in a systematic review collecting 157 cases of IA, it was found a 28% of preexisting heart conditions in the new onset IA group, compared to 8.5% in the late-onset IA group. (9). Thus, we can speculate that in our case, the hearth rate changes were primarily driven by the focal seizures, but coronary artery disease could also contribute, shifting the "tachycardia-bradycardia dichotomy" toward the bradycardia and IA.

Finally, it is convincible that the prevalence of IA or ictal bradycardia is currently underestimated (17–19). Accordingly, data from out-patient cohorts have illustrated that bradyarrhythmias may occur at a higher frequency than what was reported from video-electroencephalogram recording centers (18). In a recent study, we also depicted ECG abnormalities, most frequently bradyarrhythmia, in ~15% of patients with a confirmed diagnosis of refractory epilepsy (12). More importantly, some patients have potentially showed to have life-threatening cardiac arrhythmias, which may make them more vulnerable to seizures that may become fatal (8).

CONCLUSIONS

The present case was unique as it shows the potential association between IA and coronary stenosis, also suggesting a possible therapeutic role for coronary angioplasty. It also highlights the importance of carefully investigating falling as associated with patients with epilepsy (20) especially in the elderly, since IA-related falls can be easily misdiagnosed in older age. Thus, if IA is identified as such, a deeper cardiac evaluation should be considered. As seen in our patient, non-invasive diagnostic examinations including routine, prolonged and exercised ECG, as well as echocardiogram, are readily available and informative in diagnosing cardiac abnormalities that are amenable to specific treatment.

ETHICS STATEMENT

The studies involving human participants were reviewed and approved by Comitato Etico Sezione Area Centro, Calabria, Italy. The patients/participants provided their written informed consent to participate in this study. Written informed consent was obtained from the individual(s) for the publication of any potentially identifiable images or data included in this article.

AUTHOR CONTRIBUTIONS

FF, AL, and AG contributed to conception and design of the study. FF wrote the first draft of the manuscript. MT, CS, and CI had a major role in the acquisition, analysis, and interpretation of the data. AG and AL revised the manuscript critically for important intellectual contents. All authors contributed to manuscript review, revision, and approved the submitted version.

REFERENCES

1. Schuele SU, Bermeo AC, Alexopoulos AV, Locatelli ER, Burgess RC, Dinner DS, et al. Video-electrographic and clinical features in patients with ictal asystole. *Neurology.* (2007) 69:434–41. doi: 10.1212/01.wnl.0000266595.77885.7f
2. Nguyen-Michel VH, Adam C, Dinkelacker V, Pichit P, Boudali Y, Dupont S, et al. Characterization of seizure-induced syncopes: EEG, ECG, and clinical features. *Epilepsia.* (2014) 55:146–55. doi: 10.1111/epi.12482
3. Giovannini G, Meletti S. Ictal asystole as the first presentation of epilepsy: a case report and systematic literature review. *Epilepsy Behav Case Rep.* (2014) 2:136–41. doi: 10.1016/j.ebcr.2014.06.001
4. Brignole M, Moya A, de Lange FJ, Deharo JC, Elliott PM, Fanciulli A, et al. 2018 ESC guidelines for the diagnosis and management of syncope. *Eur Heart J.* (2018) 39:1883–948. doi: 10.5603/KP.2018.0161
5. Benditt DG, van Dijk G, Thijs RD. Ictal asystole: life-threatening vagal storm or a benign seizure self-termination mechanism? *Circ Arrhythm Electrophysiol.* (2015) 8:11–4. doi: 10.1161/CIRCEP.114.002546
6. Tinuper P, Cerullo A, Marini C, Avoni P, Rosati A, Riva R, et al. Epileptic drop attacks in partial epilepsy: clinical features, evolution, and prognosis. *J Neurol Neurosurg Psychiatry.* (1998) 64:231–7. doi: 10.1136/jnnp.64.2.231
7. Li W, Jayagopal LA, Taraschenko O. Ictal asystole with isolated syncope: a case report and literature review. *Epilepsy Behav Case Rep.* (2018) 11:47–51. doi: 10.1016/j.ebcr.2018.11.006
8. Verrier RL, Pang TD, Nearing BD, Schachter SC. Epileptic heart: a clinical syndromic approach. *Epilepsia.* (2021) 62:1780–89. doi: 10.1111/epi.16966
9. Tényi D, Gyimesi C, Kupó P, Horváth R, Bóné B, Barsi P, et al. Ictal asystole: a systematic review. *Epilepsia.* (2017) 58:356–62. doi: 10.1111/epi.13644
10. Rugg-Gunn FJ, Simister RJ, Squirrell M, Holdright DR, Duncan JS. Cardiac arrhythmias in focal epilepsy: a prospective long-term study. *Lancet.* (2004) 364:2212–9. doi: 10.1016/S0140-6736(04)17594-6
11. Strzelczyk A, Cenusa M, Bauer S, Hamer HM, Mothersill IW, Grunwald T, et al. Management and long-term outcome in patients presenting with ictal asystole or bradycardia. *Epilepsia.* (2011) 52:1160–7. doi: 10.1111/j.1528-1167.2010.02961.x
12. Labate A, Mumoli L, Curcio A, Tripepi G, D'Arrigo G, Ferlazzo E, et al. Value of clinical features to differentiate refractory epilepsy from mimics: a prospective longitudinal cohort study. *Eur J Neurol.* (2018) 25:711–17. doi: 10.1111/ene.13579
13. Nguyen-Michel VH, Bornand A, Balathazar AM, Kinugawa K, Lâm XY, Piette F, et al. Fall related to epileptic seizures in the elderly. *Epileptic Disord.* (2015) 17:287–91. doi: 10.1684/epd.2015.0752
14. Hampel KG, Thijs RD, Elger CE, Surges R. Recurrence risk of ictal asystole in epilepsy. *Neurology.* (2017) 89:785–91. doi: 10.1212/WNL.0000000000004266
15. Bestawros M, Darbar D, Arain A, Abou-Khalil B, Plummer D, Dupont WD, et al. Ictal asystole and ictal syncope: insights into clinical management. *Circ Arrhythm Electrophysiol.* (2015) 8:159–64. doi: 10.1161/CIRCEP.114.001667
16. Agewall S. Coronary artery disease and arrhythmias. *Eur Heart J Cardiovasc Pharmacother.* (2017) 3:69–70. doi: 10.1093/ehjcvp/pvx005
17. Sevcencu C, Struijk JJ. Autonomic alterations and cardiac changes in epilepsy. *Epilepsia.* (2010) 51:725–37. doi: 10.1111/j.1528-1167.2009.02479.x
18. Pang TD, Nearing BD, Krishnamurthy KB, Olin B, Schachter SC, Verrier RL. Cardiac electrical instability in newly diagnosed/chronic epilepsy tracked by Holter and ECG patch. *Neurology.* (2019) 93:450–8. doi: 10.1212/WNL.0000000000008077
19. Tinuper P, Bisulli F, Cerullo A, Carcangiu R, Marini C, Pierangeli G, et al. Ictal bradycardia in partial epileptic seizures: autonomic investigation in three cases and literature review. *Brain.* (2001) 124:2361–71. doi: 10.1093/brain/124.12.2361
20. Rubboli G, Bisulli F, Michelucci R, Meletti S, Ribani MA, Cortelli P, et al. Sudden falls due to seizure-induced cardiac asystole in drug-resistant focal epilepsy. *Neurology.* (2008) 70:1933–5. doi: 10.1212/01.wnl.0000289193.89796.83

16

Case Report: A Novel Missense Mutation c.517G>C in the *UMPS* Gene Associated with Mild Orotic Aciduria

Rui Ma[1,2], *Jing Ye*[1], *Jiaqi Han*[1,2], *Lehong Gao*[1,2*†], *Chaodong Wang*[1,3*†] and *Yuping Wang*[1,2*†]

[1] Department of Neurology, Xuanwu Hosptial, Captial Medical University, Beijing, China, [2] Beijing Key Laboratory of Neuromodulation, Beijing, China, [3] National Clinical Research Center for Geriatric Diseases, Beijing, China

***Correspondence:**
Lehong Gao
gaolehong@sina.com
Chaodong Wang
cdongwang01@126.com
Yuping Wang
mdwangyp@sina.cn

† These authors have contributed equally to this work and share senior authorship

Background: Hereditary orotic aciduria (HOA) is a rare genetic disorder of pyrimidine metabolism caused by variations in the uridine monophosphate synthetase (*UMPS*) gene and inheritance are autosomal recessive. Heterozygous *UMPS* mutations can also lead to orotic aciduria without clinical consequence.

Methods: We conducted molecular genetic analyses on proband using whole-exome sequencing (WES) and on 12 family members using Sanger sequencing for *UMPS* mutation. We analyzed the urine metabolites of family members carrying *UMPS* heterozygous variants with standard gas chromatography-mass spectrometry (GC-MS).

Results: We identified a novel *UMPS* mutation (c.517G>C) in a Chinese-origin of orotic aciduria pedigree. The proband presented with epilepsy and intellectual disability (ID). Other mutation carriers in our pedigree presented with mild orotic aciduria without relevant medical complaints except for the proband.

Conclusion: Our study further expanded the genotype of orotic aciduria and highlighted the probability of misdiagnosis in clinical practice.

Keywords: case report, orotic aciduria, *UMPS*, epilepsy, intellectual disability

INTRODUCTION

Hereditary orotic aciduria (HOA) (OMIM #258900) is a rare genetic disorder of pyrimidine metabolism characterized by early onset of megaloblastic anemia, global developmental delay, and failure to thrive, which is associated with massive urinary overexcretion of orotic acid (sometimes with orotic acid crystalluria) (1). Patients without megaloblastic anemia, but with additional manifestations such as epilepsy, have also been reported (2). The HOA is caused by variations in the uridine monophosphate synthetase (*UMPS*) gene with autosomal recessive inheritance. Heterozygous *UMPS* mutations can also lead to mild and isolated orotic aciduria without clinical consequence (1). Here, we discuss a mild orotic aciduria (OA) pedigree with a novel heterozygous *UMPS* mutation.

MATERIALS AND METHODS

Editorial Policies and Ethical Considerations

This study was approved by the Xuanwu Hospital Capital Medical University, and all participants provided written informed consent.

Patients and Family Members

We investigated a large family with 36 members spanning four generations, originating from Beijing province, China (**Figure 1A**). Five family members, including the proband (IV-5), carried a heterozygous mutation in the *UMPS* gene. Family members without an *UMPS* mutation were included as controls.

Genetic Tests

Genomic DNA was extracted from peripheral blood samples of the enrolled patient and their available family members using standard procedures. Variants were detected by next-generation sequencing using the NovaSeq600 platform by Berry Genomics (Beijing, China). Sanger sequencing with specific primers (5′-TTGAAGGTCACTGATGCCATAGT-3′ as the forward primer and 5′-GATTCGCTGCCACAAAGACA-3′ as the reverse primer) was performed to confirm the selected variant in the proband and other family members.

Metabolic Screening Tests

Urine metabolites were analyzed by standard gas chromatography-mass spectrometry (GC-MS) as previously described (3).

RESULTS

Case Report

The patient is a 16-year-old Chinese man who presented with epilepsy and intellectual disability. Pregnancy and delivery were uneventful. His parents are not consanguineous, and they had no relevant medical complaints. The first seizure, at the age of eight, was a generalized tonic-clonic seizure (GTCS) after he fell asleep. The second attack came 5 years later, presenting with limb weakness, numbness, head involuntary movement, and impaired awareness after a fever to a maximum of 38.4°C. Paroxysmal unilateral limb numbness with face numbness, dizziness, double vision, and slurred speech occurred approximately twice a year after the age of 14. Wechsler Intelligence Scale for Children (WISC) was tested at the age of eight, indicating mild intelligent disability (intelligence quotient 68). Several electroencephalograms (EEG)s showed paroxysmal generalized spike and slow-wave, prominent in the posterior head. No abnormality was observed in the head MRI. The patient did not have blood count abnormalities, relevant hyperammonemia, or altered plasma amino acid profile except a reduced level of Vitamin B12 (161 pg/ml, reference range 180-914 pg/ml). The patient's parents refused to take antiepileptic drugs and uridine triacetate except for mecobalamin. None of these episodes occurred at a one-year follow-up.

Genetic and Metabolic Screening Analysis

After obtaining informed consent, blood samples were collected and processed for genomic DNA isolation. Whole-exome sequencing (WES) was performed using a trio-based approach (patient, mother, and father). The analysis demonstrated a previously unreported heterozygous mutation inherited from his father in the *UMPS* gene (c.517G>C, p.Val173Leu, reference sequence: NM_000373.3), which have not yet been reported in the literature. These sequence data have been submitted to the GenBank databases under accession number OK605588. Parents were clinically asymptomatic. Subsequent Sanger sequencing of all available paternal family members found that III-7, II-5, III-1, and IV-2 also carried *UMPS* variant (c.517G>C, p.V173L) with no neurological symptoms (**Figures 1A,B**). The mutation located in the orotate phosphoribosyltransferase domain was not found in The Genome Aggregation (GnomAD), The Exome Aggregation (ExAC), and 1,000 Genomes (1,000G) databases. Prediction tools [Sorting Intolerant from Tolerant (SIFT) and Polymorphism Phenotyping v2 (PolyPhen-2)] were suggested for c.517G>C (p.V173L), a minor effect on enzymatic activity. Mutation Taster considered the mutation disease-causing. Based on the American College of Medical Genetics and Genomics (ACMG) standards and guidelines, c.517G>C of the *UMPS* gene was predicted to be likely pathogenic (PS3+PM1+PM2). The location of the mutation in the schematic diagram shown in **Figure 2**.

Further findings of a significant urinary excretion of orotate in our patient at the age of 16 (elevated 16.739 times of reference value) supported the diagnosis of orotic aciduria. Values of urinary excretion of orotate of family members carrying *UMPS* heterozygous variant are shown in **Table 1**. Except for III-1, our patient's paternal uncle, the ratios of analysis value to reference value of other family members with *UMPS* variant are more significant than one, indicating the diagnosis of orotic aciduria. According to the results of metabolic screening analysis, four family members (III-7, II-5, IV-2, and the proband) in this family can be diagnosed as orotic aciduria, although with no neurological symptoms.

DISCUSSION

The HOA results from deficiencies in uridine monophosphate synthetase (UMPS), which consists of two domains of the enzyme: orotate phosphoribosyl pyrophosphate transferase (OPRTase, EC 2.4.2.10) and orotidine monophosphate decarboxylase (OMPdecase, EC 4.1.1.23). According to the values of urinary orotic acid and orotidine excretion, the type of UMPS deficiency can be presented *in vivo* (4): Type I is caused by the loss of both enzyme activities of the UMP enzyme; Type II is thought to be due to the specific inactivation of OMPdecase; Type III, orotic aciduria without megaloblastic anemia (OAWA), is expected to be also secondary to the inactivation of OMPdecase. Urinary orotidine levels were not available in our pedigree, so the type of OA cannot be further classified.

To the best of our knowledge, this *UMPS* nonsynonymous mutation (c.517G>C) had never been identified in the single-nucleotide polymorphism database (dbSNP), Leiden Open Variation Database (LOVD) (v3.1), and ClinVar

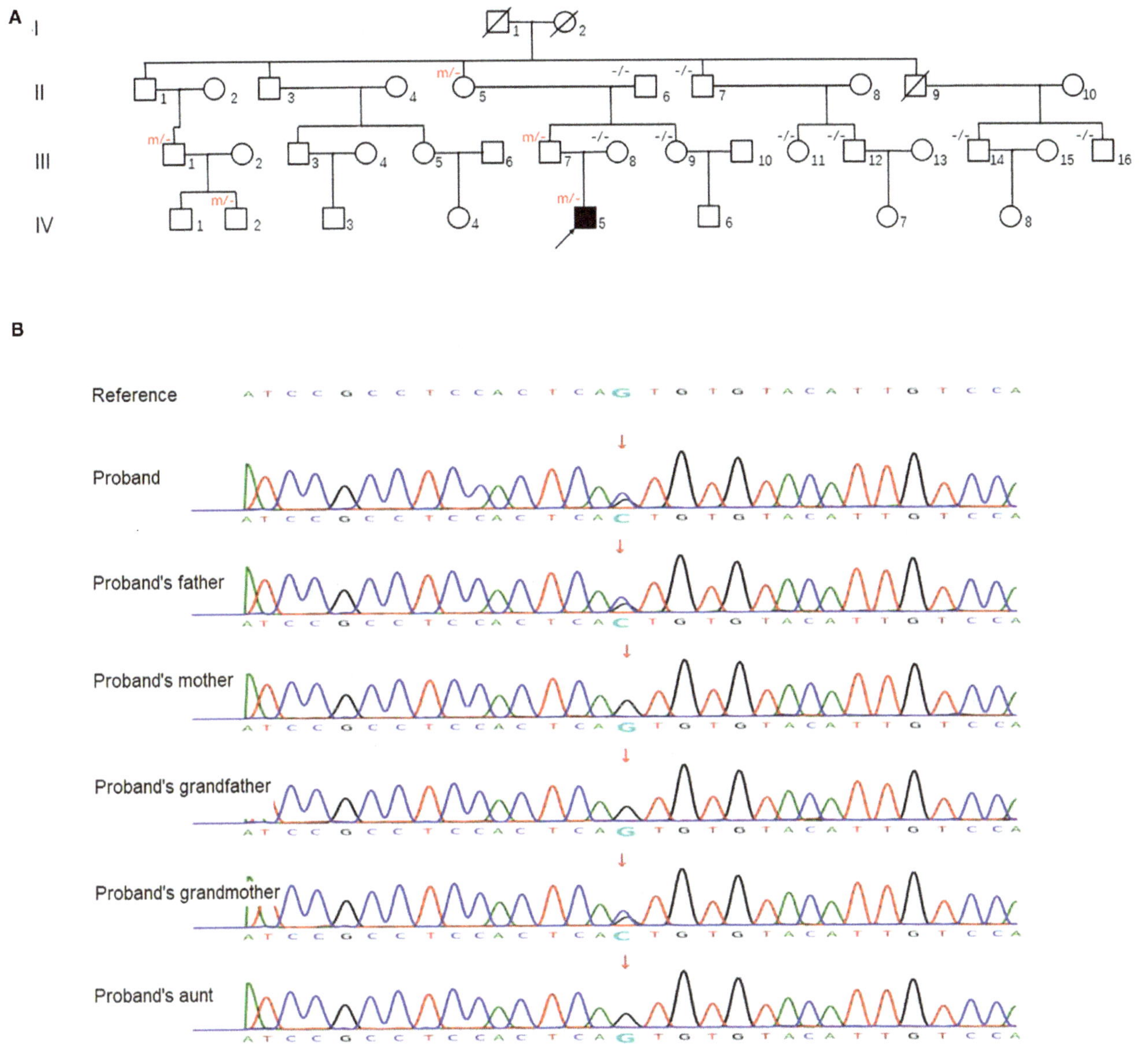

FIGURE 1 | (A) Family pedigree. An arrow denotes the proband. "m/–" and "–/–" in the upper left indicates ascertained *UMPS* heterozygous mutation carrier and wildtype subject, respectively. **(B)** Sequence analysis of human *UMPS* gene in the proband and his family members. Representative sequence electropherograms are shown.

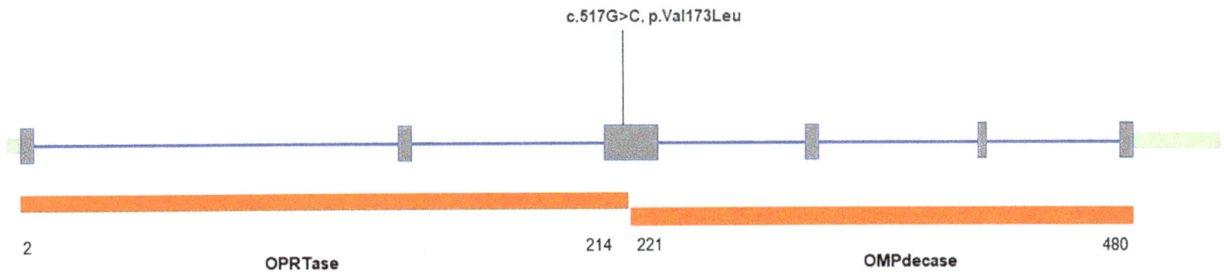

FIGURE 2 | Structure of the human uridine monophosphate synthetase (UMPS) gene with variant found in our patient.

TABLE 1 | Value of urinary excretion of orotate of family members carrying uridine monophosphate synthetase (UMPS) heterozygous variant.

Number	Clinical signs and symptoms	Age of test/year	Analysis value	Reference value	Ratio
V-5	Epilepsy and intellectual disability	13	0.0479	0.023	2.083
		16	0.3850		16.739
III-7	NRMC	43	0.0556		2.417
II-5	NRMC	70	0.0366		1.591
III-1	NRMC	45	0.011		0.483
IV-2	NRMC	12	0.027		1.174

NRMC no relevant medical complaints.

(https://www.ncbi.nlm.nih.gov/clinvar/) databases. There are previous reports of patients with seizure-associated HOA (2, 5), thus, proposing a link between UMPS deficiency and epilepsy. Intellectual disability occurs in patients with OA with homozygous and heterozygous *UPMS* mutations (1). Moreover, our OA proband presented with epilepsy, intellectual disability, and vitamin B12 deficiency, which is partly consistent with previous reports. Wortmann et al. (1) reported 11 index cases and 18 healthy heterozygous mutation carriers, revealing high phenotypic heterogeneity of *UMPS* mutations. They thought that presentation of developmental delay or intellectual disability in their patient population might be due to ascertainment bias and *in utero* exposure to elevated levels of orotic acid and/or decreased pools of pyrimidines. However, our proband had a paternally derived mutation and did not support the utero exposure hypothesis. The other four *UPMS* mutation carriers in our family all presented with no neurologic complaints. Three of them had mild orotic aciduria, which also confirms the high phenotypic heterogeneity of *UMPS*. Significant urinary excretion of orotate was detected in those members who carried this mutation by urine metabolic screening in our research. Orotate is a substrate of orotate phosphoribosyl pyrophosphate transferase and orotidine monophosphate decarboxylase, which are encoded by the *UMPS* gene. Therefore, the excessive accumulation of orotate can reflect the impaired function of the *UMPS* gene and augment the value of this case report (6).

In 2015, the U.S. Food and Drug Administration approved a treatment for HOA called uridine triacetate (Xuriden), which is a pyrimidine analog indicated for uridine replacement therapy (7). Patients who took the drug responded well (5). Although our proband only took mecobalamin, he was seizure-free for one year. We will continue to pay attention to the patient's condition and adjust the treatment plan according to the condition at any time.

CONCLUSION

Although extremely rare, hereditary orotic aciduria should be suspected in any child with neurological disorders, such as epilepsy and developmental delay, and with or without anemia. Our study characterizes a highly heterogeneous *UMPS* pedigree, expanding the mutational spectrum as we report one novel variant that is identified in the *UMPS* gene. Early diagnosis and treatment are essential for disease course.

ETHICS STATEMENT

The studies involving human participants were reviewed and approved by the Ethical Committee of Xuanwu Hospital Capital Medical University. Written informed consent to participate in this study was provided by the participants' legal guardian/next of kin. Written informed consent was obtained from the individual(s), and minor(s)' legal guardian/next of kin, for the publication of any potentially identifiable images or data included in this article.

AUTHOR CONTRIBUTIONS

RM: writing—original draft, visualization. JY: resources. JH: investigation. LG: writing—reviewing and editing, validation. CW: data curation and conceptualization. YW: supervision, project administration, and funding acquisition. All authors contributed to the article and approved the submitted version.

ACKNOWLEDGMENTS

We are grateful for the family's cooperation and permission to publish this information.

REFERENCES

1. Wortmann SB, Chen MA, Colombo R, Pontoglio A, Alhaddad B, Botto LD, et al., Mild orotic aciduria in UMPS heterozygotes: a metabolic finding without clinical consequences. *J Inherit Metab Dis.* (2017) 40:423–31. doi: 10.1007/s10545-017-0015-9
2. Grohmann K, Lauffer H, Lauenstein P, Hoffmann GF, Seidlitz G. Hereditary orotic aciduria with epilepsy and without megaloblastic anemia. *Neuropediatrics.* (2015) 46:123–5. doi: 10.1055/s-0035-1547341
3. Zhang C, Xu K, Dave UP, Wang Y, Matsumoto I. Inborn errors of metabolism discovered in Asian department of pediatrics and mental retardation research center. *J Chromatogr B Biomed Sci Appl.* (2000) 746:41–9. doi: 10.1016/S0378-4347(00)00087-6

4. Bailey CJ. Orotic aciduria and uridine monophosphate synthase: a reappraisal. *J Inherit Metab Dis.* (2009) 32:S227–33. doi: 10.1007/s10545-009-1176-y
5. Al Absi HS, Sacharow S, Al Zein N, Al Shamsi A, Al Teneiji A. Hereditary orotic aciduria (HOA): A novel uridine-5-monophosphate synthase (UMPS) mutation. *Mol Genet Metab Rep.* (2021) 26:100703. doi: 10.1016/j.ymgmr.2020.100703
6. Nykamp K, Anderson M, Powers M, Garcia J, Herrera B, Ho YY, et al. Sherloc: a comprehensive refinement of the ACMG-AMP variant classification criteria. *Genet Med.* (2017) 19:1105–17. doi: 10.1038/gim.2017.37
7. In brief: Uridine triacetate (Xuriden) for hereditary orotic aciduria. *Med Lett Drugs Ther.* (2016) 58:e49.

17

Case Report: Behavioral Disorder Following Hemispherotomy: A Valproate Effect?

Konstantin L. Makridis [1,2,3†], *Sebastian Triller* [1,2†], *Deniz A. Atalay* [1,2], *Christine Prager* [1,2], *Christian E. Elger* [1,2,4] *and Angela M. Kaindl* [1,2,3*]

[1] Charité – Universitätsmedizin Berlin, Department of Pediatric Neurology, Berlin, Germany, [2] Charité – Universitätsmedizin Berlin, Center for Chronically Sick Children, Berlin, Germany, [3] Charité – Universitätsmedizin Berlin, Institute of Cell- and Neurobiology, Berlin, Germany, [4] Beta Neurology – Competence Center for Epilepsy, Bonn, Germany

***Correspondence:**
Angela M. Kaindl
angela.kaindl@charite.de

† These authors have contributed equally to this work and share first authorship

Background: Hemispherotomy is an epilepsy surgery procedure applied to cure particularly pharmacorefractory lesional epilepsy due to unihemispheric pathologies. Such a disconnection of an entire hemisphere is followed by reorganizational processes.

Methods: We describe an acute aggravation of behavioral problems following a hemispherotomy in a patient treated with valproic acid, which subsided once valproate was discontinued.

Results: A 9-year-old boy with drug-resistant epilepsy caused by the residua of a perinatal stroke treated for several years with valproic acid and lamotrigine underwent hemispherotomy. Shortly after surgery, minimal preoperative behavioral problems intensified dramatically, and aggression occurred as a new symptom. Assuming a correlation between valproate treatment and the postoperative altered neuronal network, we tapered off valproate. The behavioral problems decreased in intensity with the reduction of valproate dose and disappeared after drug discontinuation.

Conclusion: We describe severe behavioral problems after hemispherotomy that subsided when valproate was tapered off. While we cannot rule out a spontaneous correction of a post-hemispherotomy network dysregulation, our report raises awareness to possible altered effects of the anticonvulsant valproic acid parallel to reorganizational processes after hemispherotomy.

Keywords: drug resistant epilepsy, pediatrics, behavioral problems, children, valproic acid, epilepsy surgery, hemispherotomy

INTRODUCTION

Epilepsy is one of the most common neurologic diseases in childhood and adolescence (1). Antiseizure medications (ASMs) are the primary choice of treatment. However, in about one-third of affected individuals, they fail to achieve seizure freedom (2). In patients with drug-resistant structural epilepsy, the possibility of epilepsy surgery should be considered. Children with unilateral hemispheric lesions can profit from hemispherotomy. Several studies have illustrated functional reorganization after such an anatomic disconnection of a whole hemisphere. Here, we describe an aggravation of behavioral problems following hemispherotomy in a child treated with valproate (VPA). The behavioral problems subsided when VPA was discontinued. We suggest a possible altered anticonvulsant drug effect at a time when network changes likely occur.

CASE

A 9-year-old boy was outborn at term without complications as the first child of non-consanguineous and healthy parents after a complicated course of pregnancy (vaginal bleeding on gestational week 12, gestational diabetes). Postpartum weakness of the left arm was noted. He was first presented to our Center for Chronically Sick Children at 2.6 years of age. He had spastic hemiparesis affecting particularly the left arm, hemineglect, and intermittent spontaneous nystagmus. A cranial MRI revealed a cystic parenchyma defect of the right parietotemporal side due to an ischemic stroke of his middle cerebral artery (**Figure 1A**). At this point, he had no reported seizures.

At the age of 9 years, the patient presented again because of global developmental delay, hemiparesis, and drug-refractory epilepsy with persistent seizures. ASM treatment with VPA (18.75 mg/kg/day) and lamotrigine (LTG) (0.95 mg/kg/day) failed to control the seizures. First focal-onset seizures had occurred at 4 years of age. Over time, these gradually shifted to focal-onset seizures with increasingly impaired awareness. At presentation, he had focal to tonic-clonic seizures every 8 weeks. He showed appropriate engagement during social contact with a slight decrease in proximity-distance regulation. In neuropsychological examination, difficulties in attentional control, impulse control, and inhibition, as well as slightly increased motor agitation could be observed. Furthermore, he showed reduced stress resilience and frustration tolerance in the presence of excessive emotions. Because of highly increased emotional stress of the parents, it was not possible to examine neuropsychological data *via* questionnaires.

We classified the patient as drug-resistant and included him in our epilepsy surgery program. Further investigations with congruent findings in MRI and EEG led to the indication for hemispherotomy. A vertical parasagittal hemispherotomy on the right side was performed without complications. Since then, the patient has remained seizure-free (**Figure 1B**).

Two weeks after surgery, he showed an acute increase in psychological problems. He showed an acute aggravation of neuropsychological issues: hyperactivity, inhibition, and attentional control. The patient was restless and hardly controllable during medical examinations. Furthermore, the parents and teachers reported an increased tendency to aggressive behavior, which led to an exclusion from school. Overall, the symptoms had a high impact on the well-being of the family and the patient. An EEG showed no evidence of leftward transition with no evidence of clinical seizure signs (**Figure 2A**).

We considered these behavioral problems to be related to the postoperatively changed neuronal networks of the brain. This working hypothesis was based on clinical experience by one of the senior authors (CE) on VPA-induced behavioral disturbances after epilepsy surgery that has not been reported previously. Already after VPA reduction from 18.75 to 14 mg/kg/day, the behavioral problems decreased. Once VPA was tapered-off, the behavioral problems were back at the preoperative level. Serum levels of the ASM of the patient were not measured. An EEG performed 6 months post-operatively showed no evidence of seizures (**Figure 2B**). A standardized neuropsychological follow-up assessment 6, 12, and 24 months postoperatively revealed a significant improvement in attention span, inhibitory skills, and frustration tolerance. Aggressive behavior was not detected during the medical examinations. The parents reported them to be absent during everyday life.

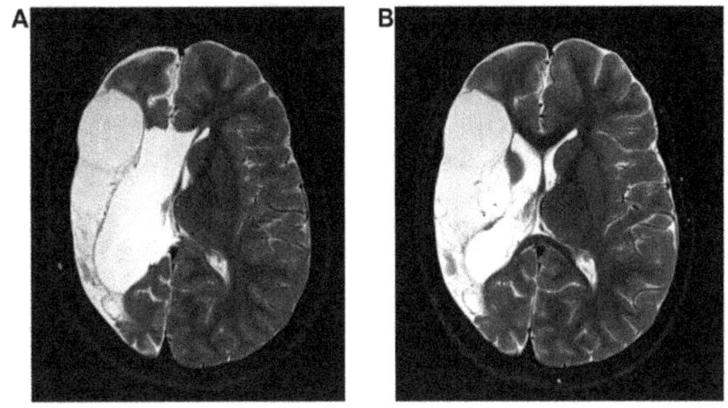

FIGURE 1 | Magnetic resonance imaging (MRI) of the patient. **(A)** Shown is the preoperative MRI of the 2; 10 year old patient. **(B)** Normal MRI of the patient 6 months after surgery showing the malacic transformed medial infarct on the right side with no evidence of hemorrhage, infarction, or liquor circulatory disturbances.

DISCUSSION

Here, we report an acute aggravation of behavioral problems in a patient following hemispherotomy, which subsided after discontinuation of VPA. VPA is an inhibitor of γ amino butyric acid degradation and of voltage-gated ion channels. In addition to its use as an ASM, it is applied as a mood stabilizer to prevent aggressive impulsive behavior (3). However, behavioral abnormalities in association with VPA are known. They usually occur after drug initiation and, as in our case, disappear with tapering-off of the drug (4). In our case, however, the patient had been taking VPA for several years without severe behavioral problems. They aggravated acutely following hemispherotomy. There are no explanations in terms of an altered social environment or acute interpersonal experiences. Therefore, we propose VPA-induced behavioral problems due to postoperative altered neuronal network function and structures. We did not reintroduce the drug to test our hypothesis for ethical reasons. We did not measure VPA and LTG serum levels.

Behavioral problems after epilepsy surgery have been described. Although behavioral abnormalities are known to occur after surgery, in our patient, they disappeared when the drug dose was tapered and have not recurred since in a follow-up period of 30 months (5). We cannot rule out the spontaneous correction of post-hemispherotomy network dysregulation and, thus, a timely coincidence with the tapering of valproic acid. In adults and children, especially those with long-standing drug resistant epilepsy, there is a phenomenon referred to as forced normalization. Forced normalization is

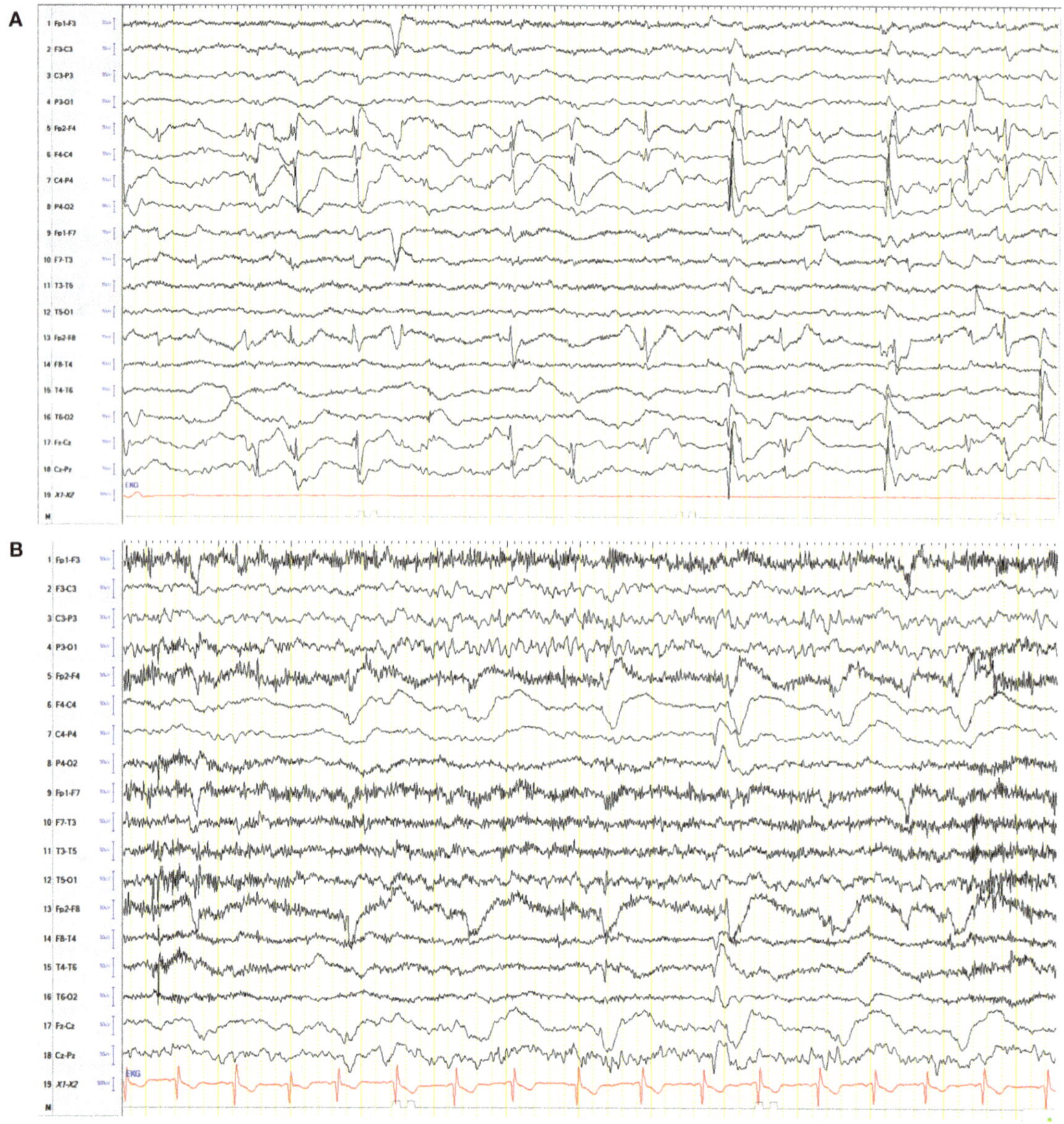

FIGURE 2 | Electroencephalogram (EEG) of the patient. **(A)** Awake EEG after hemispherotomy under VPA. Hypersynchronous activity on the right frontocentral side over the disconnected hemisphere without evidence of clinical seizure signs and without evidence of transition to the left. **(B)** Six months after surgery without VPA, the EEG showed continuous right hemispheric dysfunction, hypersynchronic right frontocentral activity, and activation during sleep without clinical signs.

characterized by the occurrence of psychiatric problems after achieving seizure freedom (6). The underlying mechanisms are not well-understood. In forced normalization, however, symptoms typically persist for an average of 111 days and require antipsychotic therapy in about 73% of all patients. Control of symptoms is achieved in only 28.5% of patients with forced normalization after epilepsy surgery (6). This phenomenon is unlikely in our patient, since the symptoms reduced already after the reduction of the VPA dose by 4.75 mg/kg/day after 4 days, and no further therapy was needed.

It is known that the combination of LTG and VPA, although effective, also increases the risk of adverse effects, e.g., through an increase in LTG serum levels (7, 8). Both VPA and LTG have been associated with behavioral problems, and, therefore, both could be putatively responsible for the described symptoms (9). Tapering off of VPA led to the resolution of symptoms quickly, arguing more for a primary VPA effect given the shorter half-life of the ASM than for a primary LTG effect. In our patient, no severe adverse effects occurred preoperatively. Changes in ASM serum levels after epilepsy surgery have been reported temporary and directly after surgery (10, 11). Theoretically, a postoperative increase in VPA in our patient may have occurred and resulted in behavioral side effects. However, in our case, the symptoms were not present directly postoperatively. The patient rather presented more than 1 month after surgery with the described symptoms, rendering a surgery-related ASM serum level change unlikely. Moreover, the symptoms rapidly resolved after the reduction of VPA dose.

To further corroborate the proposed correlation between VPA-triggered behavioral abnormalities parallel to altered neuronal networks, we assessed the probability of an adverse drug reaction with the score presented in Koh et al. (12). The reaction is considered probable.

The aim of that report is to raise awareness to possible altered effects of VPA parallel to reorganizational processes after hemispherotomy. We could not find any description of acute behavioral issues after hemispherotomy in association with VPA in the PubMed research literature. Anticipating further reports, underlying pharmacological mechanisms should be studied. Furthermore, we highlight the importance of pre- and post-operative ASM levels to better assess such interactions.

ETHICS STATEMENT

The studies involving human participants were reviewed and approved by Ethikkommission der Charité - Universitätsmedizin Berlin. Written informed consent for participation was not required for this study in accordance with the national legislation and the institutional requirements.

AUTHOR CONTRIBUTIONS

KM, CE, DA, and CP contributed to conception and design of the study. ST and KM organized the database and wrote the first draft of the manuscript. All authors contributed to manuscript revision, read, and approved the submitted version.

REFERENCES

1. Camfield P, Camfield C. Incidence, prevalence and aetiology of seizures and epilepsy in children. *Epileptic Disord.* (2015) 17:117–23. doi: 10.1684/epd.2015.0736
2. Kwan P, Brodie MJ. Early identification of refractory epilepsy. *N Engl J Med.* (2000) 342:314–9. doi: 10.1056/NEJM200002033420503
3. Huband N, Ferriter M, Nathan R, Jones H. Antiepileptics for aggression and associated impulsivity. *Cochrane Database Syst Rev.* (2010) 2010:Cd003499. doi: 10.1002/14651858.CD003499.pub3
4. Glauser TA. Behavioral and psychiatric adverse events associated with antiepileptic drugs commonly used in pediatric patients. *J Child Neurol.* (2004) 19(Suppl. 1):S25–38. doi: 10.1177/088307380401900104 01
5. Braams O, Maher C, Jennekens-Schinkel A, Braun K, van Nieuwenhuizen O, van Schooneveld M, et al. Social functioning of children after epilepsy surgery: a literature review. *Epilepsy Behav.* (2019) 96:210–8. doi: 10.1016/j.yebeh.2019.04.037
6. Calle-López Y, Ladino LD, Benjumea-Cuartas V, Castrillón-Velilla DM, Téllez-Zenteno JF, Wolf P. Forced normalization: a systematic review. *Epilepsia.* (2019) 60:1610–8. doi: 10.1111/epi.16276
7. Guberman AH, Besag FM, Brodie MJ, Dooley JM, Duchowny MS, Pellock JM, et al. Lamotrigine-associated rash: risk/benefit considerations in adults and children. *Epilepsia.* (1999) 40:985–91. doi: 10.1111/j.1528-1157.1999.tb00807.x
8. Thome-Souza S, Moreira B, Valente KD. Late adverse effects of the coadministration of valproate and lamotrigine. *Pediatr Neurol.* (2012) 47:47–50. doi: 10.1016/j.pediatrneurol.2012.04.026
9. Moavero R, Santarone ME, Galasso C, Curatolo P. Cognitive and behavioral effects of new antiepileptic drugs in pediatric epilepsy. *Brain Dev.* (2017) 39:464–9. doi: 10.1016/j.braindev.2017.01.006
10. Hiremath GK, Kotagal P, Bingaman W, Hovinga C, Wyllie E, Morris H, et al. Risk factors for carbamazepine elevation and toxicity following epilepsy surgery. *Seizure.* (2005) 14:312–7. doi: 10.1016/j.seizure.2005.04.003
11. Paul F, Veauthier C, Fritz G, Lehmann T-N, Aktas O, Zipp F, et al. Perioperative fluctuations of lamotrigine serum levels in patients undergoing epilepsy surgery. *Seizure.* (2007) 16:479–84. doi: 10.1016/j.seizure.2007.03.006
12. Koh Y, Yap CW Li SC. A quantitative approach of using genetic algorithm in designing a probability scoring system of an adverse drug reaction assessment system. *Int J Med Inform.* (2008) 77:421–30. doi: 10.1016/j.ijmedinf.2007.08.010

18

Case Report: Vortioxetine in the Treatment of Depressive Symptoms in Patients with Epilepsy—Case Series

Marcin Siwek[1], Aleksandra Gorostowicz[2], Magdalena Bosak[3] and Dominika Dudek[2]*

[1]Department of Affective Disorders, Jagiellonian University Medical College, Kraków, Poland, [2]Department of Psychiatry, Jagiellonian University Medical College, Kraków, Poland, [3]Department of Neurology, Jagiellonian University Medical College, Krakow, Poland

***Correspondence:**
Marcin Siwek
marcin.siwek@uj.edu.pl

Epilepsy and depression are both serious and potentially disabling conditions which often coexist—bidirectional relationship between the two disorders has been observed. Comorbidity between depression and epilepsy can be attributed to: underlying common pathophysiological mechanisms, psychiatric side effect of antiepileptic medications and psychological response to stress in people with chronic, neurological condition. Despite high prevalence of depressive symptoms in patients with epilepsy, current evidence of the effectiveness of antidepressant therapy in this group of patients is very limited. Vortioxetine is an antidepressant with multimodal activity, very good treatment tolerability, low risk of inducing pharmacokinetic interactions, relative safety of treatment in patients with somatic comorbidities, low risk of causing: sedation, sexual dysfunctions and metabolic side effects. Vortioxetine seems to be a promising treatment option for depressed patients with cognitive dysfunctions, anhedonia and anxiety. In this case series, we report nine cases of patients with epilepsy and depressive symptoms treated with vortioxetine. Seven cases are patients with secondary focal and generalized epilepsy and two with unclassified epilepsy. Three patients presented with depressive episode in the course of bipolar disorder and six patients had depressive symptoms due to organic mood disorder. The dose range of vortioxetine was between 10 and 20 mg. In all of the presented cases effectiveness and tolerability of treatment were very good. Remission of depressive symptoms was achieved in all patients. No epilepsy seizures after switch to vortioxetine were observed in seven cases. In two patients seizures occurred during the first months of vortioxetine treatment but this most probably was due to suboptimal antiepileptic treatment—satisfactory seizure control was achieved after optimization of antiepileptic pharmacotherapy. Vortioxetine was discontinued in two of the presented cases due to pregnancy planning. The duration of observation period during vortioxetine therapy ranged from 2 to 48 months. In conclusion, vortioxetine can be a promising treatment option in patients with epilepsy and comorbid depressive symptoms.

Keywords: vortioxetine, depression, bipolar disorder, seizure, antidepressants, epilepsy, mood disorders, depressive symptoms

INTRODUCTION

Epilepsy is a chronic, heterogenous neurological condition affecting more than 50 million people globally (Elger et al., 2017). It is defined by any of the following: (Elger et al., 2017) At least two unprovoked (or reflex) seizures occurring >24 h apart; (Fisher et al., 2014) one unprovoked (or reflex) seizure and at least 60% probability of further seizures, occurring over the next 10 years; (Josephson et al., 2017) diagnosis of an epilepsy syndrome (Fisher et al., 2014). Psychiatric disorders, especially depression, are considered to be prevalent comorbidities in patients with epilepsy. The risk of developing depression seems to be increased around twofold in epilepsy (compared to the general population) (Tellez-Zenteno et al., 2007; Josephson et al., 2017). Data considering the prevalence of depression in epilepsy patients is inconsistent, with results ranging from around 6% to more than 50% (Bosak et al., 2012; Bosak et al., 2015a; Błaszczyk and Czuczwar, 2016; Elger et al., 2017)—higher prevalence is observed in drug-refractory than in well-controlled epilepsy (Bosak et al., 2012; Garcia et al., 2015; Tao and Wang, 2016) The inter-ictal form is the most common manifestation of depression in epilepsy patients (Bosak et al., 2012; Błaszczyk and Czuczwar, 2016). Clinical presentation of mood disorders in this group of patients can be different from typical depressive episode—symptoms such as irritability, low frustration tolerance, mood lability, anxiety and fatigue are prevalent (Kwon and Park, 2014). Sometimes terms "interictal dysphoric disorder" or "dysthymic-like disorders of epilepsy" are used in the literature to describe mood disorders in epilepsy (Bosak et al., 2012; Tao and Wang, 2016).

Interestingly, bidirectional relationship between depression and epilepsy has been observed. Depression is associated with around 2.5 times increased hazard of epilepsy (Josephson et al., 2017), although some studies reported that the risk of developing epilepsy in patients with a history of depression can be even up to seven-fold higher (compared to the general population) (Kanner, 2009; Bosak et al., 2012; Błaszczyk and Czuczwar, 2016). Furthermore, more than two-fold increase in the incidence of treatment-resistant epilepsy has been observed in patients with preceding depression (Hitiris et al., 2007). Comorbid depression in epilepsy is also associated with reduced quality of life, poorer treatment adherence, premature mortality and higher risk of unemployment (Johnson et al., 2004; Taylor et al., 2011; Fazel et al., 2013; Garcia et al., 2015; Keezer et al., 2016; Henning et al., 2019). Lifetime history of psychiatric disorders may be a predictor of poor outcome after epilepsy surgery (Kanner et al., 2009). It is worth mentioning that people with epilepsy have even 5-fold increased risk of suicide (compared to controls) and this can be mediated by psychiatric disorders (Bosak et al., 2015b; Bosak et al., 2016; Hesdorffer et al., 2016).

Comorbidity between depression and epilepsy can be attributed to different underlying common pathophysiological mechanisms. Some of the suggested ones are: neuroinflammation, structural and functional brain abnormalities (in temporal and prefrontal areas), alterations in neurotransmission (particularly GABA, glutamate, serotonin, noradrenaline, dopamine transmission), hyperactivity in hypothalamic-pituitary-adrenal axis, shared genetic susceptibility (Bosak et al., 2012; Błaszczyk and Czuczwar, 2016; Mazarati and Sankar, 2016; Tao and Wang, 2016). Besides, a few antiseizure medications are known to potentially induce or exacerbate depressive symptoms, e.g., levetiracetam, topiramate, vigabatrin, barbiturates and zonisamide (Bosak et al., 2012; Błaszczyk and Czuczwar, 2016; Chen et al., 2017). Finally, depressive symptoms could potentially be an element of psychological response to stress, stigmatization and isolation due to living with epilepsy (Błaszczyk and Czuczwar, 2016).

Data considering efficacy and safety of antidepressants in treatment of depressive symptoms in epilepsy patients are relatively scarce—only a few randomized controlled trials have been published so far (Elger et al., 2017). According to the Cochrane Review from 2021, current evidence on the effectiveness of treatment with antidepressant medications in patients with epilepsy is very limited (Maguire et al., 2021). Relatively the largest amount of data refers to SSRIs (SSRI—Selective Serotonin Reuptake Inhibitors) which seem to be safe and effective (although heterogeneity of the results is significant) (Mula, 2019). Despite previous fears of a potential seizure-provoking action of antidepressants, data from more thorough analyses indicate that treatment with these medications is rather safe (with exceptions for bupropion, clomipramine and maprotiline) (Alper et al., 2007; Steinert and Fröscher, 2018; Mula, 2019). Moreover, a summary of FDA data from clinical trials showed that the incidence of seizures was lower in patients receiving antidepressants than placebo (standardized incidence ratio = 0.48) (Alper et al., 2007).

One of the latest therapeutic options for treatment of depressive symptoms is the multimodal antidepressant vortioxetine which has a very favorable safety and tolerance profile and a relatively low risk of drug interactions (Chen et al., 2018). Therefore, it seems reasonable to consider vortioxetine as a therapeutic option in patients with epilepsy and depressive symptoms.

Preclinical studies mostly indicate that vortioxetine may reduce seizure activity. Vortioxetine has been observed to reduce the number of epileptic discharges in penicillin-induced epilepsy model and to play a role in controlling epileptiform activity in pentylenetetrazole-induced kindling model in rats (Ögün et al., 2019; Taskiran and Unal, 2021). One study has shown proconvulsant activity of vortioxetine in genetic absence epileptic WAG/Rij rats (Aygun and Ayyildiz, 2021).

To the best of our knowledge, only one case of a patient with epilepsy (symptomatic occipital lobe epilepsy) successfully treated with vortioxetine has been published so far (Onder et al., 2018). In this case series, we report nine cases of patients with epilepsy and depressive symptoms treated with vortioxetine.

CASE SERIES—RESULTS

All nine cases are outpatients treated in the Department of Psychiatry, University Hospital in Cracow (Poland) during the

TABLE 1 | Presentation of nine cases of patients with depressive symptoms and epilepsy treated with vortioxetine.

Patient	1	2	3	4	5	6	7	8	9
Gender	F	M	F	M	F	M	F	M	K
Age (at VOR initiation)	24	74	28	77	43	59	39	30	59
Neurological diagnosis (with ICD-10 code) Scheffer et al. (2017)	G40 Epilepsy	G40.2 Focal epilepsy	G40.2 Focal epilepsy	G40.2 Focal epilepsy	G40.2 Focal epilepsy	G40.2 Focal epilepsy	G40 Epilepsy	G40.2 Focal epilepsy	G40.2 Focal epilepsy
Epilepsy etiology	Unknown etiology	Structural (craniotomy for brain abscess in the temporal lobe)	Structural (surgery for oligoastrocytoma)	Structural (craniotomy for brain abscess in the temporal lobe)	Structural (posttraumatic)	Structural (poststroke)	Brain injury after cardiac arrest	Structural (surgery for astrocytoma in the temporal lobe)	Unknown etiology
Type of epilepsy seizures before VOR Tx (Fisher et al., 2017)	Tonic-clonic seizures	Focal seizures with impaired awareness	Focal seizures with and without impaired awareness, remission since the age of 20	Focal seizures with and without impaired awareness, 1 per 2 months	Focal seizures with impaired awareness, last one 2 years before. Just before VOR Tx the patient had focal to bilateral tonic-clonic seizure and status epilepticus due to medication overdose (suicidal attempt)	2 epilepsy seizures in the last months. Focal seizures with impaired awareness and focal to bilateral tonic-clonic seizure 1 per 3 months	Tonic-clonic seizures	Focal seizures with impaired awareness	Daily focal seizures with and without impaired awareness
DRE	No	No	No	Yes	No	Yes	No	Yes	Yes
Duration of previous antiseizure Tx (years)	1	5	12	2	14	1	4	15	28
ASM during VOR Tx	Levetiracetam 1,000 mg daily	Lamotrigine 400 mg, Levetiracetam 3 g daily	Lamotrigine 200 mg daily	Valproate 1,000 mg, Levetiracetam 500 mg daily	Lamotrigine (doses increased from 200 to 250 mg during treatment with VOR), Valproate (doses increased from 1,000 to 1,600 mg daily)	Valproate 2,000 mg daily, then switched to lamotrigine 200 mg daily	Lamotrigine 100 mg daily	Levetiracetam 1,500 mg daily	Valproate 1,000 mg daily, topiramate 62.5 mg daily
Mood disorder ICD-10 diagnosis	F31 Bipolar affective disorder	F31 Bipolar affective disorder	F31 Bipolar affective disorder	F06.3 Mood disorder due to known physiological condition	F06.3 Mood disorder due to known physiological condition	F06.3 Mood disorder due to known physiological condition	F06.3 Mood disorder due to known physiological condition	F06.3 Mood disorder due to known physiological condition	F06.3 Mood disorder due to known physiological condition

(Continued on following page)

TABLE 1 | *(Continued)* Presentation of nine cases of patients with depressive symptoms and epilepsy treated with vortioxetine.

Total duration of psychiatric treatment	8 years	7 years	6 years	No psychiatric treatment before VOR initiation	13 years	4 years	9 years	2 months	8 years
Duration of the depressive episode before VOR initiation	3 months	3 weeks	3 weeks	6 months	3 weeks	1 month	1 month	1 month	1 year
Clinical picture of depression at VOR initiation	Fatigue, hypersomnia, cognitive dysfunctions, lowered mood	Lowered mood, apathy, anhedonia, generalized anxiety	Generalized anxiety, lowered mood, anhedonia, cognitive dysfunctions	Apathy, anhedonia, lowered mood, social withdrawal, deterioration of verbal fluency, irritability, fatigue	Anhedonia, generalized anxiety, cognitive dysfunctions, lowered mood, feeling of guilt, insomnia	Lowered mood, apathy, anhedonia, lack of energy, sexual dysfunctions	Lowered mood, apathy, anxiety	Anergy, apathy, anhedonia, amotivation, lowered mood, cognitive dysfunctions	Cognitive dysfunction, irritability, lowered mood, lack of energy, apathy, feeling of hopelessnes, anhedonia
Psychiatric comorbidity	—	F07 Personality and behavioural disorders due to brain disease, damage and dysfunction F10 Mental and behavioural disorders due to use of alcohol F13 Sedative, hypnotic, or anxiolytic related disorders	—	—	F07 Personality and behavioural disorders due to brain disease, damage and dysfunction	—	F06.2 Psychotic disorder with delusions due to known physiological condition F04 Amnestic disorder due to known physiological condition	F06.2 Psychotic disorder with delusions due to known physiological condition	— —
Previously used antidepressants	Escitalopram	Duloxetine	—	—	Venlafaxine	Sertraline, escitalopram, duloxetine	—	—	citalopram
Reason for VOR initiation	Depression with cognitive dysfunctions. Insufficient effectiveness of escitalopram	Somatic comorbidities, depressive symptoms: anhedonia, anxiety. Lack of effectiveness of duloxetine	Depression with anhedonia, anxiety and cognitive dysfunctions	Depressive symptoms: anhedonia and cognitive dysfunctions	Depressive symptoms: anhedonia, anxiety and cognitive dysfunctions Insufficient effectiveness of venlafaxine	Depressive symptoms: anhedonia, apathy, sexual dysfunctions and insufficient effectiveness of SSRI and SNRI medications	Depressive symptoms: apathy, anxiety, cognitive dysfunctions	Depressive symptoms: apathy, cognitive dysfunctions, anhedonia	Depressive symptoms: anhedonia, apathy, cognitive dysfunctions
VOR dosage (mg)	10	Initially 10 mg, increased to 20	10	10	15	10	10	10	10
Other simultaneously	Aripiprazole 10 mg	Naltrexone 50 mg 1 × 1 Trazodone XR	—	—	Trazodone CR 0-0-150 mg	—	Haloperidol depot—50 mg	Risperidone 1 mg Eszopiclone 1 mg	-

(Continued on following page)

TABLE 1 | *(Continued)* Presentation of nine cases of patients with depressive symptoms and epilepsy treated with vortioxetine.

used psychiatric medications (daily doses)		0-0-150 mg Sulpiride up to 350 mg Bromazepam up to 6 mg daily					i.m. every 3 weeks Biperiden 4 mg daily		
Somatic comorbidities	—	Non-insulin-dependent diabetes mellitus Hypertension	—	Ischemic heart disease	—	Chronic obstructive pulmonary disease, Migraine, nephrolithiasis, dyslipidemia	—	—	—
Other medications during VOR Tx	—	Amlodipine Lisinopril Hydro-chlorothiazide Eplerenone Nebivolol Dabigatran Levothyroxine Glimepiride	—	Amlodipine	—	Ciclesonide, formoterol, tiotropium, atorvastatine, acetylsalicylic acid	—	—	—

ASM, antiseizure medications, CR, controlled release, DRE, drug-resistant epilepsy [defined according to the consensus proposal of the ILAE Commission on Therapeutic Strategies as failure of adequate trials of two tolerated, appropriately chosen and used antiepileptic drug schedules (whether as monotherapies or in combination) to achieve sustained seizure freedom (Kwan et al., 2010)] F, female, ICD-10, International Classification of Diseases Version 10, i.m., intramuscular, M, male, SNRI, Serotonin Norepinephrine Reuptake Inhibitor, SSRI, Selective Serotonin Reuptake Inhibitor, Tx, treatment, VOR, vortioxetine, XR, extended release.

last 5 years. The cases were identified by thorough analysis of records from patient visits since 2015 until September 2021. Relevant socio-demographic and clinical data are presented in **Table 1**.

The presented group of cases includes five female and four male patients, aged between 24 and 77 year-old. Seven cases are patients with secondary focal and generalized epilepsy and two with unclassified epilepsy, with mostly satisfactory control of the neurological disease. In most cases (5/9) lamotrigine was used as part of the antiseizure pharmacotherapy, but four patients were treated with levetiracetam and one with topiramate—medications with, as already mentioned in the introduction, know potential to induce psychiatric side effects. However, due to good antiseizure effect, the attending neurologists decided to maintain treatment with the use of these medications. Before starting treatment with vortioxetine three patients presented with depressive episode in the course of bipolar disorder and six patients had depressive symptoms due to organic mood disorder (i.e., due to known physiological condition). Vortioxetine was the first line of antidepressant treatment in four patients, second line in four patients and the fourth line in one case. Vortioxetine was preferred either because of the clinical presentation (depression with anhedonia, anxiety and cognitive dysfunctions—in all patients), insufficient effectiveness of previously used antidepressants (in five patients) or somatic comorbidities and high risk of drug interactions due to polytherapy (in three patient). In the subgroup of patients with bipolar disorder, vortioxetine was chosen after analysis of the history of previous lack of antidepressant effectiveness of other agents (such as mood-stabilizers or antipsychotics) and taking into consideration relative safety of different pharmacological options when treating patients with epilepsy. Moreover, results of a naturalistic, open-label, add-on study of vortioxetine in bipolar depression indicate that this medication can be an efficient and well-tolerated therapeutic option in bipolar patients (Siwek et al., 2021a). It is also worth noticing that two out of three bipolar patients in our case series were treated with lamotrigine which was used not only due to its antiseizure but also antidepressant properties.

The dose range of vortioxetine was between 10 and 20 mg. In all presented cases remission of depressive symptoms was achieved and tolerability of the treatment was good. Time needed to reach remission ranged from 3 weeks to 3 months. No epilepsy seizures after introduction of vortioxetine were observed in seven cases. In two cases seizures occurred during the observation period. In one patient (Patient 5) epileptic seizure appeared after 7 months of the treatment and this could have been attributed to inadequately low doses of lamotrigine (which was previously used in doses up to 600 mg with optimal seizure control, but during the first months of vortioxetine treatment daily dose of lamotrigine was reduced by neurologists to only 200 mg)—after lamotrigine dose adjustments no seizures were observed for the following 5 months of observation. In another patient (Patient 6) epileptic seizure occurred after 2 months of

TABLE 2 | Effectiveness and tolerability of vortioxetine treatment in nine presented cases.

Patient	1	2	3	4	5	6	7	8	9
Psychiatric outcome of VOR Tx	remission	remission	remission	remission	remission	remission	remission	remission	Remission
Time to remission	3 months	2 months	2 months	2 months	3 weeks	2 months	1 month	2 months	2 months
Epilepsy course during VOR Tx	No epilepsy seizures	No epilepsy seizures	No epilepsy seizures	No epilepsy seizures	One epileptic seizure after 7 months of treatment (lamotrigine dose was increased consequently)	One epileptic seizure after approximately 2 months of treatment (valproate was afterwards switched to lamotrigine)	No epilepsy seizures	No epilepsy seizures	No epilepsy seizures
Duration of observation (months)	5 (VOR discontinued due to pregnancy planning)	38	6 (VOR discontinued due to pregnancy planning)	2	12	48	26	4	6
Treatment tolerability	good	good	good	good	good	Good	good	good	Good

Tx, treatment, VOR, vortioxetine.

vortioxetine treatment—antiseizure medication was switched afterwards (from valproate to lamotrigine) with optimal control: no other epileptic seizure was observed during nearly 4 following years of antidepressant treatment. It is worth noticing that possibly in these two cases no optimal control of epileptic seizures was reached prior to vortioxetine treatment—both patients had seizure episodes requiring hospitalization shortly before vortioxetine initiation. Vortioxetine was discontinued in two of the presented cases due to pregnancy planning, taking into consideration scarcity of data regarding safety of vortioxetine use in pregnant women. Duration of observation period ranged from 2 to 48 months.

Table 2 presents clinical data on the effectiveness and tolerability of treatment with vortioxetine.

DISCUSSION

In the presented cases vortioxetine was very well tolerated and effective (remission of depressive symptoms was reached in all patients), despite the fact that all patients were treated with polytherapy and three had somatic comorbidities (apart from epilepsy). It is worth mentioning that the majority of cases included patients with symptomatic epilepsy due to brain lesion (after stroke, cardiac arrest, brain injury or neurosurgery)—current data on effectiveness and tolerability of antidepressants in patients with depression following brain damage (due to, e.g., stroke or traumatic brain injury) is limited, which makes any reports of successful treatment of depressive episodes in this group of patients especially valuable (Qin et al., 2018; Kreitzer et al., 2019). Besides, two of the presented cases were elderly patients (74 and 77 year-old)—both reached remission in 2 months and tolerated vortioxetine very well, even though possible reduced tolerability and effectiveness of antidepressants in patients over the age of 65 has been observed (Cleare et al., 2015).

As already mentioned in the introduction, current evidence on the treatment of depression in epilepsy is limited and inconclusive. According to the available clinical recommendations, SSRI and SNRI (Serotonin Norepinephrine Reuptake Inhibitors) are the first-line pharmacological treatment options, while tricyclic antidepressants or NDRI (norepinephrine-dopamine reuptake inhibitors) should be avoided (Elger et al., 2017; Mula, 2019).

Vortioxetine is a relatively new antidepressant (approved by FDA—Food and Drug Administration, in 2013) with multimodal activity—it is an inhibitor of serotonin transporter, an agonist of 5HT1A receptor, a partial agonist of 5HT1B receptor, and an antagonist of 5HT1D, 5HT3 and 5HT7 receptors. Antidepressant efficacy has been demonstrated in doses 5–20 mg daily. It is metabolized primarily by CYP2D6 isoenzyme of P450 cytochrome (to inactive metabolites). Vortioxetine does not seem to impact activity of the liver enzymes in a clinically relevant way which potentially lowers the risk of pharmacokinetic drug interactions (Chen et al., 2018). Results of the network meta-analysis comparing efficacy and acceptability of 21 antidepressants in patients with MDD (Major Depressive Disorder) indicate that vortioxetine was in the group of more effective and more tolerable agents (Cipriani et al., 2018). Data from clinical trials has shown that vortioxetine carries relatively (compared to other antidepressants) low risk of inducing sexual dysfunctions, weight gain and sleep disturbance (Jacobsen et al., 2015; Jacobsen et al., 2016; D'Agostino et al., 2015; Liguori et al., 2019; Baldwin et al.,

2016a). Besides, efficacy of vortioxetine on anhedonia and anxiety symptoms in patients with MDD has been observed (Baldwin et al., 2016b; Cao et al., 2019). Vortioxetine also appears to have relatively good tolerability and safety profile in depressed elderly patients (Borhannejad et al., 2020; Danielak, 2021).

Vortioxetine seems to be a promising treatment option for cognitive dysfunctions in MDD patients—it has been observed to improve cognition (both objectively and subjectively) independently of the alleviation of depression severity and to induce greater improvement in different cognitive domains compared to other antidepressants (Bennabi et al., 2019). Moreover, it has been demonstrated that vortioxetine added to a mood stabilizing agents can be an effective and well-tolerated treatment option in patients with bipolar depression (Siwek et al., 2021a). Finally, it is worth remembering that vortioxetine withdrawal can be associated with occurrence of discontinuation symptoms (although, contrary to the majority of SSRI and SNRI medications, the risk of withdrawal syndrome seems to be low) (Siwek et al., 2021b).

Seizures were very rarely observed in the published results of clinical trials of vortioxetine in MDD patients—only one randomized, double-blind 8-week trial reported 1 case of seizure occurrence in a patient receiving 5 mg of vortioxetine (out of 153 patients in this group and compared to no seizures observed in the placebo arm) (Mahableshwarkar et al., 2013).

Data considering use of vortioxetine in epilepsy patients is scarce. To the best of our knowledge, only one case of a 52-year-old female patient with secondary epilepsy and depressive symptoms has been presented—the authors reported excellent response to vortioxetine (in dose of 20 mg daily) and, interestingly, reduction of visual scotomas after initiation of antidepressant treatment (Onder et al., 2018). As patients with epilepsy often suffer from somatic and psychiatric comorbidities and thus may frequently require polytherapy, vortioxetine as a relatively safe, well-tolerated antidepressant with low risk of inducing pharmacokinetic interactions seems to be a valid treatment option in this group of patients (Baldwin et al., 2016a; Bosak et al., 2019). Besides, patients with epilepsy commonly suffer from cognitive impairment and it would be interesting to find out whether cognition enhancing properties of vortioxetine may additionally improve effects of treatment with this medication (Holmes, 2015).

CONCLUSION

Vortioxetine, as an effective and relatively well-tolerated antidepressant with potentially lower risk of pharmacokinetic drug interactions and additional cognitive benefits in depression, seems to be a promising treatment option for patients with epilepsy and depressive symptoms (especially in the view of current limited evidence on the effectiveness of antidepressants in epilepsy patients). We have presented 9 cases of patients successfully treated with this medication—symptomatic remission was achieved with good treatment tolerance. Further studies regarding vortioxetine use in larger populations of patients with epilepsy and depression are definitely needed in order to broaden our knowledge and improve clinical management of this group of patients.

AUTHOR CONTRIBUTIONS

Conceptualization: MS, AG, MB, and DD. Data acquisition: MS, MB, and DD. Formal analysis: MS, AG, and MB. Supervision: DD. Writing–original draft: AG and MS. Writing–review & editing: MS, AG, MB, and DD.

REFERENCES

1. Alper, K., Schwartz, K. A., Kolts, R. L., and Khan, A. (2007). Seizure Incidence in Psychopharmacological Clinical Trials: An Analysis of Food and Drug Administration (FDA) Summary Basis of Approval Reports. *Biol. Psychiatry* 62 (4), 345–354. doi:10.1016/j.biopsych.2006.09.023
2. Aygun, H., and Ayyildiz, M. (2021). Vortioxetine Increases Absence-like Seizures in WAG/Rij Rats but Decreases Penicillin- and Pentylenetetrazole-Induced Seizures in Wistar Rats. *Epilepsy Behav.* 116, 107797. doi:10.1016/j.yebeh.2021.107797
3. Baldwin, D. S., Chrones, L., Florea, I., Nielsen, R., Nomikos, G. G., Palo, W., et al. (2016). The Safety and Tolerability of Vortioxetine: Analysis of Data from Randomized Placebo-Controlled Trials and Open-Label Extension Studies. *J. Psychopharmacol.* 30 (3), 242–252. doi:10.1177/ 0269881116628440
4. Baldwin, D. S., Florea, I., Jacobsen, P. L., Zhong, W., and Nomikos, G. G. (2016). A Meta-Analysis of the Efficacy of Vortioxetine in Patients with Major Depressive Disorder (MDD) and High Levels of Anxiety Symptoms. *J. Affect Disord.* 206, 140–150. doi:10.1016/j.jad.2016.07.015
5. Bennabi, D., Haffen, E., and Van Waes, V. (2019). Vortioxetine for Cognitive Enhancement in Major Depression: From Animal Models to Clinical Research. *Front. Psychiatry* 1010, 771. doi:10.3389/fpsyt.2019.00771
6. Błaszczyk, B., and Czuczwar, S. J. (2016). Epilepsy Coexisting with Depression. *Pharmacol. Rep.* 68 (5), 1084–1092. doi:10.1016/j.pharep.2016.06.011
7. Borhannejad, F., Shariati, B., Naderi, S., Shalbafan, M., Mortezaei, A., Sahebolzamani, E., et al. (2020). Comparison of Vortioxetine and Sertraline for Treatment of Major Depressive Disorder in Elderly Patients: A Double-Blind Randomized Trial. *J. Clin. Pharm. Ther.* 45 (4), 804–811. doi:10.1111/jcpt.13177
8. Bosak, M., Dudek, D., and Siwek, M. (2012). Depresja U Chorych Z Padaczka [Depression in Patients with Epilepsy]. *Psychiatr. Pol.* 46 (5), 891–902.
9. Bosak, M., Dudek, D., Siwek, M., and Szczudlik, A. (2015). Subtypes of Interictal Depressive Disorders According to ICD-10 in Patients with Epilepsy. *Neurol. Neurochir Pol.* 49 (2), 90–94. doi:10.1016/j.pjnns.2015.01.008
10. Bosak, M., Kowalik, M., Mołek, P., and Słowik, A. (2019). Somatic Comorbidity in Polish Patients with Epilepsy. *Pol. Arch. Intern. Med.* 129 (5), 303–307. doi:10. 20452/pamw.14794
11. Bosak, M., Turaj, W., Dudek, D., Siwek, M., and Szczudlik, A. (2015). Depressogenic Medications and Other Risk Factors for Depression Among Polish Patients with Epilepsy. *Neuropsychiatr. Dis. Treat.* 11, 2509–2517. doi:10. 2147/NDT.S91538
12. Bosak, M., Turaj, W., Dudek, D., Siwek, M., and Szczudlik, A. (2016). Suicidality and its Determinants Among Polish Patients with Epilepsy. *Neurol. Neurochir Pol.* 50 (6), 432–438. doi:10.1016/j.pjnns.2016.07.009
13. Cao, B., Park, C., Subramaniapillai, M., Lee, Y., Iacobucci, M., Mansur, R. B., et al. (2019). The Efficacy of Vortioxetine on Anhedonia in Patients with Major Depressive Disorder. *Front. Psychiatry* 10, 17. doi:10.3389/fpsyt.2019.00017
14. Chen, B., Choi, H., Hirsch, L. J., Katz, A., Legge, A., Buchsbaum, R., et al. (2017). Psychiatric and Behavioral Side Effects of Antiepileptic Drugs in Adults with Epilepsy. *Epilepsy Behav.* 76, 24–31. doi:10.1016/j.yebeh.2017. 08.039
15. Chen, G., Højer, A.-M., Areberg, J., and Nomikos, G. (2018). Vortioxetine: Clinical Pharmacokinetics and Drug Interactions. *Clin. Pharmacokinet.* 57, 673–686. doi:10.1007/s40262-017-0612-7
16. Cipriani, A., Furukawa, T. A., Salanti, G., Chaimani, A., Atkinson, L. Z., Ogawa, Y., et al. (2018). Comparative Efficacy and Acceptability of 21 Antidepressant Drugs for the Acute Treatment of Adults with Major Depressive Disorder: a Systematic Review and Network Meta-Analysis. *Lancet* 391 (10128), 1357–1366. doi:10.1016/S0140-6736(17)32802-7

17. Cleare, A., Pariante, C. M., Young, A. H., Anderson, I. M., Christmas, D., Cowen, P. J., et al. (2015). Evidence-based Guidelines for Treating Depressive Disorders with Antidepressants: A Revision of the 2008 British Association for Psychopharmacology Guidelines. *J. Psychopharmacol.* 29 (5), 459–525. doi:10.1177/0269881115581093
18. D'Agostino, A., English, C. D., and Rey, J. A. (2015). Vortioxetine (Brintellix): A New Serotonergic Antidepressant. *P T* 40 (1), 36–40.
19. Danielak, D. (2021). Vortioxetine in Management of Major Depressive Disorder - a Favorable Alternative for Elderly Patients? *Expert Opin. Pharmacother.* 22 (9), 1167–1177. doi:10.1080/14656566.2021.1880567
20. Elger, C. E., Johnston, S. A., and Hoppe, C. (2017). Diagnosing and Treating Depression in Epilepsy. *Seizure* 44, 184–193. doi:10.1016/j.seizure.2016.10.018
21. Fazel, S., Wolf, A., Långström, N., Newton, C. R., and Lichtenstein, P. (2013). Premature Mortality in Epilepsy and the Role of Psychiatric Comorbidity: A Total Population Study. *Lancet* 382 (9905), 1646–1654. doi:10.1016/S0140-6736(13)60899-5
22. Fisher, R. S., Acevedo, C., Arzimanoglou, A., Bogacz, A., Cross, J. H., Elger, C. E., et al. (2014). ILAE Official Report: A Practical Clinical Definition of Epilepsy. *Epilepsia* 55 (4), 475–482. doi:10.1111/epi.12550
23. Fisher, R. S., Cross, J. H., French, J. A., Higurashi, N., Hirsch, E., Jansen, F. E., et al. (2017). Operational Classification of Seizure Types by the International League against Epilepsy: Position Paper of the ILAE Commission for Classification and Terminology. *Epilepsia* 58 (4), 522–530. doi:10.1111/epi.13670
24. Garcia, M. E., Garcia-Morales, I., and Gil-Nagel, A. (2015). Prevalence of Depressive Symptoms and Their Impact on Quality of Life in Patients with Drug-Resistant Focal Epilepsy (IMDYVA Study). *Epilepsy Res.* 110, 157–165. doi:10.1016/j.eplepsyres.2014.11.003
25. Henning, O., Lossius, M. I., Lima, M., Mevåg, M., Villagran, A., Nakken, K. O., et al. (2019). Refractory Epilepsy and Nonadherence to Drug Treatment. *Epilepsia Open* 4 (4), 618–623. doi:10.1002/epi4.12367
26. Hesdorffer, D. C., Ishihara, L., Webb, D. J., Mynepalli, L., Galwey, N. W., and Hauser, W. A. (2016). Occurrence and Recurrence of Attempted Suicide Among People with Epilepsy. *JAMA Psychiatry* 73 (1), 80–86. doi:10.1001/jamapsychiatry.2015.2516
27. Hitiris, N., Mohanraj, R., Norrie, J., Sills, G. J., and Brodie, M. J. (2007). Predictors of Pharmacoresistant Epilepsy. *Epilepsy Res.* 75 (2-3), 192–196. doi:10.1016/j. eplepsyres.2007.06.003
28. Holmes, G. L. (2015). Cognitive Impairment in Epilepsy: The Role of Network Abnormalities. *Epileptic Disord.* 17 (2), 101–116. doi:10.1684/epd.2015.0739
29. Jacobsen, P. L., Mahableshwarkar, A. R., Chen, Y., Chrones, L., and Clayton, A. H. (2015). Effect of Vortioxetine vs. Escitalopram on Sexual Functioning in Adults with Well-Treated Major Depressive Disorder Experiencing SSRI-Induced Sexual Dysfunction. *J. Sex. Med.* 12 (10), 2036–2048. doi:10.1111/jsm.12980
30. Jacobsen, P. L., Mahableshwarkar, A. R., Palo, W. A., Chen, Y., Dragheim, M., and Clayton, A. H. (2016). Treatment-emergent Sexual Dysfunction in Randomized Trials of Vortioxetine for Major Depressive Disorder or Generalized Anxiety Disorder: A Pooled Analysis. *CNS Spectr.* 21 (5), 367–378. doi:10.1017/ S1092852915000553
31. Johnson, E. K., Jones, J. E., Seidenberg, M., and Hermann, B. P. (2004). The Relative Impact of Anxiety, Depression, and Clinical Seizure Features on Health-Related Quality of Life in Epilepsy. *Epilepsia* 45 (5), 544–550. doi:10.1111/j.0013-9580. 2004.47003.x
32. Josephson, C. B., Lowerison, M., Vallerand, I., Sajobi, T. T., Patten, S., Jette, N., et al. (2017). Association of Depression and Treated Depression with Epilepsy and Seizure Outcomes: A Multicohort Analysis. *JAMA Neurol.* 74 (5), 533–539. doi:10.1001/jamaneurol.2016.5042
33. Kanner, A. M., Byrne, R., Chicharro, A., Wuu, J., and Frey, M. (2009). A Lifetime Psychiatric History Predicts a Worse Seizure Outcome Following Temporal Lobectomy. *Neurology* 72 (9), 793–799. doi:10.1212/01.wnl.0000343850.85763.9c
34. Kanner, A. M. (2009). Suicidality and Epilepsy: A Complex Relationship that Remains Misunderstood and Underestimated. *Epilepsy Curr.* 9 (3), 63–66. doi:10.1111/j.1535-7511.2009.01294.x
35. Keezer, M. R., Sisodiya, S. M., and Sander, J. W. (2016). Comorbidities of Epilepsy: Current Concepts and Future Perspectives. *Lancet Neurol.* 15 (1), 106–115. doi:10.1016/S1474-4422(15)00225-2
36. Kreitzer, N., Ancona, R., Mccullumsmith, C., Kurowski, B. G., Foreman, B., Ngwenya, L. B., et al. (2019). The Effect of Antidepressants on Depression after Traumatic Brain Injury: A Meta-Analysis. *J. Head Trauma Rehabil.* 34 (3), E47–E54. doi:10.1097/HTR.0000000000000439
37. Kwan, P., Arzimanoglou, A., Berg, A. T., Brodie, M. J., Hauser, W. A., Mathern, G., et al. (2010). Definition of Drug Resistant Epilepsy: Consensus Proposal by the Ad Hoc Task Force of the ILAE Commission on Therapeutic Strategies. *Epilepsia* 51, 1069–1077. doi:10.1111/j.1528-1167.2009.02397.x
38. Kwon, O. Y., and Park, S. P. (2014). Depression and Anxiety in People with Epilepsy. *J. Clin. Neurol.* 10 (3), 175–188. doi:10.3988/jcn.2014.10.3.175
39. Liguori, C., Ferini-Strambi, L., Izzi, F., Mari, L., Manfredi, N., D'Elia, A., et al. (2019). Preliminary Evidence that Vortioxetine May Improve Sleep Quality in Depressed Patients with Insomnia: a Retrospective Questionnaire Analysis. *Br. J. Clin. Pharmacol.* 85 (1), 240–244. doi:10.1111/bcp.13772
40. Maguire, M. J., Weston, J., Singh, J., and Marson, A. G. (2021). Antidepressants for People with Epilepsy and Depression. *Cochrane Database Syst. Rev.* 4, CD010682. doi:10.1002/14651858.CD010682.pub2
41. Mahableshwarkar, A. R., Jacobsen, P. L., and Chen, Y. (2013). A Randomized, Double-Blind Trial of 2.5 Mg and 5 Mg Vortioxetine (Lu AA21004) versus Placebo for 8 Weeks in Adults with Major Depressive Disorder. *Curr. Med. Res. Opin.* 29 (3), 217–226. doi:10.1185/03007995.2012.761600
42. Mazarati, A., and Sankar, R. (2016). Common Mechanisms Underlying Epileptogenesis and the Comorbidities of Epilepsy. *Cold Spring Harb Perspect. Med.* 6 (7), a022798. doi:10.1101/cshperspect.a022798
43. Mula, M. (2019). Developments in Depression in Epilepsy: Screening, Diagnosis, and Treatment. *Expert Rev. Neurother* 19 (3), 269–276. doi:10.1080/14737175. 2019.1585244
44. Ögün, M. N., Çetinkaya, A., and Beyazçiçek, E. (2019). The Effect of Vortioxetine on Penicillin-Induced Epileptiform Activity in Rats. *Arq Neuropsiquiatr* 77 (6), 412–417. doi:10.1590/0004-282X20190064
45. Onder, H., Coskun, A., and Goksungur, M. T. (2018). Recovery of Visual Scotomas by Vortioxetine in a Patient with Symptomatic Occipital Lobe Epilepsy. *Ann. Indian Acad. Neurol.* 21 (1), 88–90. doi:10.4103/aian.AIAN_291_17
46. Qin, B., Chen, H., Gao, W., Zhao, L. B., Zhao, M. J., Qin, H. X., et al. (2018). Efficacy, Acceptability, and Tolerability of Antidepressant Treatments for Patients with post-stroke Depression: A Network Meta-Analysis. *Braz. J. Med. Biol. Res.* 51 (7), e7218. doi:10.1590/1414-431x20187218
47. Scheffer, I. E., Berkovic, S., Capovilla, G., Connolly, M. B., French, J., Guilhoto, L., et al. (2017). ILAE Classification of the Epilepsies: Position Paper of the ILAE Commission for Classification and Terminology. *Epilepsia* 58 (4), 512–521. doi:10.1111/epi.13709
48. Siwek, M., Chrobak, A., Sołtys, Z., Dudek, D., Krupa, A., and Rybakowski, J. (2021). A Naturalistic, 24-week, Open-Label, Add-On Study of Vortioxetine in Bipolar Depression. *Psychiatr. Pol.* ONLINE FIRST Nr 222: 1–14. doi:10.12740/pp/ onlinefirst/132962
49. Siwek, M., Chrobak, A. A., Gorostowicz, A., Krupa, A. J., and Dudek, D. (2021). Withdrawal Symptoms Following Discontinuation of Vortioxetine-Retrospective Chart Review. *Pharmaceuticals (Basel)* 14 (5), 451. doi:10. 3390/ph14050451
50. Steinert, T., and Fröscher, W. (2018). Epileptic Seizures under Antidepressive Drug Treatment: Systematic Review. *Pharmacopsychiatry* 51 (4), 121–135. doi:10. 1055/s-0043-117962
51. Tao, K., and Wang, X. (2016). The Comorbidity of Epilepsy and Depression: Diagnosis and Treatment. *Expert Rev. Neurother* 16 (11), 1321–1333. doi:10.1080/14737175.2016.1204233
52. Taskiran, M., and Unal, G. (2021). Vortioxetine Suppresses Epileptiform Activity and Cognition Deficits in a Chronic PTZ-Induced Kindling Rat Model. *Epileptic Disord.* 23 (6), 893–900. doi:10.1684/epd.2021.1344
53. Taylor, R. S., Sander, J. W., Taylor, R. J., and Baker, G. A. (2011). Predictors of Health-Related Quality of Life and Costs in Adults with Epilepsy: A Systematic Review. *Epilepsia* 52 (12), 2168–2180. doi:10.1111/j.1528- 1167.2011.03213.x
54. Tellez-Zenteno, J. F., Patten, S. B., Jetté, N., Williams, J., and Wiebe, S. (2007). Psychiatric Comorbidity in Epilepsy: A Population-Based Analysis. *Epilepsia* 48 (12), 2336–2344. doi:10.1111/j.1528-1167.2007.01222.x

19

Case Report: Migralepsy: The Two-Faced Janus of Neurology

*Giorgia Sforza [1], Claudia Ruscitto [2], Romina Moavero [2], Fabiana Ursitti [1], Michela Ada Noris Ferilli [1], Samuela Tarantino [1], Martina Balestri [3], Federico Vigevano [3], Massimiliano Valeriani [1,4] and Laura Papetti [1]**

[1] Pediatric Headache Center, Department of Neuroscience, Bambino Gesù Children Hospital, Istituto di Ricovero e Cura a Carattere Scientifico, Rome, Italy, [2] Child Neurology and Psychiatry Unit, Tor Vergata University of Rome, Rome, Italy, [3] Child Neurology Unit, Bambino Gesù Children's Hospital, Istituto di Ricovero e Cura a Carattere Scientifico, Rome, Italy, [4] Center for Sensory-Motor Interaction, Aalborg University, Aalborg, Denmark

***Correspondence:**
Laura Papetti
laura.papetti@opbg.net

We report three cases of pediatric patients suffering from migraine aura triggered seizures. This entity, also called migralepsy, still does not have a unique definition today. Migraine and epilepsy are both episodic neurological disorders with periods of interictal well-being; this is indicative of similar pathophysiological mechanisms, such as increased neuronal excitation and ion channel dysfunction. The purpose of this paper is to discuss the clinical and instrumental features of migralepsy through the description of three clinical cases in which the symptoms of the usual migraine aura developed into a generalized tonic–clonic or focal seizure.

Keywords: migralepsy, migraine, epilepsy, seizure, aura

INTRODUCTION

Migraine is the most common type of primary headache in pediatric population and the prevalence varies according to presenting age, going from 3% in younger children to ~20% in adolescents (1, 2). Pediatric epilepsy is another frequent neurological condition, with a prevalence of approximately 3.2–5.5/1,000 in developed countries (3). There is a large range of comorbidity between migraine and epilepsy: among patients with migraine, epilepsy can occur in 1–17% of the cases (as in the healthy pediatric population) while, among epileptic patients, the prevalence of migraine ranges from 7 to 26% (4).

The International Headache Society (IHS) in the International Classification of Headache Disorders (ICHD-3 edition) identified three main associations between headache and epilepsy, including migraine-triggered seizure (migralepsy), hemicrania epileptica, and postictal headache (5).

Migralepsy is defined as a seizure triggered by a migraine attack with aura: in particular, the seizure must fulfill the diagnostic criteria for a specific seizure, it has to occur in a patient suffering from migraine with aura (MA), during, or within 1 h of a migraine attack with aura (5). To date several cases of patients with migralepsy have been described, many of which have turned out to be cases of occipital epilepsy (6, 7).

Therefore, the purpose of this study is to discuss the clinical and instrumental features of migralepsy through the description of three clinical cases in which the symptoms of the usual migraine aura developed into a generalized tonic–clonic or focal seizure.

CASE SERIES

Clinical characteristics of our patients are reported in **Table 1**. The parents of the patients signed informed consent for the publication of the data. Furthermore, the submission of the paper was validated by the ethics committee of the Bambino Gesù Hospital.

Patient 1

An 11-year-old girl was followed at our headache center, suffering from MA and without aura (MO) since the age of 7 according to the ICHD-3 criteria (5). She was born full term with a normal delivery and had normal developmental milestones. Her father suffered from MO, but no family member had a history of epilepsy.

When she was 7 years old, she developed MO attacks, which occurred once a week. Three years later, she began experiencing MA attacks. Her aura was characterized by the appearance of a black circle in the center of the visual field, which subsequently became a scintillating scotoma. These symptoms occurred for about 5–10 min, with the subsequent onset of a headache that persisted for a few hours. The headache had migraine characteristics with throbbing pain contralateral to the site of the visited aura and associated with photophobia, phonophobia, and vomiting. These attacks occurred two or three times a month, almost exclusively in the evening after studying.

At age 11, she presented two episodes characterized by her usual visual aura followed by a loss of consciousness, staring, falling to the ground, and subsequent evolution into tonic–clonic seizures.

The patient was hospitalized, and she underwent a magnetic resonance imaging (MRI) of the brain that was normal. An interictal EEG was also performed showing bilateral temporal occipital epileptic spike anomalies and photo paroxysmal response.

The girl reported that the visual aura that preceded the seizures was the same as the aura that used to precede her migraine attacks in the past. Long-term therapy with topiramate was initiated at a dose of 2 mg/kg/day. Control interictal-EEG performed 1 month after the beginning of the therapy did not show anomalies, but only photo paroxysmal response. She was diagnosed with MA and migralepsy or migraine aura-triggered seizure.

After 1 year, control EEGs subsequently showed rare occipital spike-wave anomalies predominantly right or bilateral.

Since starting treatment, the girl has no longer had seizures or headaches, but only recurrent aura episodes without migraine.

At the age of 13, she started having migraine attacks with aura with sporadic frequency again, she had no further seizures and her last EEG was normal.

Patient 2

A 6-year-old girl was born premature (gestational age of 27 weeks), suffering from MA and MO since the age of 5 according to ICHD-3 criteria (5). The headache had migraine characteristics with throbbing and severe pain associated with photophobia, phonophobia, and nausea. Rarely, her migraine attacks were preceded by a visual aura characterized by the vision of a colored and scintillating cube. The frequency of the attacks was about two for a month.

She was admitted at the age of 6 to our hospital for a first epileptic seizure characterized by a visual phenomenon, with

TABLE 1 | Main features of clinical cases and Visual Aura Rating Scale (VARS).

	Patient 1	Patient 2	Patient 3
Gender	Female	Female	Female
Migraine age onset	7	5	8
Seizure age onset	11	6	12
Visual Aura Rating Scale (VARS):			
Duration 5–60 min (three points)	Yes	Yes	Yes
Temporal development ≥5 min (two points)	Yes	Yes	Yes
Scotoma (two points)	Yes	Yes	Yes
Fortification (two points)	No	No	No
Homonymus character (one point)	No	No	No
Brain MRI findings	None	None	None
Treatment	Topiramate 2 mg/kg/day	Valproic acid 20 mg/kg/day, replaced for side effects and poor efficacy with Topiramate 2 mg/kg/day	Topiramate 2 mg/kg/day
Outcome	Migraine	Migraine	Migraine/Isolated visual aura

vision of a colored cube, together with confusion, dizziness, and malaise, followed by loss of consciousness, deviation of the eyes to the right, and stiffening of the limbs. The episode lasted about 20 min and was followed by a migraine attack.

The interictal-EEG performed during the hospitalization showed left posterior slow electrical activity, while brain MRI showed no pathological sign. She was discharged with a diagnosis of idiopathic occipital epilepsy and endorectal diazepam therapy as needed.

Over the next 2 months, she had two more episodes with the same visual and epileptics features; one of the episodes lasted 30 min during which diazepam e.r. and ibuprofen were administered with no effect.

All the episodes were followed by a migraine attack. Control interictal EEGs showed epileptiform potentials with high-voltage spikes are observed in the right temporo occipital region and sporadic slow waves in the left temporo occipital region. The girl was then discharged and diagnosed with migralepsy or migraine aura-triggered seizure.

The patient subsequently presented two other prolonged seizures with the same characteristics, so she was treated with valproic acid 600 mg per day (20 mg/kg/day), then replaced for side effects and poor efficacy with topiramate at a dose of 75 mg per day (2 mg/kg/day). With topiramate, the girl began to have fewer migraine attacks with aura and no longer had seizures.

Patient 3

A 12-year-old girl was admitted in our hospital for a first epileptic episode.

Until the age of 8 she suffered from MO and MA according to the ICH-3 criteria. Her visual aura was characterized by the vision of "pulsating spots" (scintillating scotoma). The episodes were usually followed by headache with migraine features such as photo- and phonophobia and vomiting.

The first epileptic episode was characterized by her typical migraine aura (vision of a scintillating scotoma) in the left visual half field, progressive loss of consciousness and posture with semi-flexed limbs, followed, after 15 min, by deviation of the head and gaze to the left, and subsequent evolution in tonic-clonic seizure. The crisis subsided at the emergency department with the administration of 2 mg of intravenous midazolam. In the postictal phase, blurring of vision followed until the next day.

Brain MRI was normal. Interictal-EEG showed epileptic alterations with right occipital spikes. She was discharged with diagnosis of probable migraine aura-triggered seizure and with oromucosal midazolam as needed. After 4 years, at the age of 16, she presented a further episode characterized by a scintillating circle-shaped scotoma visualized in the left half field without headache. She then presented progressive loss of consciousness with staring and tonic-clonic seizure. The scotoma phase was quite long (10–15 min), with a short seizure (2–3 min), followed by severe drowsiness and headache that lasted for about an hour. An EEG was then performed, which was normal.

In later years, the patient experienced further migraine attacks with and without aura or, possibly, isolated aura episodes, without having seizures anymore.

DISCUSSION

In this case series, we present three patients affected by migraine aura-triggered seizure, also known as migralepsy. We consider these cases representative of this type of manifestation for the following reasons: (1) a history of migraine with typical aura that precedes the onset of epilepsy, (2) the same visual symptoms that have always characterized the migraine aura, also induce epileptic seizures, and (3) a recurring association of the phenomena and the ability of antiepileptic therapy to completely control epilepsy while only partially controlling migraine and/or aura.

Migraine and epilepsy are both relatively frequent paroxysmal neurological disorders which can therefore often coexist and their association could thus be attributed to coincidence. However, these conditions also seem to share pathogenic mechanisms such as increased neuronal excitation and ion channels dysfunction (3). Although the possibility of a closer relationship between these two conditions in both clinical and pathophysiological terms has always been a hot topic, there is still no real consensus for the definition of this relationship (8).

In particular, there are two open issues: (1) the need of a more specific/accurate definition of migralepsy, and (2) the boundary between MA and epilepsy with visual symptoms (e.g., occipital epilepsy).

The term "migralepsy" literally derives from the combination of the words migraine and epilepsy and the definition was introduced by Lennox and Lennox in 1960 to describe a disorder in which "ophthalmic migraine (now called MA) with nausea and vomiting is followed by characteristic features of epilepsy" (9). The term "migralepsy" was originally used to define the condition of visual symptoms followed by migraine and subsequently by an epileptic seizure. However, this term may be applied both to an epileptic phenomenon resembling migraine and to a real migraine attack followed by a seizure (10). Therefore, it is a term requiring a better and consensual definition. In fact, migralepsy is described in the headache classification (ICHD-3), but not in the classification of the epilepsies [International Classification of Epileptic Seizures of the League Against Epilepsy (ILAE)] (8–10). Several cases have been presented with the diagnosis of migralepsy or possible migralepsy (6, 7). However, some of them appeared to be occipital seizures (7), or possible ictal focal visual manifestations followed by a generalized tonic–clonic seizure (6). Sances et al. (6) reviewed 50 cases reported in literature and only two cases presented features supporting the diagnosis of migralepsy. Noteworthy, in none of the described cases was an ictal EEG recording available which included the onset of the seizure. Furthermore, it is also important to point out that the term "migralepsy" does not clearly refer to a seizure, that begins with a migraine aura, or to an actual migraine attack followed by (and/or possibly triggering) a seizure, thus, not indicating a specific reference to one of these two clinical entities (10). In view of all this, in our opinion until a consensus is reached to define its meaning, the term "migralepsy" should be replaced by the more appropriate definition of "migraine aura-triggered seizure." In the ICHD-3, the term "migraine aura-triggered seizure" is proposed for a condition in which an epileptic seizure occurs "during, or within 1 h after, an attack of migraine with aura" in a patient suffering from MA. However, it should be proven that the seizure is really "triggered" by migraine, the association may be in fact be due to the activation of putatively similar mechanisms, or simply be a random association. A triggering effect of migraine, rather than an occasional association, is suggested when a history of epilepsy is lacking or in cases of repeated occurrence (10).

Another important point is the distinction between a migraine visual aura and an epileptic seizure presenting with visual symptoms. Visual auras can occur in migraine or in focal epilepsy (11). The diagnosis is usually based on clinical elements, but this might be challenging in isolated auras. Besides the ICHD-3 (8), the Visual Aura Rating Scale (VARS) provides parameters to facilitate the clinical identification of migraine auras (12). It includes a visual aura duration of 5-60 min (three points) and gradual temporal development ≥5 min (two points), the presence of scotomas (two points) and fortifications (two points), and the homonymous character of the visual sensations (one point). A total score of at least five points is supposed to identify migraine with visual aura with a sensitivity of 91–96% and a specificity of 96–98%. Visual Aura Rating Scale might be helpful in patients presenting with typical migraine or epilepsy, but it can lead to misdiagnosis especially in cases of isolated auras (12). In **Table 1**, we summarized the characteristics of our patients, including the VARS parameters. To the best of our knowledge, most reported cases of migrainous visual aura followed by epileptic seizures are based merely on the clinical history of the patient or observation. An EEG video monitoring evaluation proved the epileptic nature of a visual aura, which was previously diagnosed as migraine aura fulfilling the diagnostic criteria for migralepsy (13). Epileptic auras may also be associated with a lack of EEG ictal patterns and in addition to this, most patients with occipital lobe epilepsy lack occipital lobe EEG seizure patterns in non-invasive EEG examinations (13). On the other hand, migraine attacks may be associated with EEG slowing but not with epileptiform discharges. Thus, patients with suspected migraine-triggered epilepsy should be studied carefully with EEG-video monitoring as the clinical findings of visual aura that precede both conditions can be ambiguous (14). Unfortunately, ICDH-3 diagnostic criteria do not include EEG evaluation (8).

A final point of discussion is the definition of the ictal epileptic headache (IEH) as defined in the ICHD-3 (5). Ictal epileptic headache is defined as a headache caused by and occurring during a partial epileptic seizure, ipsilateral to the epileptic discharge, and remitting immediately or soon after the seizure has terminated. Ictal epileptic headache may be followed by other epileptic manifestations (motor, sensory, or autonomic). This condition should be differentiated from "pure" or "isolated" IEH occurring as the sole epileptic manifestation and requiring differential diagnosis from other headache types. Finally, "hemicrania epileptica" is a very rare variant of IEH characterized by ipsilateral location of headache and ictal EEG paroxysms (5). In the previously reported cases of migralepsy or IEH, no specific EEG picture was detected: (a) high voltage, rhythmic, 11–12 Hz activity with intermingled spikes over the right temporo-occipital regions; (b) high voltage theta activity intermingled with sharp waves over occipital region; and (c) bilateral continuous spike- and slow-wave discharges (15).

More recently Parisi et al. have proposed to include as main IEH criterion the ictal EEG and clinical response to antiepileptic intravenous administration. In the absence of this last data, IEH should be classified as "probable IEH" diagnosis (16). The definition of IEH should be used to classify the events in which headache represents the only ictal epileptic feature (15) while the term "hemicrania epileptica" should be maintained for all cases in which an IEH "coexist" and is associated synchronously or sequentially with other ictal sensory-motor events (15).

The same authors supported the theory that the concept of migralepsy is potentially confusing and should not be used to describe the sequence of migraine aura seizure and an ictal EEG recording is mandatory to confirm diagnosis (15, 17).

CONCLUSION

The term migralepsy should be replaced by migraine aura-triggered seizure. However, the criteria for diagnosis should be specified better. In particular, the recording of the visual phenomenon with an EEG should be considered a major diagnostic criterion. However, considering that the episodes can be very rare, thus, difficult to be recorded by EEG, some clinical elements should be necessary for the diagnosis: (1) previous history of MA before the onset of epilepsy, (2) the visual aura triggering the epileptic seizure must have the same clinical features as the migraine visual auras not followed by epileptic manifestations, (3) there must be a recurrence in the association between the visual aura and the epileptic fit, and (4) visual symptoms should meet the VARS criteria. In our cohort of patients, all the aforementioned criteria are met at the same time, and we think that this may be congruous with the diagnosis of "migraine aura-triggered seizure."

AUTHOR CONTRIBUTIONS

GS, MB, and CR contributed to the writing of the paper. RM, MF, FU, and ST collected the cases. MV conceptualized the study. FV and LP provided supervision. LP wrote the paper. All authors contributed to the article and approved the submitted version.

REFERENCES

1. Papetti L, Ursitti F, Moavero R, Ferilli MAN, Sforza G, Tarantino S, et al. Prophylactic treatment of pediatric migraine: is there anything new in the last decade? *Front Neurol.* (2019) 10:771. doi: 10.3389/fneur.2019.00771
2. Lewis D. Pediatric migraine. *Neurol Clin.* (2009) 27:481–501. doi: 10.1016/j.ncl.2008.11.003
3. Papetti L, Nicita F, Parisi P, Spalice A, Villa MP, Kasteleijn-Nolst Trenité DG. "Headache and epilepsy"—how are they connected? *Epilepsy Behav.* (2013) 26:386–93. doi: 10.1016/j.yebeh.2012.09.025
4. Kasteleijn-Nolst Trenité D, Parisi P. Migraine in the borderland of epilepsy: "migralepsy" an overlapping syndrome of children and adults? *Epilepsia.* (2012) 7:20–5. doi: 10.1111/j.1528-1167.2012.03711.x
5. Headache Classification Committee of the International Headache Society (IHS). The International Classification of Headache Disorders, 3rd edition. *Cephalalgia.* (2018); 38:1-211. doi: 10.1177/0333102417738202
6. Sances G, Guaschino E, Perucca P, Allena M, Ghiotto N, Manni R. Migralepsy: a call for a revision of the definition. *Epilepsia.* (2009) 50:2487–96. doi: 10.1111/j.1528-1167.2009.02265.x

7. Verrotti A, Coppola G, Di Fonzo A, Tozzi E, Spalice A, Aloisi P, et al. Should "migralepsy" be considered an obsolete concept? A multicenter retrospective clinical/EEG study and review of the literature. *Epilepsy Behav.* (2011) 21:52–9. doi: 10.1016/j.yebeh.2011.03.004
8. Belcastro V, Striano P, Parisi P. Migraine and epilepsy terminology and classification: opening Pandora's box. *Epileptic Disord.* (2013) 15:216–7. doi: 10.1684/epd.2013.0582
9. Lennox WGLM. *Epilepsy and Related Disorders.* Boston, MA: Little, Brown and Company (1960).
10. Cianchetti C, Pruna D, Ledda M. Epileptic seizures and headache/migraine: a review of types of association and terminology. *Seizure.* (2013) 22:679–85. doi: 10.1016/j.seizure.2013.05.017
11. Panayiotopoulos CP. Visual phenomena and headache in occipital epilepsy: a review, a systematic study and differentiation from migraine. *Epilep Disord.* (1999) 1:205–16.
12. Eriksen MK, Thomsen LL, Olesen J. The Visual Aura Rating Scale (VARS) for migraine aura diagnosis. *Cephalalgia.* (2005) 25:801–10. doi: 10.1111/j.1468-2982.2005.00955.x
13. Hartl E, Rémi J, Noachtar S. Two patients with visual aura - migraine, epilepsy, or migralepsy? *Headache.* (2015) 55:1148–51. doi: 10.1111/head.12615
14. Belcastro V, Striano P, Parisi P. Is it migralepsy? Still don't know. *Headache.* (2015) 55:1446–7. doi: 10.1111/head.12696
15. Belcastro V, Striano P, Kasteleijn-Nolst Trenité DG, Villa MP, Parisi P. Migralepsy, hemicrania epileptica, post-ictal headache and "ictal epileptic headache": a proposal for terminology and classification revision. *J Headache Pain.* (2011) 12:289–94. doi: 10.1007/s10194-011-0318-4
16. Parisi P, Paolino MC, Raucci U, Della Vecchia N, Belcastro V, Villa MP, et al. Ictal epileptic headache: when terminology is not a moot question. *Front Neurol.* (2019) 10:785. doi: 10.3389/fneur.2019.00785
17. Parisi P, Striano P, Negro A, Martelletti P, Belcastro V. Ictal epileptic headache: an old story with courses and appeals. *J Headache Pain.* (2012) 13:607–13. doi: 10.1007/s10194-012-0485-y

20

Myoclonic Epilepsy: Case Report of a Mild Phenotype in a Pediatric Patient Expanding Clinical Spectrum of *KCNA2* Pathogenic Variants

Lorenzo Perilli [1], Gioia Mastromoro [2], Manuel Murciano [1,3], Ilaria Amedeo [1], Federica Avenoso [1], Antonio Pizzuti [2], Cristiana Alessia Guido [1] and Alberto Spalice [1]*

[1] Department of Mother and Child and Urological Sciences, Sapienza University of Rome, Rome, Italy, [2] Faculty of Medicine and Dentistry, Department of Experimental Medicine, Sapienza University of Rome, Rome, Italy, [3] Department of Emergency Pediatrics, Bambino Gesù Children's Hospital, IRCCS, Rome, Italy

***Correspondence:**
Lorenzo Perilli
dottorperilli@gmail.com

We report on the rare case of a male toddler presenting with myoclonic epilepsy characterized by daily episodes of upward movements of the eyebrows, and myoclonic jerks of both head and upper limbs. In addition, the child showed speech delay, tremors, and lack of motor coordination. Next Generation Sequencing analysis (NGS) performed in trio revealed in the proband the c.889C>T *de novo* missense variant in the *KCNA2* gene in heterozygous state. This is the first case of myoclonic epilepsy in a toddler due to a c.889C>T *KCNA2* missense variant. The patient was treated with valproic acid and ethosuximide with a good clinical response. At 6 years old, follow-up revealed that the proband was seizure-free with tremors and clumsiness in movements. According to the literature, this case supports the correlation between myoclonic epilepsy and *KCNA2* alterations. This evidence suggests that performing genomic testing including the *KCNA2* gene in preschool patients affected by myoclonic epilepsy, especially when associated with delayed neurodevelopment. Our goal is to expand the phenotypical spectrum of this rare condition and adding clinical features following a genotype-first approach.

Keywords: epilepsy, *KCNA2*, epileptic encephalopathies, genetic variants, genotype-first approach, epilepsy—abnormalities, classification, drug therapy

INTRODUCTION

Among the genetically determined forms of epilepsy, many genes remain unknown. Cases of epilepsy caused by a *KCNA2* mutation are known in literature (as shown in **Table 1**) different from the one reported in this manuscript. In 2017, Sachdev et al. (8) described a case of genetically determined epilepsy carrying the same mutation of our patient, but with different phenotype, described in **Table 2**. We report for the first time a pediatric patient affected by myoclonic epilepsy due to the heterozygous c.889C>T missense variant in the *KCNA2* gene. According to the literature, this case supports the correlation between myoclonic epilepsy and *KCNA2* alterations. This evidence suggests that performing genomic testing including the *KCNA2* gene in preschool patients affected by myoclonic epilepsy, especially when associated with delayed neurodevelopment. Our goal is to expand the phenotypical spectrum of this rare condition and adding clinical features following a genotype-first approach.

TABLE 1 | Comparison between the characteristics of patients reported in the literature with mutation in the same triplet encoding an amino acid as the patient analyzed in this study.

	Pena and Coimbra (1)	**Syrbe et al. (2)**	**Corbett et al. (3)**	**Masnada et al. (4)**	**Masnada et al. (4)**	**Masnada et al. (4)**	**Masnada et al. (4)**	**Masnada et al. (4)**	**Canafoglia et al. (5)**	**Nashabat et al. (6)**	**Costain et al. (7)**
Case number	Case 1	Case 1	Case 1	Case 1	Case 2	Case 3	Case 4	Case 5	Case 1	Case 1	Case 1
Variant	c.890G>A, p.Arg297Gln *De novo*	c.890G>A, p.Arg297Gln *De novo*	c.890G>A, p.Arg297Gln *De novo*	c.890G>A, p.Arg297Gln *De novo*	c.890G>A, p.Arg297Gln (ovodonation)	c.890G>A, p.Arg297Gln *De novo*	c.890G>A, p.Arg297Gln *De novo*	c.890G>A, p.Arg297Gln (NR)	c.890G>A, p.Arg297Gln *De novo*	c.890 G > A, p.Arg297Gln (consanguinity)	c.890G>A, p.Arg297Gln *De novo*
Functional analisys	NR	Gain of function	Gain of function	NR	NR	NR	NR	NR	NR	NR	NR
Age of onset	15 m	5 m	12 m	10 m	15 m	since birth	6 m	12 m	36 m	20 m	8 m
Seizure type at onset	FS	Febrile SE	T, MC, AS	FS	FS	Infantile spasms	GTCS	GTCS	T	GTCS	T, GTCS, AS, MC
Other seizure types	MC, AS, GTCS	GTCS, AS	NR	GTCS, MC	MC, AS, GTCS	AS w/o MC, GTCS	AAS w/o MC	No	Prominent cortical myoclonus	No	NR
Clinical features	hypotonia and mild ataxia	Moderate-severe ataxia	psychomotor delay	Aggressiveness, stubbornness, psychomotor delay	Moderate ID, language delay, Stubbornness, difficulty of concentration, psychomotor delay	Moderate-severe ID and language delay, psychomotor delay (since birth)	Psychom. dev. delay (8–9 mo), ASD	Learning difficulties	Psychomotor delay, jerky movements of the upper limbs, clumsiness	N	N
Development at onset	Normal	Normal	N	N	Delayed	Delayed	N	Delayed	NR	N	N
EEG findings	BGS, irregular GSW; sleep activation	GSW and poly-Sp-W	GSW and polySp-W; bilateral posterior SW, BGS;	GSW, theta-beta activity + Sp in the midline	Slow background activity, Irregular GSW; sleep activation	BGS, GSW, posterior SW	BGS, right Occipital Sh-W, disorganized BG; irregular 2H GSW	BGS, GSW, Multifocal Epileptiform discharges	GSW; BGS, Sp on the posterior derivations, bilateral Sp during light sleep.	NR	Sp, SpW
Magnetic Resonance Imaging	NR	Normal	mild cerebellar atrophy	Severe cerebellar atrophy, small hippocampi	Severe cerebellar atrophy	N	Hyperintense subcortical white matter lesions	Cerebellar atrophy	Mild cerebellar atrophy, cisterna magna	Brain atrophy+cerebellar hypoplasia	Cerebellar atrophy
Neurological examination	ataxia and obvious delay of development	Moderate-severe ataxia, hyper-reflexia	Ataxia, cerebellar signs on examination, normal eye movement	Tremor, impaired coordination of fine motor skills, ataxia, dysarthria, myoclonia, pyramidal signs	N	Ataxia, finger tremor, impaired coordination	Tremor, ataxia, head titubation, axial hypotonia, pyramidal signs, impaired motor coordination	Impaired incoordination, mild dysdiadochokinesia, mild-moderate ataxia, dysarthria	Ataxia, irregularly repetitive myoclonic jerks during active hand movements	Ataxia	NR
Development at follow up	tremor of the extremities, loss of sphincter control and hyperkinetic behavior	Moderate ID	Slowing at 12 months	NR	NR	NR	NR	NR	Worsening of the movement disorder	Refractory to medications, still having seizure	NR

NR, Not reported; GSW, generalized spike waves; Sp-W, spike-waves; Sp, spikes; Sh-W, sharp waves; BGS, background slowing; N, normal; ID, intellectual disability; ASD, autism spectrum disorder; S, febrile seizure; MC, Myoclonic convulsion; AS, absence seizures; T, tonic; AAS, atypical absence seizures; GTCS, generalized tonic seizures; SE, status epilepticus; EEG, electroencephalogram.

TABLE 2 | Comparison between the characteristics of the patient studied with the only previous case reported in the literature with the same mutation.

	Sachdev et al. (8)	Our patient
Variant	c.889 C>T, p.Arg297Trp *de novo*	c.889 C>T, p.Arg297Trp *de novo*
Functional analisys	Not reported	Not performed
Age of onset	4 years	4 years
Seizure type at onset	Generalized tonic seizures	Absence seizures
Other seizure types	Status epilepticus	Myoclonic convulsion
Development at onset	Normal	Speech delay
EEG findings	Slow posterior dominant rhythm activity, delta activity with Sp, Spike and Slow Waves in the bioccipital regions, Parasagittal ShW and Sp during activity, GSW, bifrontal ShW; GBS	Slow posterior dominant rhythm activity, theta activity with Sp on the parieto-occipital regions, GSW
MRI	Normal	Ectopy of the cerebellar tonsils (6 mm), hyperintensity of the deep white matter in the suvra/paratrigonal, in subcortical area and in the temporal area bilaterally
Neurological examination	Non-fluent language	Tremor of the hands, clumsiness in movement and in fine motricity
Development at follow up	Normal	Normal

GSW, generalized spike waves; Sp, spikes; Sh-W, sharp waves; GBS, global background slowing; EEG, electroencephalogram.

CASE DESCRIPTION

The proband was born at 38 weeks of gestational age through Cesarean section, performed due to maternal-fetal disproportion. Psychomotor development was characterized by autonomous walking at 16 months (referred balance disorder) and mild language delay improved at the age of 30 months after schooling. The patient has been fed with homogenized food up to 24 months of age and showed selectivity in choosing new ones. The parents reported frequent episodes of vomiting (once a week) without nausea, mostly after physical activity. At the age of 2, the boy experienced head trauma after loss of consciousness. Subsequently, the child showed generalized hypertonus, cyanosis, and deviation of the buccal rhyme that lasted about 2 min with self-resolution. The CT scan highlighted a skull fracture without encephalic lesions and a Chiari type 1 malformation, confirmed during the MRI that showed caudal ectopia of cerebellar tonsils (6 mm from Foramen Magnum), hyperintensity of the deep white matter in the suvra/paratrigonal, in subcortical area, and in the temporal area bilaterally, compatible with terminal areas of myelination. Based on the evidence of cerebellar tonsils ectopia, the toddler underwent clinic evaluation for hypermobility, but did not meet Beighton Criteria for Ehlers Danlos Syndrome diagnosis.

At the age of 4 years (**Figure 1A**), the child started experiencing daily episodes of upward movements of the eyebrows associated with staring spells. The first neurological examination showed tremor of both hands at the end of the index-nose test. The toddler asks for support while climbing stairs and when walking. Electroencephalogram (EEG) recordings while awake showed a trace characterized by poorly organized brain electrical activity and differentiated by age, slow anomalies with interictal paroxysmal abnormalities on bilateral parieto-occipital regions, and abundant epileptiform anomalies with diffuse expression, the most prolonged associated with clinical correlates (**Figures 1B,C**). The physical examination does not underline any dysmorphism except for the presence of flaring of the lateral side of the eyebrows. After 3 months, frequency and duration of the seizures had increased (up to 20 episodes/day in clusters), subsequently associated with massive ictal myoclonus of the upper limbs or head of very short duration (80 episodes/day in clusters). A 48-h EEG recording showed multiple episodes of myoclonus and pathologic graphoelements.

Next Generation Sequencing analysis (NGS) performed in trio on a panel of 77 genes related to epilepsy revealed the missense variant c.889C>T; p.Arg297Trp: NM_004974 in the third exon of the KCNA2 gene (potassium channel, voltage-gated, shaker-related subfamily, member 2, chr1:110,593,579-110,631,535;GRCh38, MIM *176262) in a heterozygous state. Sanger sequencing did not detect this variant in parental DNA, suggesting a *de novo* origin of the alteration.

So, the toddler started antiepileptic therapy with sodium valproate at a dosage of 15 mg/kg/day which required, given the poor control of events, a raise to 21 mg/kg/day. This therapy did not result in any change of the clinical picture and EEG pattern. Therefore, after about 2 months of treatment, ethosuximide was added at a dosage of 25 mg/day with a reduction in the seizures and EEG abnormalities. Approximately a year later, due to the poor control of the therapy, valproic acid was raised to 30 mg/Kg/day and ethosuximide to 30 mg/Kg/day with complete resolution of the pathological picture.

At the age of 5 years and 11 months, the toddler has been tested with WPPSI-III, CPM, CBCL, and ABAS II. Based on the evaluation carried out, a normal cognitive functioning emerges (IQ 91), with abilities adequate to the expected level in the verbal performance and general language scale.

There is a significant decline in the domain that evaluates the processing speed. Non-verbal intelligence is adequate for the chronological age. Assessment of the adaptive profile, as reported by the mother of child, showed subnormal scores in

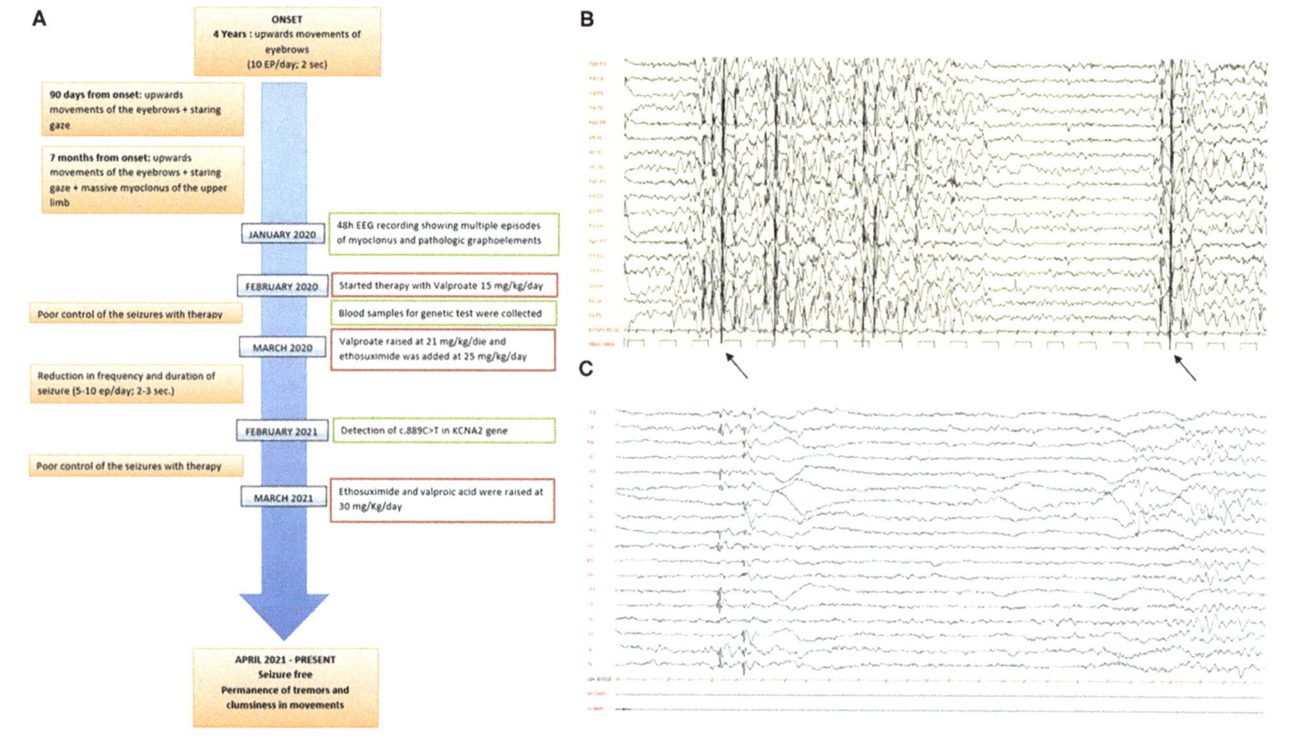

FIGURE 1 | (A) Timeline of clinical features, instrumental characteristics, and therapy approaches in the proband since the toddler started showing epilepsy. **(B,C)** Electroencephalogram (EEG) performed when the child was 4 years old. The trace is characterized by poorly organized brain electrical activity, slow anomalies with interictal paroxysmal abnormalities on bilateral parieto-occipital sites, and abundant epileptiform anomalies with diffuse expression.

the conceptual, social, and practical domains. Critical issues were observed in the categories related to preschool skills, communication, self-control, play, and use of the environment. Currently, the proband presents no epileptic events and improvement in the EEG picture, which still maintains theta-delta slow wave bursts in the occipital regions. Neurological examination appears to be normal, except for tremor of the hands and mild fine motor skills deficit. Some behavioral problems persist. In the EEG assessments carried out from 2017 to 2021, it was evident that the permanence of the slow theta-delta variable rhythm anomalies in the posterior regions, with isolated spike-and-wave complexes on the parieto-occipital sites bilaterally, sometimes fronto- or temporo-central that tend to present in diffuse paroxysms with diffuse expression of varying duration. The associated clinical correlation consists in a reduction in contact, ideomotor slowdown with spontaneous resolution, and asynchronous four-limb myoclonus. Overall, the EEG picture appeared disorganized for the age of child. After 7 months being seizure free, in the latest evaluation, the child no longer presents generalized epileptiform abnormalities.

The psychological tests carried out showed performance at the normal range in the ability to analyze and synthesize visual stimuli based on correct visual perception and visuomotor coordination. In addition, they highlighted results in the average range in logical reasoning and in the ability to abstract reason and categorize visual stimuli. The child showed good expressive and receptive language skills. The scale that assesses skills related to comprehension of verbal terms and instructions associated with long-term memory reached levels above normal. There was a decline in the ability to perform cognitive tasks smoothly and automatically especially under the pressure to maintain focused attention and concentration. Scores showed significantly below normal abilities related to the visual discrimination associated with visual short-term memory and visual-motor coordination and cognitive flexibility; even the ability to work quickly with unusual material achieved below normal performance. The toddler presented a cognitive profile that is adequate to the expected level for gender and age, although there is a significant drop in the domain that assesses the speed of processing. The adaptive framework presents criticalities that currently do not seem to affect the life of the child.

DISCUSSION

This is the first case of a toddler affected by myoclonic epilepsy due to a *de novo* missense pathogenic variant (c.889C>T) in the *KCNA2* gene in the heterozygous state.

The *KCNA2* gene encodes for 2 NCBI Refseq transcripts (NM_004974.4 and NM_001204269.2). Monoallelic *KCNA2* pathogenic variants, encoding the voltage-gated K+ channel Kv1.2, have been reported as a cause of developmental delay and seizures (Developmental and epileptic encephalopathy 32, MIM #616366) (1–3, 9–13).

Mice models, carrying a *KCNA2* mutation, show motor incoordination, myoclonic jerks, tremor, and small body size (14), while null animals present increased seizure susceptibility (15). Previous functional studies showed that *KCNA2* mutations cause either a dominant-negative loss-of-function, or a drastic gain-of function (2), determining distinct phenotypes in patients (4, 16). Alterations, causing loss-of-function, are characterized by a better prognosis than gain-of-function and mixed forms. In dominant-negative loss-of-function, focal predominant seizures with greater sleep activation are reported in literature. In gain-of-function, critical events seem to be prevalently severe generalized seizures, most frequently are problems in neurodevelopment, such as ataxia. At a structural level, the cerebellar or whole brain atrophy has been frequently reported. Severe early onset epilepsies appear to be more frequent in mixed forms. Neonatal onset epilepsies with developmental impairments or generalized ictal events are rare (4, 16, 17). Recently the phenotypic spectrum has been expanded to include forms of progressive myoclonus epilepsy and myoclonic-atonic epilepsy (18) and functional studies of pathogenic variants had been performed (19).

The p.Arg297Trp variant, detected in the present case, is ranked as "Likely Pathogenic" according to the American College of Medical Genetics guidelines and "Pathogenic" according to ClinVar. Allele frequency is not available. The case we describe here represents the first in pediatric age and the second overall case of myoclonic epilepsy caused by this heterozygous pathogenic variant in *KCNA2*.

The toddler presented at the onset generalized epileptiform abnormalities that were often associated with upward movements of the eyebrows, fixation gaze, and ictal myoclonus of head and upper limbs. The toddler still presents difficulties in autonomous walking and while climbing stairs. The parents reported weekly vomiting episodes not preceded by nausea mostly associated with physical exercise, that could represent a clinical manifestation of seizure. After the therapeutical adjustments, given the considerable reduction in ictal events and the inability to perform a functional analysis of the gene, it has not been possible to attempt therapeutic strategies as recently suggested by the literature, such as 4-aminopyridine (20).

During sleep EEG showed fast/slow wave and polypoint/slow wave of medium- or large-voltage, on the fronto-central regions bilaterally, electrical status epilepticus during sleep (ESES) was not present as described by previous authors (21).

A literature review was conducted to identify the characteristics of reported patients who presented a mutation at the same triplet encoding an amino acid (as shown in **Table 1**). A case with the same mutation was described (8): the patient, differently from our toddler, was diagnosed with unprovoked generalized tonic-clonic seizures. Age of onset was 4 years old in a normal psychomotor neurodevelopment. After carbamazepine treatment, the boy showed seizure remittance. The toddler was worsened from 19 years old, when started presenting episodes of refractory status epilepticus strongly drug resistant. Similarly to our patient, EEG at the age of 4 was characterized by continuous polymorphic delta and theta slowing of the posterior dominant rhythm, intermittent bursts of rhythmic 2–2.5 Hz delta activity intermixed with spikes, spike-and-slow wave discharges over the bi-occipital regions, and isolated parasagittal sharp wave and spike activity during sleep.

Sachdev et al. (8) compared the similar clinical picture of their patient carrying the c.889 C>T mutation, to the reported cases detected with the c.890 G>A mutation in the same amino acidic site, differently from our patient that presents a mild clinical history. In **Table 2**, we compare the characteristics of the patient analyzed in this study with the only previous case reported in the literature with the same mutation (8).

Several cases detected with the c.890G>A p.(Arg297Gln) variant in the KCNA2 gene had been reported, expanding the clinical spectrum of developmental and epileptic encephalopathy and highlighting the variable expressivity. Progressive myoclonic epilepsy was described in one of the patients described by Canafoglia (5). This case showed ataxia and psychomotor delay, whereas epilepsy was delayed and limited to relatively rare tonic seizures, associated with prominent cortical myoclonus, occurred at 3 years. Syrbe et al. (2) reported the case of a toddler carrying a c.890G>A p.(Arg297Gln) *de novo* mutation in the *KCNA2* gene, whose functional analysis showed a gain-of-function alteration. The patient, differently from the reported case, experienced generalized tonic-clonic seizures, absences, status epilepticus often during febrile events. Moreover, the patient presented moderate-severe ataxia and moderate intellectual disability. The same nucleotidic variant was described in a patient with myoclonic and absence seizures. The age of onset, the clinical, and the neuropsychological deterioration was different from our case, resulting in a progressive worsening and drug resistance.

Masnada et al. (4) enrolled five patients carrying this mutation in the KCNA2 gene. Differently from the present case, all of them showed generalized tonic-clonic seizures, but they all presented tremors, ataxia, and a moderate intellectual disability. Two of them experienced myoclonic seizures associated with absences. Only one was seizure-free from 18 months of age. Corbett et al. (3) reported a patient that started having tonic seizures at 12 months, progressing in erratic myoclonic tremors. The proband showed different ictal phenotypes, while EEG and the neuropsychological evaluation showed similar results. Nashabat et al. (6) described the case of a patient that, differently from the present case, experienced earlier onset of generalized tonic-clonic seizures in a good global development, but with poor response to therapy. Costain et al. (7) reported a patient showing various ictal events, such as generalized tonic and tonic-clonic seizures, absences, and myoclonic seizures. This toddler presented an earlier age of onset, a good global development, and ataxia. Ngo et al. (22) described a case with apparently isolated ataxia as primary symptom, but no more clinical information was provided.

Interestingly, an unusual case of mosaicism of two novel missense variants in *KCNA2* had been reported, expanding the phenotypic spectrum associated with this mutations of gene, but not presenting with myoclonic epilepsy (23).

CONCLUSIONS

The present case aims to expand the clinical spectrum associated with heterozygous *KCNA2* pathogenic variants. This evidence suggests a genotype-first approach, performing genomic tests that include the *KCNA2* gene, in patients with myoclonic epilepsy diagnosis. According to the literature, we highlight the variability in expression that can be clinically observed in patients with heterogeneous ictal events (15), even in those who show mutations in the same triplet encoding an amino acid. Indeed, the patient we describe presented a good prognosis characterized by a good response to therapy, and an improved neurodevelopment, in contrast with the previously reported cases, presenting with a more severe clinical picture (1, 2, 11).

We suggest that an accurate clinical examination improve the detection of genotype-phenotype correlations and expand the possibility of predicting the functional impact of *KCNA2* variants (18). Even if it is a rare condition, a *KCNA2* gene mutation test should be performed in patients over 3 years of age.

ETHICS STATEMENT

Ethical review and approval was not required for the study on human participants in accordance with the local legislation and institutional requirements. Written informed consent to participate in this study was provided by the participants' legal guardian/next of kin.

AUTHOR CONTRIBUTIONS

LP, GM, MM, IA, FA, AP, CG, and AS: conceptualization, data curation, resources, investigation, writing—original draft, methodology, visualization, supervision, and writing—review and editing. All authors contributed to the article and approved the submitted version.

REFERENCES

1. Pena SD, Coimbra RL. Ataxia and myoclonic epilepsy due to a heterozygous new mutation in KCNA2: proposal for a new channelopathy. *Clin Genet.* (2015) 87:e1–3. doi: 10.1111/cge.12542
2. Syrbe S, Hedrich UBS, Riesch E, Djémié T, Müller S, Møller RS, et al. *De novo* loss- or gain-of function mutations in KCNA2 cause epileptic encephalopathy. *Nat Genet.* (2015) 47:393–9. doi: 10.1038/ng.3239
3. Corbett MA, Bellows ST, Li M, Carroll R, Micallef S, Carvill GL, et al. Dominant KCNA2 mutation causes episodic ataxia and pharmacoresponsive epilepsy. *Neurology.* (2016) 87:1975–84. doi: 10.1212/WNL.0000000000003309
4. Masnada S, Hedrich UBS, Gardella E, Schubert J, Kaiwar C, Klee EW, et al. Clinical spectrum and genotype-phenotype associations of KCNA2-related encephalopathies. *Brain.* (2017) 140:2337–54. doi: 10.1093/brain/awx184
5. Canafoglia L, Castellotti B, Ragona F, Freri E, Granata T, Chiapparini L, et al. Progressive myoclonus epilepsy caused by a gain-of-function KCNA2 mutation. *Seizure.* (2019) 65:106–8. doi: 10.1016/j.seizure.2019.01.005
6. Nashabat M, Al Qahtani XS, Almakdob S, Altwaijri W, Ba-Armah DM, Hundallah K, et al. The landscape of early infantile epileptic encephalopathy in a consanguineous population. *Seizure.* (2019) 69:154–72. doi: 10.1016/j.seizure.2019.04.018
7. Costain G, Cordeiro D, Matviychuk D, Mercimek-Andrews S. Clinical application of targeted next-generation sequencing panels and whole exome sequencing in childhood epilepsy. *Neuroscience.* (2019) 418:291–310. doi: 10.1016/j.neuroscience.2019.08.016
8. Sachdev M, Gaínza-Lein M, Tchapyjnikov D, Jiang YH, Loddenkemper T, Mikati MA. Novel clinical manifestations in patients with KCNA2 mutations. *Seizure.* (2017) 51:74–6. doi: 10.1016/j.seizure.2017.07.018
9. Tang S, Addis L, Smith A, Topp SD, Pendziwiat M, Mei D, et al. Phenotypic and genetic spectrum of epilepsy with myoclonic atonic seizures. *Epilepsia.* (2020) 61:995–1007. doi: 10.1111/epi.16508
10. Allen NM, Conroy J, Shahwan A, Lynch B, Correa RG, Pena SD, et al. Unexplained early onset epileptic encephalopathy: exome screening and phenotype expansion. *Epilepsia.* (2016) 57:e12–7. doi: 10.1111/epi.13250
11. Hundallah K, Alenizi A, AlHashem A, Tabarki B. Severe early-onset epileptic encephalopathy due to mutations in the KCNA2 gene: expansion of the genotypic and phenotypic spectrum. *Eur J Paediatr Neurol.* (2016) 20:657–60. doi: 10.1016/j.ejpn.2016.03.011
12. Drögemöller BI. Maintaining the balance: both gain- and loss-of-function KCNA2 mutants cause epileptic encephalopathy. *Clin Genet.* (2015) 88:137–9. doi: 10.1111/cge.12615
13. Allou L, Julia S, Amsallem D, El Chehadeh S, Lambert L, Thevenon J, et al. Rett-like phenotypes: expanding the genetic heterogeneity to the KCNA2 gene and first familial case of CDKL5-related disease. *Clin Genet.* (2017) 91:431–40. doi: 10.1111/cge.12784
14. Xie G, Harrison J, Clapcote SJ, Huang Y, Zhang JY, Wang LY, et al. A new Kv1.2 channelopathy underlying cerebellar ataxia. *J Biol Chem.* (2010) 285:32160–73. doi: 10.1074/jbc.M110.153676
15. Brew HM, Gittelman JX, Silverstein RS, Hanks TD, Demas VP, Robinson LC, et al. Seizures and reduced life span in mice lacking the potassium channel subunit Kv1.2, but hypoexcitability and enlarged Kv1 currents in auditory neurons. *J Neurophysiol.* (2007) 98:1501–25. doi: 10.1152/jn.00640.2006
16. Morrison-Levy N, Borlot F, Jain P, Whitney R. Early-onset developmental and epileptic encephalopathies of infancy: an overview of the genetic basis and clinical features. *Pediatr Neurol.* (2021) 116:85–94. doi: 10.1016/j.pediatrneurol.2020.12.001
17. Steel D, Symonds JD, Zuberi SM, Brunklaus A. Dravet syndrome and its mimics: beyond SCN1A. *Epilepsia.* (2017) 58:1807–16. doi: 10.1111/epi.13889
18. Döring JH, Schröter J, Jüngling J, Biskup S, Klotz KA, Bast T, et al. Refining genotypes and phenotypes in KCNA2-related neurological disorders. *Int J Mol Sci.* (2021) 22:2824. doi: 10.3390/ijms22062824ijms22062824
19. Arbini A, Gilmore J, King MD, Gorman KM, Krawczyk J, McInerney V, et al. Generation of three induced pluripotent stem cell (iPSC) lines from a patient with developmental epileptic encephalopathy due to the pathogenic KCNA2 variant c.869T>G; p.Leu290Arg (NUIGi052-A, NUIGi052-B, NUIGi052-C). *Stem Cell Res.* (2020) 46:101853. doi: 10.1016/j.scr.2020.101853
20. Imbrici P, Conte E, Blunck R, Stregapede F, Liantonio A, Tosi M, et al. A novel *KCNA2* variant in a patient with non-progressive congenital ataxia and epilepsy: functional characterization and sensitivity to 4-aminopyridine. *Int J Mol Sci.* (2021) 22:9913. doi: 10.3390/ijms22189913
21. Gong P, Xue J, Jiao X, Zhang Y, Yang Z. Genetic etiologies in developmental and/or epileptic encephalopathy with electrical status epilepticus during sleep: cohort study. *Front Genet.* (2021) 12:607965. doi: 10.3389/fgene.2021.607965
22. Ngo KJ, Rexach JE, Lee H, Petty LE, Perlman S, Valera JM, et al. A diagnostic ceiling for exome sequencing in cerebellar ataxia and related neurological disorders. *Hum Mutat.* (2020) 41:487–501. doi: 10.1002/humu.23946
23. Gong P, Jiao X, Zhang Y, Yang Z. Complex mosaicism of two distinct mutations in a female patient with *KCNA2*-related encephalopathy: a case report. *Front Genet.* (2020) 11:911. doi: 10.3389/fgene.2020.

21

Case Report: Hypopituitarism Presenting with Nonconvulsive Status Epilepticus

Huimin Li, Lina Xu, Fengbing Yang, Longbin Jia, Hongjiang Cheng and Wei Liu*

Jincheng People's Hospital Affiliated to Shanxi Medical University, Jincheng, China

Correspondence:
Longbin Jia
sxjcjlb@163.com

Introduction: Hypopituitarism is defined as one or more partial or complete pituitary hormone deficiencies. Nonconvulsive status epilepticus (NCSE) refers to a state of continuous or repetitive seizures without convulsions. In this paper, we review a case of an old female patient with hypopituitarism who presented with NCSE, which is rare in the clinic.

Case Report: This paper describes a 67-year-old female patient with hypopituitarism who presented as NCSE. She had surgical resection of pituitary tumor half a year before the seizures and did not get regular hormone replacement therapy. She presented general convulsive status epilepsy as the initial symptom and got sedation and antiepileptic drug in the emergency room. The seizure was terminated but the patient fell in coma in the following days. The patient had magnetic resonance imaging (MRI) and other inspects, and EEG showed epileptic discharges. Combining these clinical symptoms and examinations, we made the diagnosis of NCSE. Finally, she regained consciousness after the treatment with diazepam.

Conclusion: This case report and literature review investigated the possible mechanism of hypopituitarism presenting with NCSE.

Keywords: nonconvulsive status epilepticus, hypopituitarism, hormone, seizure, case report

INTRODUCTION

Status epilepticus (SE) refers to a condition caused either by the failure of seizure termination or by the initiation of prolonged seizures. According to the classification of SE proposed by the International League Against Epilepsy (ILAE), NCSE is defined as SE without prominent motor symptoms, including NCSE with coma and NCSE without coma (1). The role of hormones in the pathophysiology of epilepsy has been gradually recognized (2, 3). In this paper, we report a patient with hypopituitarism presenting with NCSE.

CASE REPORT

A 67-year-old woman with diabetes was admitted to the emergency department due to two generalized tonic-clonic seizures and loss of awareness in the interictal period. The patient had never experienced seizures before. Half a year ago she had surgical resection of pituitary tumor and did not get regular hormone replacement treatment. In the days leading up to the seizures, she did not have any signs of discomfort such as fever or headache. In the emergency room diazepam (5 mg, i.v.) and sodium valproate (50 mg, intravenous pumped at the rate of 160 mg/h) were given immediately as antiepileptic therapy, the seizures were terminated in several minutes and the patient fell in state of sedation shortly after, during which the patient could gradually open her eyes, answer simple questions and no more convulsions were observed. Routine blood tests in the emergency department showed hyperglycaemia (13.0 mmol/L), mild hypernatremia (151.7 mmol/L), and hyperchloremia (111.3 mmol/L). Then she was admitted to the neurology department and rescue measures including oxygen inhalation, antiepileptic therapy with sodium valproate (56 mg/h, 1 mg/kg/h), rehydration, maintaining water, and electrolyte balance were continued. About 3 h later, the patient passed into a lethargic state and she could only open her eyes on hearing our call but could not respond in words (GCS score of 8). The lethargic state continued for several hours and the patient fell in coma then (GCS score of 5), which lasted for the following 3 days. During this period the sodium valproate was pumped for 36 h continuously (56 mg/h for 24 h, 50 mg/h for 12 h, 24 mg/h for 12 h, total dose of 2,232 mg) and no remarkable facial or limb spasms or convulsions were recorded from admission. Tests of thyroid function, adrenocorticotropic hormone (ACTH), growth hormone (GH), cortisol, and sex hormone were conducted and the results supported the diagnosis of hypopituitarism (**Table 1**). MRI of the head was performed and no acute cerebral infarction, cerebral hemorrhage, and inflammatory changes were found (**Figure 1**). A lumbar puncture was performed to the patient on the 2nd day of admission. The cerebrospinal fluid (CSF) showed elevated protein levels (0.60/L, reference range 0.15–0.45 g/L) and increased chloride (137.8 mmol/L, reference range 118–132 mmol/L) and normal glucose levels and CSF pressure (**Table 1**). Autoimmune encephalitis and viral encephalitis tests were both negative, and thus the diagnosis of encephalitis was ruled out. A 24-h electroencephalogram (EEG) revealed sharp waves, spike waves, sharp-slow waves, spike-slow waves in the bilateral frontal region on a continuous slow-wave background with a trend of evolution, and the EEG also recorded paroxysmal electrical activities in this region (**Figure 2**). Combining the symptoms and examinations, the diagnosis of NCSE was considered. On the 3rd day of admission, diazepam (10 mg) was intravenously injected and the patient turned to a state of lethargy gradually and could open her eyes under painful stimulation, confirming the diagnosis of NCSE. Unfortunately, her family refused further treatment and she was discharged on the 3rd day, and she died of respiratory failure induced by epilepsy 5 days after her discharge from our hospital.

DISCUSSION

NCSE refers to a continuous nonconvulsive seizure that lasts for more than 30 min, or multiple nonconvulsive seizures happening during a period of more than 30 min and between which cognitive, motor, and/or sensory disorders is not fully recovered (4). Patients with NCSE can present as a variety of clinical manifestations, among which altered mental status is the most common (5). As the symptoms of NCSE are various, the diagnosis of NCSE relies on the combination of clinical presentation, electroencephalography findings, and clinical and electrographical reactions to antiepileptic treatments (4). The transition from generalized convulsive status epilepticus (GCSE) to NCSE is common: studies found that NCSE was quite common in patients in the ICU, accounting for about 50% (4). In our case, the patient initially presented as GCSE and went into coma which was diagnosed as NCSE finally.

The aetiology and risk factors of NCSE are complex, including acute and chronic pathological conditions (4). The role of endocrine system diseases in the pathogenesis and treatment of epilepsy has been studied continuously.

TABLE 1 | Laboratory data.

Test	Result	Normal range of value	Test	Result	Normal range of value
GH	0.031 ng/ml	(0.126–9.880)	FT3	2.40 pmol/L	(3.28–6.47)
Cortisol (00:00)	18.67 nmol/L	(185–624)	FT4	9.51 pmol/L	(7.64–16.03)
Cortisol (08:00)	17.28 nmol/L	(185–624)	TT3	0.24 nmol/L	(1.01–2.48)
Cortisol (16:00)	25.54 nmol/L	(185–624)	TT4	54.30 nmol/L	(69.97–152.52)
ACTH (00:00)	<1.00 pg/ml	(7.20–63.40)	TSH	0.04 uIU/ml	(0.56–5.91)
ACTH (08:00)	<1.00 pg/ml	(7.20–63.40)	Estradiol	0.02 pg/ml	(10–30)
ACTH (16:00)	<1.00 pg/ml	(7.20–63.40)	Testosterone	<0.1 ng/ml	(0.1–0.75)
Prolactin	28.67 ng/ml	(2.74–19.64)	Progesterone	<0.08 ng/ml	(<1.0 ng/ml)
LH	0.30 mIU/ml	(10.87–58.64)	FSH	10.87 mIU/ml	(16.74–113.5)
CSF protein	0.60 g/L	(0.15–0.45)	CSF chloride	137.8 mmol/L	(118–132)
CSF glucose	3.82 mmol/L	(2.5–4.2)	CSF white blood cell	0.002 × 10^9/L	(0–8)
CSF red blood cell	0.002 × 10^{12}/L	0			

Tests of hormone levels support the diagnosis of hypopituitarism.

GH, growth hormone; ACTH, adrenocorticotropic hormone; LH, luteinising hormone; FSH, folliclestimulating hormone; TSH, thyroid-stimulating hormone; FT3, free triiodothyronine; FT4, free thyroxine; TT3, total triiodothyronine; TT4, total thyroxine.

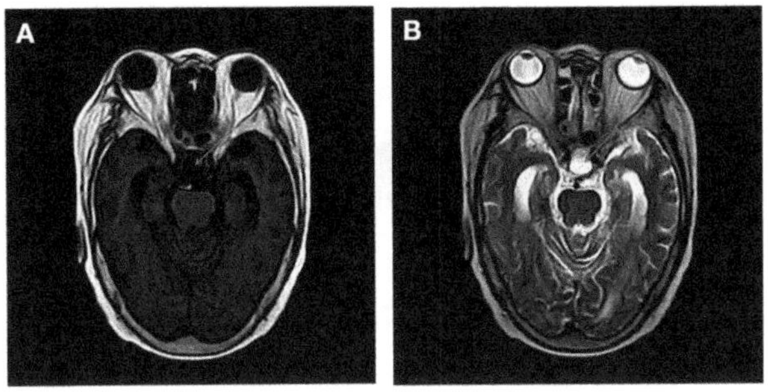

FIGURE 1 | MRI of the brain revealed change after removal of pituitary tumor and no acute cerebral infarction, cerebral hemorrhage, and inflammatory changes were found on T1 and T2 sequences [T1, T1-Weighted Magnetic Resonance Imaging; T2, T2-Weighted Magnetic Resonance Imaging **(A)** T1, **(B)** T2].

Hypopituitarism is defined as deficiency of one or more pituitary hormones produced in the anterior lobe and posterior lobe, including GH, the gonadotropins follicle stimulating hormone (FSH) and luteinizing hormone (LH), ACTH, thyroid stimulating hormone (TSH), prolactin, oxytocin, and antidiuretic hormone (ADH) (6).

Metabolic encephalopathy can also present with disorders of consciousness and it can be differentiated from NCSE by etiology, laboratory examination, and EEG. While increasing slowing of the waking background frequency was observed in hyperglycemia and hypoglycemia, hyponatremia may initially produce posterior slowing followed by more diffuse delta activity (7), hypopituitarism and hypoadrenalism may cause diffuse theta and delta activity. Furthermore, diffuse suppression with scant activity may be found in patients with hypothyroidism (8).

The relation between hormones and epilepsy is complicated. Concerning sex hormones, while androgens, progesterone and its metabolites have been found to have anticonvulsant effects, proconvulsant effects of estrogens were well-described (9). Studies have found that changes in hormone levels correspond to changes in seizures' frequency, which was considered as the effect of hormones on brain excitability (9), and this association was well-documented in catamenial epilepsy, in which the distribution of seizure numbers varied across the days of the menstrual cycle (10). Our patient showed remarkably low level of sex hormones including estradiol, FSH, LH, progesterone, and testosterone, making the evaluation of the role of any single hormone in the seizures complicated. Studies have found increased serum prolactin in about 67% of cases after complex-partial seizures or generalized tonic-clonic seizures (11, 12). Our patient had a relatively high level of prolactin, which was consistent with the previous reports.

The use of sex steroid hormones or their analogs for the treatment of epilepsy has been studied (13). It has been shown that supplementation of progesterone was effective in the management of seizure in patients with anovulatory cycles (14). Indeed, studies have confirmed that hormones including corticosteroids and ACTH were effective in the management of pediatric epilepsies including West syndrome, the Landau–Kleffner syndrome, other epilepsies, and epilepsy syndromes (15, 16).

It has been reported increasingly that stress plays a role in precipitating seizures (17, 18). Preclinical models of epilepsy showed that neuronal excitability and seizure susceptibility were both influenced by stress hormones (19). The hypothalamic-pituitary-adrenal axis is the main neuroendocrine system activated by stress (20). Studies on animal models revealed that neuronal excitability and seizure threshold were affected by stress hormones including corticotrophic hormone and corticosterone (21). It was reported that excitability of neurons was increased under the influence of corticotropin-releasing hormone (CRH) both *in vivo* and *in vitro*, and thus seizure activity was induced (22). Given the negative feedback effect of the hypothalamus-pituitary-adrenal axis, our patient should theoretically have high levels of CRH which may induce seizures.

Under basal conditions, stress hormones can also affect disease activity in seizures (23). In most of the studies, it was shown that increases in cortisol levels were a promoter during epileptogenesis (24, 25). But Ostrowska's team had the opposite conclusion and they found that patients with epilepsy had lower cortisol levels than those without epilepsy (26). Pritchard et al. (27) found that before generalized tonic-clonic seizures and complex partial seizures, the cortisol levels increased, while before simple partial seizures and secondary generalized seizures, the results were opposite (28). More importantly, patients with epilepsy often showed increased cortisol levels (29, 30). While the mechanisms of interaction between stress and seizures are not entirely clear, both of the two would have impact on cortisol levels.

Zhang and Liu (28) conducted a study analysing ACTH and cortisol levels during sleep seizures had found that during and after an epileptic seizure, the ACTH and cortisol levels were higher than those before a seizure. The researchers believed that epileptic seizures may be induced by decrease in ACTH and cortisol levels. A possible explanation may be that at night the decrease in ACTH levels triggers the release of CRH through negative feedback regulation, and the release of CRH increase epilepsy susceptibility and lower epilepsy threshold (21, 31).

Although the mechanisms of epileptogenesis still remain to be unclear, it is well-proved that mitochondrial dysfunction (32, 33) and oxidative stress (34) play important roles in this process. Molecular evidences have revealed that thyroid hormones are involved in normal mitochondrial biogenesis and function (35) and decreased activity of thyroid hormones is related to mitochondrial dysfunction (36). As to oxidative stress, both hyperthyroidism and hypothyroidism can affect antioxidant/oxidant balance (37). The impact of thyroid hormones in different aspects of epilepsy has been demonstrated (37). Thyroid function tests showed obvious hypothyroidism in our patient, which may also play an important role in the occurrence of epilepsy.

Treatments of NCSE should be based on expert opinions as well as individual aetiology including critical illness, subtherapeutic AED levels, etc. Recommendations for first-line

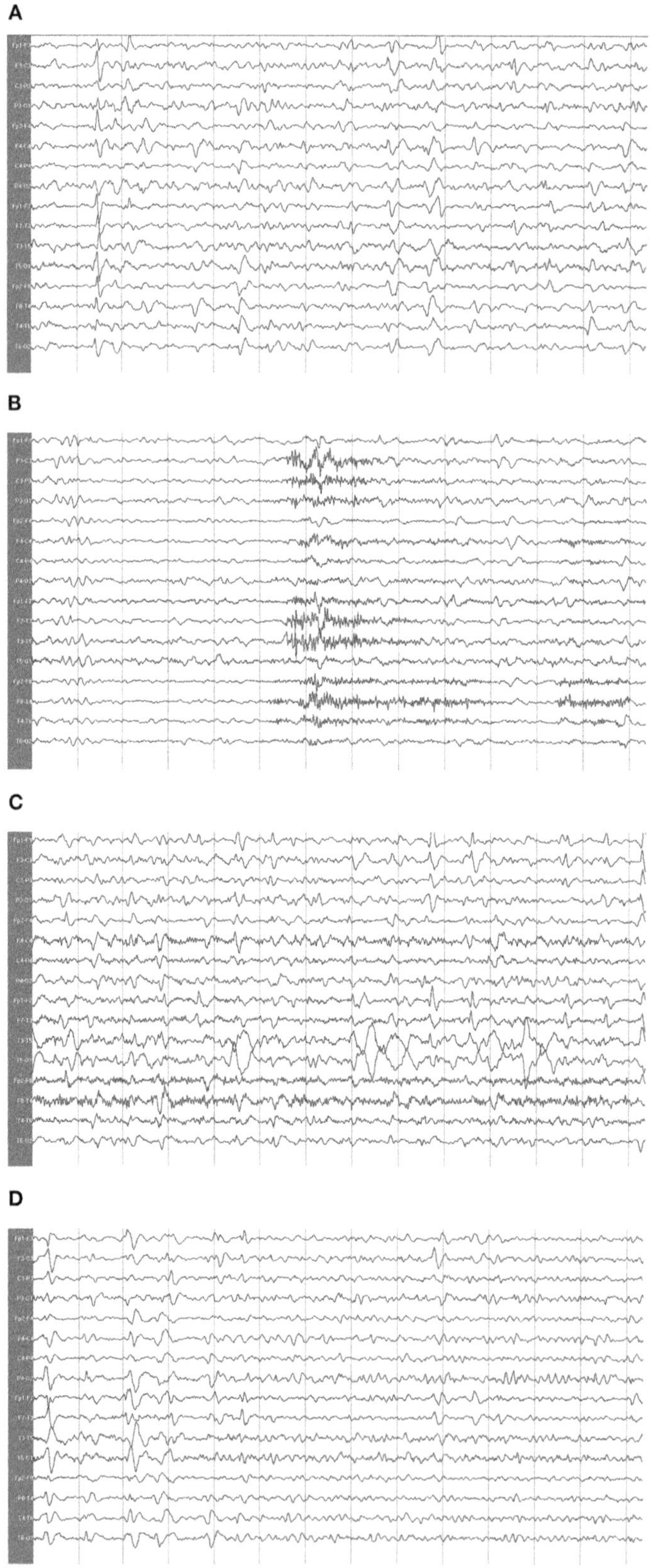

FIGURE 2 | Electroencephalogram recorded. EEG demonstrates δ and θ waves in each lead as background, mingled with sharp waves, spike waves, sharp-slow waves **(A)**. EEG shows a large number of sharp waves, spike waves, sharp-slow waves, spike-slow waves in the bilateral frontal pole, frontal and anterior temporal areas, paroxysmal or continuous, sometimes accompanied by evolution trend **(B–D)** (paper speed: 30 mm/s, high-frequency filter (HF): 30 Hz, low-frequency filter (LF): 0.53 Hz, notchfilers: 50 Hz, sensitivity:7 μv/mm. EEG A provided EEG background and the EEG B showed epileptic discharges).

treatment of NCSE are usually benzodiazepines (4). In our patient, recovery of impaired consciousness after the use of diazepam confirmed the diagnosis of NCSE. Regrettably, the patient did not receive systemic therapy and passed away finally.

CONCLUSION

In summary, our case, an old woman with hypopituitarism presenting with NCSE, led us to further explore the complex relationship between epilepsy and hormones, which contributes to the accurate diagnosis and treatment.

ETHICS STATEMENT

The study involving a human participant was reviewed and approved by the Ethics committee of Jincheng People's Hospital, Jincheng, China. The patient provided her written informed consent to participate in this study. Written informed consent was obtained from the individual for the publication of any potentially identifiable images or data included in this article.

AUTHOR CONTRIBUTIONS

LJ put forward research ideas. LX took the responsibility of communicating with the patient's family and obtaining the authorization in this paper. HL was responsible for drafting articles. FY revised the article. HC and WL were responsible for literature searches and final proofreading. All authors contributed to the article and approved the submitted version.

REFERENCES

1. Trinka E, Cock H, Hesdorffer D, Rossetti A, Scheffer I, Shinnar S, et al. A definition and classification of status epilepticus–Report of the ILAE Task Force on Classification of Status Epilepticus. *Epilepsia.* (2015) 56:1515–23. doi: 10.1111/epi.13121
2. Harden C, Pennell P. Neuroendocrine considerations in the treatment of men and women with epilepsy. *Lancet Neurol.* (2013) 12:72–83. doi: 10.1016/S1474-4422(12)70239-9
3. Pack A, Reddy D, Duncan S, Herzog A. Neuroendocrinological aspects of epilepsy: important issues and trends in future research. *Epilepsy Behav.* (2011) 22:94–102. doi: 10.1016/j.yebeh.2011.02.009
4. Sutter R, Semmlack S, Kaplan PW. Nonconvulsive status epilepticus in adults - insights into the invisible. *Nat Rev Neurol.* (2016) 12:281–93. doi: 10.1038/nrneurol.2016.45
5. Sutter R, Ruegg S, Kaplan PW. Epidemiology, diagnosis, and management of nonconvulsive status epilepticus: opening Pandora's box. *Neurol Clin Pract.* (2012) 2:275–86. doi: 10.1212/CPJ.0b013e318278be75
6. Higham CE, Johannsson G, Shalet SM. Hypopituitarism. *Lancet.* (2016) 388:2403–15. doi: 10.1016/S0140-6736(16)30053-8
7. Reddy V, Moorthy S. Electroencephalographic and clinical correlation of hyponatremia induced during transurethral resection of the prostate. *Ann Neurol.* (2001) 50:554–5. doi: 10.1002/ana.1241
8. Kaplan P. The EEG in metabolic encephalopathy and coma. *J Clin Neurophysiol.* (2004) 21:307–18. doi: 10.1080/13803390490509574
9. Taubøll E, Sveberg L, Svalheim S. Interactions between hormones and epilepsy. *Seizure.* (2015) 28:3–11. doi: 10.1016/j.seizure.2015.02.012
10. Herzog A. Catamenial epilepsy: update on prevalence, pathophysiology and treatment from the findings of the NIH Progesterone Treatment Trial. *Seizure.* (2015) 28:18–25. doi: 10.1016/j.seizure.2015.02.024
11. Trimble M. Serum prolactin in epilepsy and hysteria. *Br Med J.* (1978) 2:1682. doi: 10.1136/bmj.2.6153.1682
12. Bauer J. Epilepsy and prolactin in adults: a clinical review. *Epilepsy Res.* (1996) 24:1–7. doi: 10.1016/0920-1211(96)00009-5
13. Pennell PB. Hormonal aspects of epilepsy. *Neurol Clin.* (2009) 27:941–65. doi: 10.1016/j.ncl.2009.08.005
14. Bauer J. Interactions between hormones and epilepsy in female patients. *Epilepsia.* (2001) 42(Suppl. 3):20–2. doi: 10.1046/j.1528-1157.2001.042suppl.3020.x
15. Gupta R, Appleton R. Corticosteroids in the management of the paediatric epilepsies. *Arch Dis Childhood.* (2005) 90:379–84. doi: 10.1136/adc.2004.051375
16. Brunson K, Avishai-Eliner S, Baram T. ACTH treatment of infantile spasms: mechanisms of its effects in modulation of neuronal excitability. *Int Rev Neurobiol.* (2002) 49:185–97. doi: 10.1016/S0074-7742(02)49013-7
17. Lang J, Taylor D, Kasper B. Stress, seizures, and epilepsy: patient narratives. *Epilepsy Behav.* (2018) 80:163–72. doi: 10.1016/j.yebeh.2018.01.005
18. Novakova B, Harris P, Ponnusamy A, Reuber M. The role of stress as a trigger for epileptic seizures: a narrative review of evidence from human and animal studies. *Epilepsia.* (2013) 54:1866–76. doi: 10.1111/epi.12377
19. van Campen J, Jansen F, de Graan P, Braun K, Joels M. Early life stress in epilepsy: a seizure precipitant and risk factor for epileptogenesis. *Epilepsy Behav.* (2014) 38:160–71. doi: 10.1016/j.yebeh.2013.09.029
20. van Campen JS, Hompe EL, Jansen FE, Velis DN, Otte WM, van de Berg F, et al. Cortisol fluctuations relate to interictal epileptiform discharges in stress sensitive epilepsy. *Brain.* (2016) 139:1673–9. doi: 10.1093/brain/aww071
21. Joëls M. Stress, the hippocampus, and epilepsy. *Epilepsia.* (2009) 50:586–97. doi: 10.1111/j.1528-1167.2008.01902.x
22. Baram T, Schultz L. Corticotropin-releasing hormone is a rapid and potent convulsant in the infant rat. *Brain Res Dev Brain Res.* (1991) 61:97–101. doi: 10.1016/0165-3806(91)90118-3
23. Cano-López I, González-Bono E. Cortisol levels and seizures in adults with epilepsy: a systematic review. *Neurosci Biobehav Rev.* (2019) 103:216–29. doi: 10.1016/j.neubiorev.2019.05.023
24. Galimberti C, Magri F, Copello F, Arbasino C, Cravello L, Casu M, et al. Seizure frequency and cortisol and dehydroepiandrosterone sulfate (DHEAS) levels in women with epilepsy receiving antiepileptic drug treatment. *Epilepsia.* (2005) 46:517–23. doi: 10.1111/j.0013-9580.2005.59704.x
25. Gallagher B, Murvin A, Flanigin H, King D, Luney D. Pituitary and adrenal function in epileptic patients. *Epilepsia.* (1984) 25:683–9. doi: 10.1111/j.1528-1157.1984.tb03477.x
26. Ostrowska Z, Buntner B, Rościszewska D, Guz I. Adrenal cortex hormones in male epileptic patients before and during a 2-year phenytoin treatment. *J Neurol Neurosurg Psychiatry.* (1988) 51:374–8. doi: 10.1136/jnnp.51.3.374
27. Pritchard P, Wannamaker B, Sagel J, Daniel C. Serum prolactin and cortisol levels in evaluation of pseudoepileptic seizures. *Ann Neurol.* (1985) 18:87–9. doi: 10.1002/ana.410180115
28. Zhang S, Liu Y. Changes of serum adrenocorticotropic hormone and cortisol levels during sleep seizures. *Neurosci Bull.* (2008) 24:84–8. doi: 10.1007/s12264-008-0084-8
29. Bazil C, Short D, Crispin D, Zheng W. Patients with intractable epilepsy have low melatonin, which increases following seizures. *Neurology.* (2000) 55:1746–8. doi: 10.1212/WNL.55.11.1746
30. Abbott R, Browning M, Davidson D. Serum prolactin and cortisol concentrations after grand mal seizures. *J Neurol Neurosurg Psychiatry.* (1980) 43:163–7. doi: 10.1136/jnnp.43.2.163
31. Hooper A, Paracha R, Maguire J. Seizure-induced activation of the HPA axis increases seizure frequency and comorbid depression-like behaviors. *Epilepsy Behav.* (2018) 78:124–33. doi: 10.1016/j.yebeh.2017.10.025
32. Jarrett S, Liang L, Hellier J, Staley K, Patel M. Mitochondrial DNA damage and impaired base excision repair during epileptogenesis. *Neurobiol Dis.* (2008) 30:130–8. doi: 10.1016/j.nbd.2007.12.009

33. Kudin A, Zsurka G, Elger C, Kunz W. Mitochondrial involvement in temporal lobe epilepsy. *Exp Neurol.* (2009) 218:326–32. doi: 10.1016/j.expneurol.2009.02.014
34. Tsai H, Chang C, Chang S. The effects of pilocarpine-induced status epilepticus on oxidative stress/damage in developing animals. *Brain Dev.* (2010) 32:25–31. doi: 10.1016/j.braindev.2009.02.013
35. Yuen A, Sander J. Impaired mitochondrial energy production: the basis of pharmacoresistance in epilepsy. *Med Hypotheses.* (2011) 77:536–40. doi: 10.1016/j.mehy.2011.06.025
36. Wilms L, Larsen J, Pedersen P, Kvetny J. Evidence of mitochondrial dysfunction in obese adolescents. *Acta Paediatr.* (2010) 99:906–11. doi: 10.1111/j.1651-2227.2009.01635.x
37. Tamijani SMS, Karimi B, Amini E, Golpich M, Dargahi L, Ali RA, et al. Thyroid hormones: possible roles in epilepsy pathology. *Seizure.* (2015) 31:155–64. doi: 10.1016/j.seizure.2015.07.021

22

Targeting Inflammatory Mediators in Epilepsy: A Systematic Review of its Molecular Basis and Clinical Applications

Giorgio Costagliola [1†], Greta Depietri [2†], Alexandre Michev [3], Antonella Riva [4], Thomas Foiadelli [3], Salvatore Savasta [3], Alice Bonuccelli [2], Diego Peroni [1,2], Rita Consolini [1], Gian Luigi Marseglia [3], Alessandro Orsini [2] and Pasquale Striano [4,5]*

[1] Pediatric Immunology, Pediatric University Department, Azienda Ospedaliero Universitaria Pisana, University of Pisa, Pisa, Italy, [2] Pediatric Neurology, Pediatric University Department, Azienda Ospedaliero Universitaria Pisana, University of Pisa, Pisa, Italy, [3] Pediatric Clinic, Istituto di Ricovero e Cura a Carattere Scientifico (IRCCS) Policlinico San Matteo Foundation, University of Pavia, Pavia, Italy, [4] Pediatric Neurology and Muscular Diseases Unit, IRCCS Istituto "Giannina Gaslini", Genova, Italy, [5] Department of Neurosciences, Rehabilitation, Ophthalmology, Genetics, Maternal and Child Health, University of Genova, Genova, Italy

***Correspondence:**
Alexandre Michev
a.michev@aol.com

† These authors have contributed equally to this work

Introduction: Recent studies prompted the identification of neuroinflammation as a potential target for the treatment of epilepsy, particularly drug-resistant epilepsy, and refractory status epilepticus. This work provides a systematic review of the clinical experience with anti-cytokine agents and agents targeting lymphocytes and aims to evaluate their efficacy and safety for the treatment of refractory epilepsy. Moreover, the review analyzes the main therapeutic perspectives in this field.

Methods: A systematic review of the literature was conducted on MEDLINE database. Search terminology was constructed using the name of the specific drug (anakinra, canakinumab, tocilizumab, adalimumab, rituximab, and natalizumab) and the terms "status epilepticus," "epilepsy," and "seizure." The review included clinical trials, prospective studies, case series, and reports published in English between January 2016 and August 2021. The number of patients and their age, study design, specific drugs used, dosage, route, and timing of administration, and patients outcomes were extracted. The data were synthesized through quantitative and qualitative analysis.

Results: Our search identified 12 articles on anakinra and canakinumab, for a total of 37 patients with epilepsy (86% febrile infection-related epilepsy syndrome), with reduced seizure frequency or seizure arrest in more than 50% of the patients. The search identified nine articles on the use of tocilizumab (16 patients, 75% refractory status epilepticus), with a high response rate. Only one reference on the use of adalimumab in 11 patients with Rasmussen encephalitis showed complete response in 45% of the cases. Eight articles on rituximab employment sowed a reduced seizure burden in 16/26 patients. Finally, one trial concerning natalizumab evidenced a response in 10/32 participants.

Conclusion: The experience with anti-cytokine agents and drugs targeting lymphocytes in epilepsy derives mostly from case reports or series. The use of anti-IL-1, anti-IL-6, and anti-CD20 agents in patients with drug-resistant epilepsy and refractory status epilepticus has shown promising results and a good safety profile. The experience with TNF inhibitors is limited to Rasmussen encephalitis. The use of anti-α4-integrin agents did not show significant effects in refractory focal seizures. Concerning research perspectives, there is increasing interest in the potential use of anti-chemokine and anti-HMGB-1 agents.

Keywords: adalimumab, anakinra, canakinumab, cytokines, neuroinflammation, epilepsy, tocilizumab, rituximab

INTRODUCTION

Epilepsy affects more than 50 million people worldwide and represents an unsolved public health problem (1). In 2017 ILEA published an operational classification of seizures ad epilepsies which gave a remarkable contribution in improving epilepsy diagnosis and treatment (2, 3) (**Figure 1**). Despite the significant advances made in its treatment, about 7–20% of the children and 30–40% of the adults develop drug-resistant epilepsy (DRE) (4), which can be reasonably defined as an incompletely controlled disease despite the trial with two appropriate antiseizure medications (ASM; whether as monotherapy or in combination) at the correct posology) (5, 6). One of the most severe clinical complications observed in epileptic individuals is status epilepticus (SE), defined by ILEA (7) (**Table 1**). Refractory status epilepticus (RSE) is defined by a SE in which the administration of a benzodiazepine bolus and another ASM does not resolve the clinical picture (13). Among the research areas to improve the therapeutic strategy against drug-resistant epilepsy and RSE, there is increasing interest in the role of agents targeting neuroinflammation. Neuroinflammation is a non-specific biologic response of the brain and spinal cord innate immune system (14), which shows a bidirectional relationship with seizures. Indeed, seizures themselves can be responsible for neuronal and glial damage followed by an inflammatory response, while experimental studies investigating the effects of the administration of pro-inflammatory molecules in the central nervous system (CNS) evidenced that inflammation significantly reduces the seizure threshold (15). Although different authors have focused on the identification of the molecular mechanisms responsible for the inflammatory-dependent induction of seizures and the research for potential therapeutic agents targeting neuroinflammation for the treatment of epilepsy (16, 17), there is no uniform agreement on their use, and data from large cohorts of patients and randomized studies are missing.

In this work, we review the known molecular mechanisms linking neuroinflammation and epilepsy, including the role of the main inflammatory mediators involved in the process of epileptogenesis. For epileptic syndromes cited and terminology related to epilepsy we used the new ILEA operational practical clinical definition of epilepsy (**Table 1**) (8). Moreover, we provide a systematic review of the clinical experience with anti-cytokine agents (anti-IL-1, anti-IL-6, and anti-TNF agents) and with agents targeting the effectors of adaptive immunity in the treatment of epilepsy, with a focus on DRE and RSE. Finally, in the last section of this work, we discuss the main research perspectives in this field, including anti-chemokine agents. This paper aims to help reduce the knowledge gap in the field of neuroinflammation in epileptic individuals and represents the first systematic review performed on the role of anti-cytokine and anti-lymphocyte agents.

SEIZURES AND NEUROINFLAMMATION—AN OVERVIEW

Neuroinflammation develops as a consequence of different stimuli, such as CNS trauma, infection, ischemic and hemorrhagic diseases, and seizures, although it can be also the consequence of a systemic inflammatory response spreading to CNS (14). Additionally, neuroinflammation is partly responsible for the neuronal damage and clinical manifestations of CNS disorders primarily featured by uncontrolled adaptive immune function, including autoimmune encephalitis (Anti-NMDR, Anti-AMPAR, Anti-GABA/AR and Anti-GABA/BR, Anti-VGKC, Anti-GAD, Anti-GlyR, Anti-DPPX, Anti-mGluR5, Anti-IgLON5) (18, 19) and Rasmussen syndrome (10) (**Table 1**), and others. Although inflammatory mediators are central in maintaining brain homeostasis, being implicated in the initiation of tissue repair after CNS injury, the process of neurogenesis, neuronal plasticity, and in the behavioral responses related to stress, neuroinflammation can be responsible for neuronal damage, altered cellular function, and impaired secretion and response to neurotransmitters, thus participating to the process of epileptogenesis (14). The CNS inflammatory response depends on the activity of the resident innate immune cells (particularly, microglial cells and astrocytes) and the release of inflammatory mediators, including cytokines, chemokines, prostaglandin, nitric oxide (NO), and reactive oxygen species (ROS) (17). Among the cellular effectors of neuroinflammation, microglial cells play a central role. They function as sensors for different triggers, having macrophage-like activity, and are implicated in the recognition of pathogens and cellular debris, and the secretion of cytokines and chemokines (20). The function of immune surveillance of microglial cells depends on multiple cellular receptors, with toll-like receptors (TLR) being directly involved in the recognition of pathogen-associated molecular patterns (PAMPS) (21). Other cellular subtypes are involved in CNS inflammation and include endothelial cells and perivascular macrophages, which can act increasing vascular permeability and, through the expression of adhesion molecules, contribute to leukocyte chemotaxis (14, 22). The main cytokines participating in the CNS inflammatory response and epileptogenesis are interleukin 1β (IL-1β), IL-6, and tumor necrosis factor-α (TNF-α) (**Figure 2**). An elevation of the serum

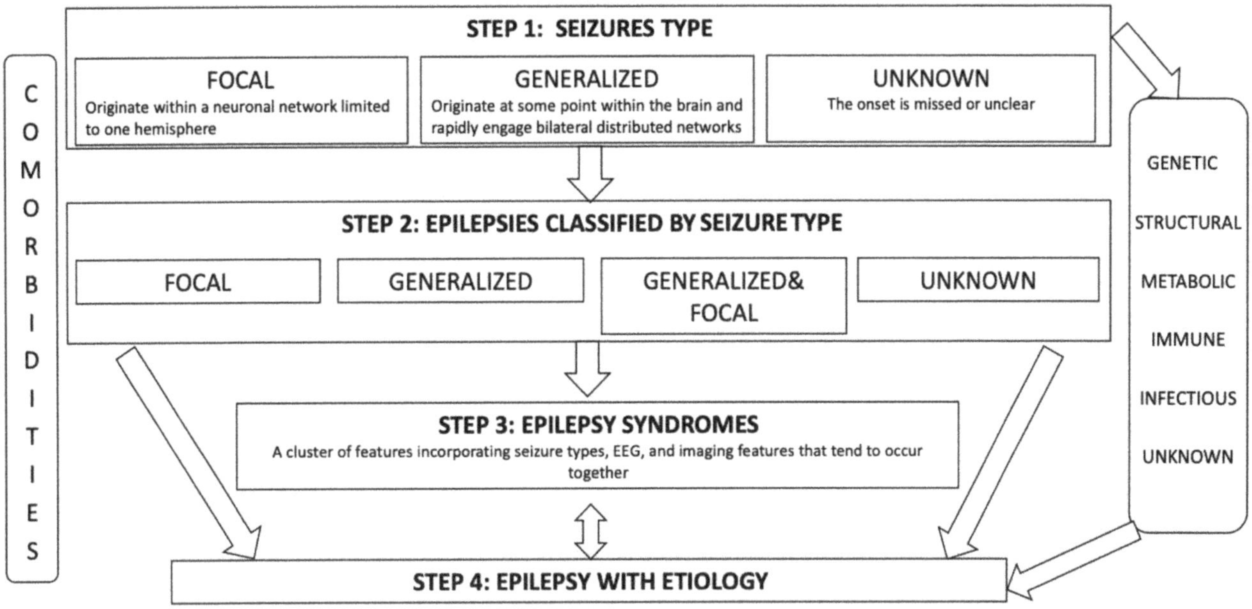

FIGURE 1 | Framework for epilepsy classification designed to allow diagnosis at multiple levels depending on the informationand resources available. At all levels of diagnosis, we should consider more broadly the etiology of the patient's epilepsy. A range of six etiological groups has been recognized: genetic, structural, metabolic, immune, infectious, and unknown.

and cerebrospinal (CSF) levels of these cytokines in individuals with epilepsy has been demonstrated in different studies (23), as well as the higher expression of genes encoding for these mediators in the brain tissue from patients who underwent brain resection for drug-resistant focal epilepsy (17). Interestingly, the levels of inflammatory mediators are higher in patients with drug-resistant epilepsy (24), suggesting a contribution of neuroinflammation in the development of drug resistance. Additionally, the demonstration that in animal models the intrathecal administration of IL-1β causes a reduction of the seizure threshold pointed out the direct role of cytokines in seizure and epileptogenesis (15).

Among soluble inflammatory mediators, the danger signal molecule high-mobility group box-1 (HMGB-1) also plays a central role in neuroinflammation, being involved in the TLR4-IL-1β axis, and in the enhancement of the CNS inflammatory response (25). Chemokines and their receptors participate in CNS inflammation favoring leukocyte migration to the site of inflammation and endothelial adhesion but are also directly implicated in epileptogenesis through the interaction with neurotransmitters and neuropeptides (26), as further discussed. Finally, the role of the blood-brain barrier (BBB) in neuroinflammation and epileptogenesis is of extreme clinical and research interest (25). Inflammatory mediators, produced both in CNS and systemically, can enhance its permeability and BBB leakage allows the spread of systemic inflammatory mediators within the CNS, thus amplifying the inflammatory process (17).

IL-1 and Epilepsy: Molecular Basis

IL-1β is mostly produced by cells of the innate immune system, including monocytes, macrophages, and dendritic cells, following a wide range of triggers, such as infections and cellular damage (i.e., oxidative stress) (27). In CNS, IL-1β is produced by glial cells and other cellular sources, including endothelial cells (28). The main molecular mechanism leading to the synthesis of IL-1β is the assembly and function of the macromolecular complex of the inflammasome, in a process that requires the recognition of the inflammatory trigger (i.e., *via* toll-like receptors) leading to the activation of caspase-1, finally allowing the release of active IL-1β (29). Once released, IL-1β acts as an initiator of the inflammatory response, promoting the synthesis of other pro-inflammatory cytokines (such as IL-6), induces fever, and acts as a direct effector of inflammatory organ damage (30). High serum and CSF levels of IL-1β have been demonstrated in individuals suffering from epilepsy, including those affected by developmental epileptic encephalopathies, with even higher concentrations in patients with drug-resistant epilepsy (17). Although the mechanisms linking IL-1β and epileptogenesis are far to be fully understood, pieces of evidence suggest that neuronal excitation and excitotoxicity secondary to the enhanced effect of glutamate play a significant role (31). Indeed, IL-1β has been demonstrated to influence the calcium influx across the N-methyl-D-aspartate (NMDA) receptor, reduce glutamate uptake by astrocytes and increase glutamate release by glial cells (32). On the other hand, studies on the influence of IL-1β on GABA-ergic transmission show conflicting results (32).

Currently, the agents targeting IL-1β comprise the IL-1 receptor antagonist anakinra, the anti-IL-1 monoclonal antibodies canakinumab (human antibody) and gevokizumab (humanized antibody), and the IL-1 inhibitor rilonacept, which consists of a fusion protein composed of the Fc portion of human IgG and the extracellular domain of IL-1 receptor (33,

TABLE 1 | Definitions.

Operational (practical) clinical definition of epilepsy (8)
Epilepsy is a disease of the brain defined by any of the following conditions: • 1. At least two unprovoked (or reflex) seizures occurring >24 h apart • 2. One unprovoked (or reflex) seizure and a probability of further seizures similar to the general recurrence risk (at least 60%) after two unprovoked seizures, occurring over the next 10 years • 3. Diagnosis of an epilepsy syndrome
Epilepsy is considered to be resolved for individuals who had an age-dependent epilepsy syndrome but are now past the applicable age or those who have remained seizure-free for the last 10 years, with no seizure medicines for the last 5 years.
Status epilepticus (7)
"A condition resulting either from the failure of the mechanisms responsible for seizure termination or from the initiation of mechanisms, which lead to abnormally, prolonged seizures (after time point t_1). It is a condition, which can have long-term consequences (after time point t_2), including neuronal death, neuronal injury, and alteration of neuronal networks, depending on the type and duration of seizures."
Super refractory status epilepticus (7)
SE continues for more than 24 h after the first administration of general anesthesia.
Autoimmune encephalitis (9)
Autoimmune encephalitis encompasses a wide variety of protean pathologic processes associated with the presence of antibodies against neuronal intracellular proteins, synaptic receptors, ion channels and/or neuronal surface proteins.
Rasmussen encephalitis (10)
Unilateral hemispheric encephalitis whose main clinical features include refractory focal epilepsy or epilepsia partialis continua, hemiparesis, and progressive cognitive decline.
New-onset refractory status epilepticus (NORSE) (11)
NORSE is a clinical presentation, not a specific diagnosis, in a patient without active epilepsy or other preexisting relevant neurological disorder, with new onset of refractory status epilepticus without a clear acute or active structural, toxic or metabolic cause.
Febrile infection-related epilepsy syndrome (FIRES) (11)
FIRES is a subcategory of NORSE, applicable for all ages, that requires a prior febrile infection starting between 2 weeks and 24 h prior to onset of refractory status epilepticus, with or without fever at onset of status epilepticus.
Electrical status epilepticus in sleep (ESES) (12)
Electrical status epilepticus in sleep (ESES), a childhood-onset epileptic encephalopathy, is characterized by epilepsy, cognitive regression, and marked activation of epileptiform activity during non-rapid eye movement (NREM) sleep to produce an electroencephalography (EEG) pattern of near-continuous spike-wave discharges.

34). Since their introduction, anti-IL-1 agents have become a cornerstone in the treatment of autoinflammatory disorders, and have also been used in other rheumatologic disorders, such as rheumatoid arthritis (RA), gout, adult-onset Still diseases and systemic juvenile idiopathic arthritis (sJIA), and cytokine storm syndromes (35), with anakinra and canakinumab being the most widely used drugs. The use of gevokizumab is still experimental, since the drug has not been approved by the Food and Drug Administration.

IL-6 and Epilepsy: Molecular Basis

IL-6 has a pivotal role in enhancing and maintaining the inflammatory response and activating adaptive immunity. Systemically, the release of IL-6 is followed by the production of acute-phase proteins (C-reactive protein, serum amyloid protein, fibrinogen), the release of platelets, angiogenesis, and an increase in vascular permeability (36). Additionally, IL-6 participates in driving the differentiation of T CD4+ cells in T helper 17 (Th17) cells, promotes the differentiation and expansion of T CD8+ cytotoxic cells, and inhibits the proliferation of regulatory T cells (Tregs) (36). In the CNS, this cytokine is mostly produced by glial cells, with a mechanism triggered by multiple factors, including the binding of IL-1β and TNF-α to specific surface receptors on glial cells (37). Additionally, IL-6 can be secreted by astrocytes and neurons and can be released by perivascular and brain endothelial cells in response to inflammatory and infectious stimuli (37). Increased serum and CFS levels of IL-6 have been demonstrated in patients with refractory epilepsy, and an association between IL-6 levels and the degree of neuronal apoptosis was evidenced in patients undergoing surgery for refractory temporal lobe epilepsy (38). Notably, the serum cytokine levels have been shown to decrease after surgery (38). Apart from the induction of apoptosis, a direct role of IL-6 in epileptogenesis has been suggested (31). It is known that IL-6 interferes with GABA-A receptor functioning, while recent data suggest that the cytokine could reduce glutamate signaling and consequent neuronal toxicity (32).

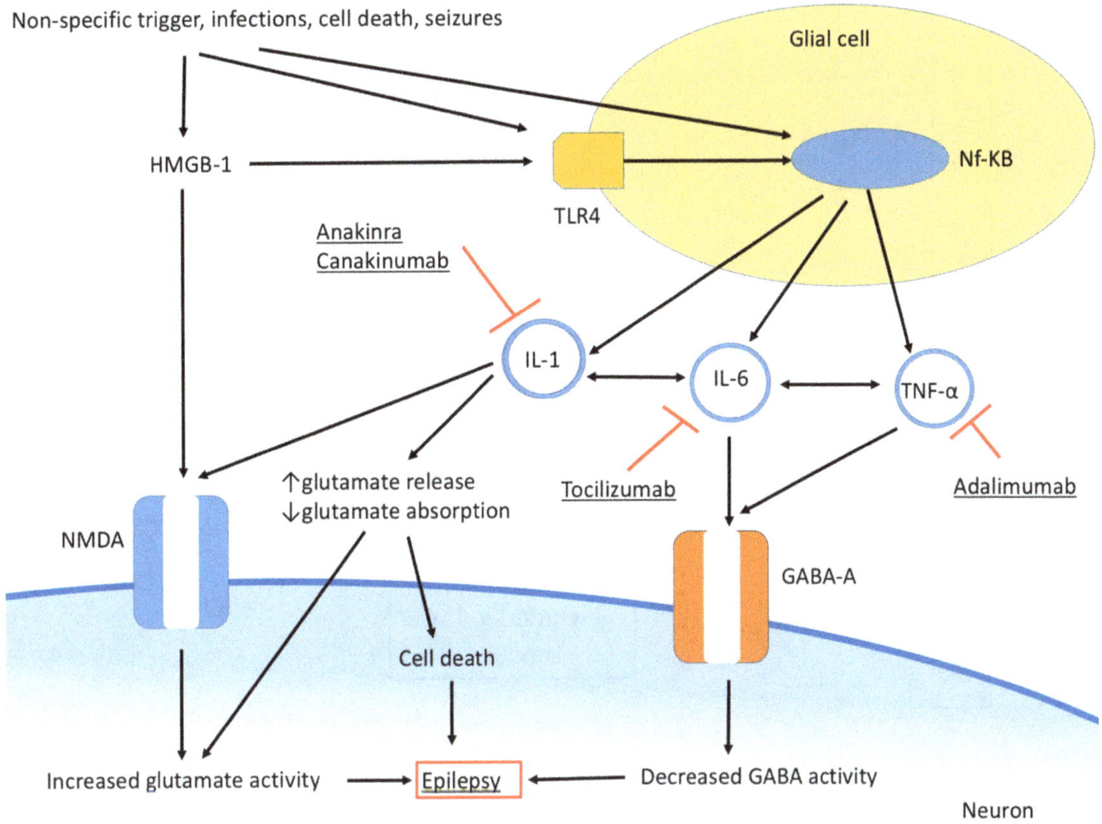

FIGURE 2 | Overview of inflammatory pathways involved in epilepsy and main therapeutic targets.

The most widely used anti-IL-6 therapeutic agent is tocilizumab, a humanized monoclonal anti-IL-6 receptor antibody that is part of the therapeutic armamentarium against autoinflammatory disorders, cytokine storm syndromes, and autoimmune diseases (36, 39). Concerning neurological diseases, tocilizumab is used in autoimmune encephalitis and different systemic inflammatory disorders with CNS involvement, including linear scleroderma "*en coup de sabre*" (LSCS), and neuro-Behcet's disease (40, 41). The human monoclonal anti-IL-6 antibody sarilumab is a therapeutic option in patients with RA and different authors suggested a role in the treatment of severe COVID-19 (42, 43).

TNF-α and Epilepsy: Molecular Basis

Tumor necrosis factor-alpha (TNF-α) is a pleiotropic effector cytokine of the TNF superfamily that plays a role in the regulation of cell homeostasis and of the immune-inflammatory pathways (28). TNF-α is produced by a wide range of cells (including microglia, astrocytes, and neurons) (44, 45) and interacts with two transmembrane glycoprotein receptors, TNF receptor 1 (TNFR1) and TNF receptor 2 (TNFR2), that differ in their cellular expression profiles, ligand affinities and signaling pathways (45). The main downstream effectors are Nuclear Factor Kappa-B, C-Jun N-terminal Kinase, p38, and the pathway of sphingomyelinase/ceramide. The exact role of TNF-α in epileptogenesis is not yet understood (46). The cytokine may operate by direct interaction with neurons or by influencing the expression of neurotransmitter receptors on glial cells (47, 48). TNF-α can also alter the permeability of the blood-brain barrier (28, 49). Reportedly, the expression of TNF-α in astrocytes may promote an inflammatory and degenerative outcome, while the cytokine expression in neuronal and microglial cells would be associated with tissue repair and remyelination (50–52). This dual role of TNF-α reflects the subtype of receptor that is preferentially involved in the signaling: TNFR1 is thought to induce an epileptogenic and proinflammatory phenotype through a series of post-translational mechanisms that regulate the expression and the turnover of AMPA, GABAA, and NMDA-NR1 receptors, while TNFR2 shows an anticonvulsant and neurotrophic orientation. Indeed, a study conducted on hippocampal tissues from patients with intractable temporal lobe epilepsy documented the predominance of TNFR1 pathways. Specifically, the involvement of TNFR1 caused the activation of apoptosis pathways capable to perpetrate the seizure-induced brain injury (53).

All molecules with TNF-inhibitory action that are currently approved for therapeutic use are monoclonal antibodies (mAbs) obtained by mutation and gene-splicing techniques (54, 55). These drugs can act both with an antagonistic effect, blocking the cellular functions mediated by TNF-receptors, or with an

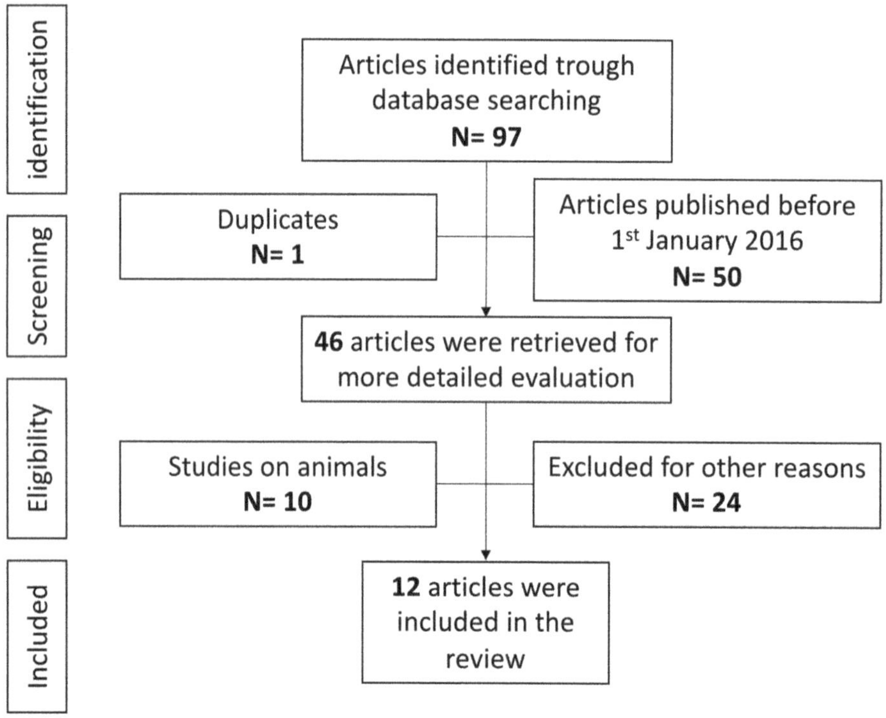

FIGURE 3 | Anti-IL-1 agents and epilepsy, literature review.

agonistic function through reverse signaling mediated by the transmembrane portion of TNF-α (56). In the spectrum of CNS disorders, the use of anti TNF-α agents has been specifically studied for multiple sclerosis (MS) (57, 58). However, two clinical trials evidenced discouraging results, since patients showed clinical and radiological signs of progression of the disease during treatment (57, 58). Moreover, a possible correlation between the exposure to anti-TNF-α agents and the occurrence of inflammatory demyelinating and non-demyelinating events emerges from different cases and case-series of patients treated for non-CNS related disorders (59–69). We speculate that the adverse neurological effects observed in patients treated with TNF-inhibitors for other diseases influence and limit the choice of these therapies for the treatment of many neurological conditions. Despite a causal correlation between demyelination and the use of anti TNF-α agents is uncertain, some mechanisms have been proposed to explain the pathogenesis of the adverse events observed, including the fact that the use of TNF-inhibitors may reduce the expression of TNFR2 receptors within the brain tissues, impairing the course of reparative processes (70–73). In the particular case of epilepsy, animal models highlighted how the effects of the TNF-α can be different depending on which receptor subtype governs the signaling pathway. Hence, future therapeutic agents may be targeted to the mechanisms that govern the predominance between TNFR1 and TNFR2, to downregulate the former without reducing the expression of the latter (74).

Adaptive Immunity and Epilepsy: Molecular Basis

Adaptive immunity plays an important role in the immune surveillance within the CNS through a series of mechanisms, considering the status of immune privilege of the CNS (75). Nonetheless, cells of adaptive immunity have also been implied in the pathogenesis of different immune-mediated diseases of the CNS (76). Moreover, experimental studies conducted in models of epilepsy suggested that adaptive immunity is actively involved in this process (77). Following seizures, the alteration of the BBB leads to the release of chemokines and drives the infiltration of lymphocytes and other cells of the innate immunity (i.e., monocytes) (78). Within the CNS, B and T cells exert their effector functions with different mechanisms. The understanding of the pathogenesis of certain forms of immune-mediated epilepsy revealed that B and T cells can respond to stimuli originating directly by neuronal antigens or by molecular mimicry between the antigens of infectious agents (mainly viruses) and components of the CNS tissues (79, 80). To date, a wide range of antibodies directed toward extracellular domains have been described and reunited under the term "Neuronal Surface Antibodies." The presence of such antibodies underlies several CNS syndromes characterized by seizures (81). In other conditions, identified as paraneoplastic syndromes, the production of antibodies is rather an epiphenomenon and the pathogenesis recognizes a role of cytotoxic T cells (82). Xu et al. investigated the involvement of cell-mediated immunity in patients with intractable forms of epilepsy and demonstrated

TABLE 2 | Systematic review of anti-IL-1 agents in epilepsy.

References	Disease	*N*, (age)	Study design	Intervention	Timing	Efficacy	Safety
Sa et al. (105)	FIRES	2 Pt 1: 1.9 years Pt 2. 2.5 years	Case Report	Pt 1 Anakinra 5 mg/Kg/day s.c for 14 days	Start: Day 43	From Day 51 seizures decreased in frequency and on Day 60 these stopped. After 3 weeks new onset of seizures (2–5/month)	No adverse effects
				Pt 2 Anakinra 10 mg/Kg/day s.c for 90 days	Start: day 22 Discontinued after 3 months of treatment	No improvement	No adverse effects
Yang et al. (106)	FIRES	1 (6 years old)	Case Report	Anakinka 100 mg s.c. twice daily for 1 year	Start: Day 28	Resolution of seizures after 4 days. Stop ketogenic diet after 9 months. Follow-up: 1 seizure/month	No adverse effects
Kern-Smith et al. (107)	NORSE	1 (5 years old)	Case Report	Anakinra for 13 days (posology not specified)	Start: Day 12 Stop: Day 24	Stop midazolam infusion, without return of electrographic status epilepticus, after 2 days	No adverse effects
Dilena et al. (108)	FIRES	1 (10 years old)	Case Report	Anankinra 2.5 mg/kg/day (100 mg) s.c and, 3 days after, 2.5 mg/kg twice daily	Start: after 18 months from diagnosis Stop: 7 months after	Full seizure control after 3 days	No adverse effects
Jyonouchi and Geng (109)	ESES	1 (6 years old)	Case Report	Anakinra 100 mg/day s.c.	Start: 25 months after diagnosis	Despite the improvement of behavioral symptoms, ESES pattern persisted.	No adverse effects
Lai et al. (110)	FIRES	25, (5–11 years old)	Retrospective	Anakinra 3–5 mg/kg/day (initial dose) Anakinra 4–9 mg/kg/day (final dose)	Start: 20 days after the onset of FIRES Stop: 86 days after	Earlier anakinra initiation after seizure onset was associated with shorter duration of mechanical ventilation, and ICU and hospital LOS. Amongst children with available seizure frequency data, 11/15 (73.3%) exhibited> 50% seizure reduction at 1 week of anakinra treatment. 3/25 (12%) died	3/25 (12%) developed DRESS 2/25 (8%) developed cytopenia 10/25 (40%) developed infections (1 discontinued anakinra for infections)
Westbrook et al. (111)	FIRES	1 (21 years old)	Case Report	Anakinra 100 mg 3 times daily s.c (Initial dose) Anakinra 100 mg twice daily s.c (after 10 days) Anakinra 100 mg once daily s.c. (after 25 days)	Start: 32 days after the diagnosis of FIRES Stop: 1 year after at which time discontinuation will be discussed	Full seizure control after 24 h	No adverse effects

(Continued)

TABLE 2 | Continued

References	Disease	*N*, (age)	Study design	Intervention	Timing	Efficacy	Safety
Kenney- Jung et al. (112)	FIRES	1 (32 months old)	Case Report	Anakinra 5 mg/kg/twice daily s.c. Anakinra 5 mg/kg/twice daily s.c.	2 cycles: Day 6–23 Day 54-ongoing	Improved seizure control in both cycles (from 5.8 to 1.3 seizure/day in the first cycle; from 8 to 0.17 seizure/day in the second). Twelve months after initial presentation, the patient experiences rare focal seizures.	Development of DRESS (day 22, followed by discontinuation)
DeSena et al. (113)	DRE	1 (14 years old)	Case Report	Anakinra 100 mg daily Anakinra 100 mg twice daily Canakinumab 300 mg every 4 weeks	Start: 2 years Stop: After 4 weeks After: 2 months	Rapid ∼80% reduction in seizure frequency (from 4 to 15/day to 4/week). No clinically evident seizures. Improvements in her fatigue, general malaise, quality of life, and academic performance. Long periods of being seizure-free, currently averaging one seizure per several months.	No adverse effects
Stredny et al. (114)	FIRES	1 (6 years old)	Case Report	Anakinra 20 mg/kg daily	From day 6 to 20 of hospitalization	No clinical response	No adverse effects
Mochol et al. (115)	RE	1 (43 years old)	Case Report	Anakinra 100 mg daily sc	26 years after disease presentation. 1st cycle: 2 months 2nd cycle: 7 months	Complete seizure control after 1 week of treatment. Relapse after 2 weeks of withdrawal 2nd cycle: full seizure control after 10 days 13 months seizure-free	Pneumonia
Choi et al. (116)	SRSE in AE	1 (38 years old)	Case Report	Anakinra 100 mg daily s.c	From week 12 Duration: 12 days	Resolution of status epilepticus Recovery in communication and walking)	No adverse effects

AE, autoimmune encephalitis; DRE, drug-resistant epilepsy; DRESS, Drug rash with eosinophilia and systemic symptoms; ESES, Encephalopathy with electrical status epilepticus in sleep; FIRES, Febrile infection-related epilepsy syndrome; NORSE, New-onset refractory status epilepticus; RE, Rasmussen encephalitis; SRSE, super-refractory status epilepticus.

localization of blood-derived, antigen-specific CD8+ and γδ T cells in the epileptogenic zone, showing how the amount of infiltrated cells correlated with seizure severity (83). Interestingly, the majority of T cells detected resulted to be memory T cells, capable to sustain an inflammatory response even in the absence of costimulatory signals. Additionally, the amount of brain infiltrating T reg cells resulted inversely correlated with seizure severity (83). The role of CD8+ cells is peculiar since under inflammatory conditions neurons can express MHC class I and II molecules perpetrating cell-mediated brain damage (84).

Studies conducted in the past years raised the awareness of how targeting the mechanisms of action of B and T cells could be of therapeutic interest. The use of monoclonal antibodies as immune modulators has substantially changed the approach to many inflammatory diseases, including some autoimmune disorders of the CNS (85). The activity of these agents consists mainly in inhibiting the production of antibodies and blocking the intrusion of effector lymphocytes in the CNS. Rituximab is a chimeric anti-CD20 mAb engineered to reduce the pool of B cells that undergo maturation and that produce antibodies, hence decreasing the entity of humoral immune response (86). Originally approved for the treatment of B cell lymphoma, to date rituximab is employed in the treatment of many immune-mediated diseases of the CNS, including multiple sclerosis and other forms of autoimmune demyelinating disorders (87, 88). This molecule represents also an off-label second line of treatment for several forms of autoimmune encephalitis (89). Particularly, the use of rituximab for the treatment of anti-NMDR has been the object of studies that evidenced a good response in terms of outcome and a lower frequency of relapses (19, 90). With a more heterogeneous degree of clinical response, the use of rituximab is also reported in cases of encephalitis associated with anti-GAD, anti-myelin oligodendrocyte glycoprotein, and anti-leucine-rich glioma inactivated 1 (LGI1) antibodies (91–93). Additionally, occasional reports in patients with RE and one patient with FIRES sustain a possible therapeutical application for rituximab in these diseases (94, 95). Natalizumab is a humanized monoclonal antibody targeting α4-integrin (CD49d) on the surface of lymphocytes (96). The interaction between this integrin and the VCAM receptor is involved in the process of diapedesis and hence crucial to lymphocyte extravasation to the CNS. Natalizumab has been prominently employed in patients with multiple sclerosis, with good therapeutic results despite the onset of progressive multifocal leukoencephalopathy (96, 97). The use of natalizumab has been studied in animal models of RE (98) and one patient with RE treated with natalizumab is reported in literature (99).

SYSTEMATIC REVIEW OF THE LITERATURE

Objective of the Systematic Review

This systematic review aims to assess whether anti-cytokine (anti-IL-1, anti-IL-6, anti-TNF), anti-CD20, and anti-α4-integrin agents could be effective and safe for the treatment of DRE and RSE.

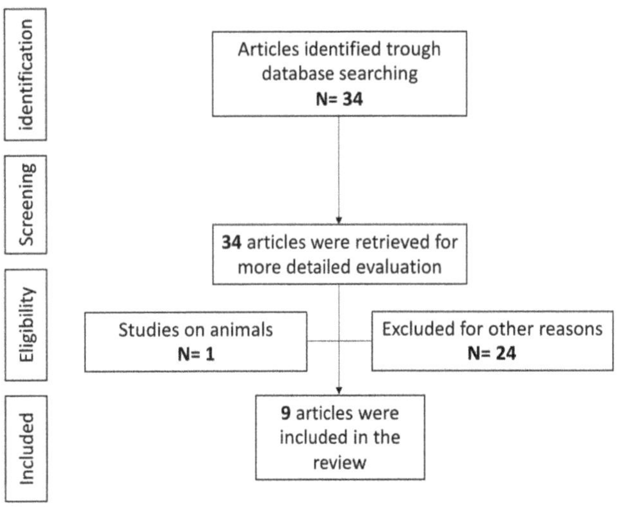

FIGURE 4 | Anti-IL-6 agents and epilepsy, literature review.

Methods

Protocol

This systematic review was performed following the preferred reporting items for systematic reviews and meta-analysis protocol (PRISMA-P) reporting guidelines (100). The review protocol has not been registered.

Inclusion Criteria

Population

The study included patients with no age restriction and diagnosed with DRE or RSE. Patients with DRE or RSE caused by specific syndromes (autoimmune encephalitis, LSCS, RE) were included.

Intervention

We included patients receiving treatment with anti-IL-1 (anakinra, canakinumab), anti-IL-6 (tocilizumab), anti-TNF (infliximab, adalimumab, etanercept), anti-CD20 (rituximab), anti- anti-α4-integrin (natalizumab) agents.

Comparators

Patients receiving ASM, corticosteroids, and other conventional immunosuppressive agents or placebo were included. Studies not including a comparator arm have also been included.

Outcomes

The primary outcomes for this review were the efficacy in decreasing or arresting seizures in RSE, controlling the epileptic phenotype in DRE, and the safety of the therapeutic agents in epileptic individuals. The secondary outcome was (when available) the analysis of the motor, behavioral, and cognitive function and recovery after treatment.

Study Types

We included all the case reports, case series, retrospective, prospective studies, and clinical trials in which the following

TABLE 3 | Systematic review of anti-IL-6 agents in epilepsy.

References	Disease	PTS *N* Age	Study design	Intervention	Timing	Efficacy	Safety
Magro et al. (117)	CNS disease and DRE associated with LSCS.	1 (22 years old)	Case Report	Tocilizumab 162 mg S.C. once a week	Start: 6 months after	Noticeable improvement in cognitive and affective symptoms with decrease in seizure frequency. Resolution of many of the enhancing lesions on brain MRI	No adverse effects
Stredny et al. (114)	FIRES	1 (6 years old)	Case Report	Tocilizumab 12 mg/kg S.C. every 2 weeks	Start: Day 20 Stop: Day 76	Reduction of seizure	No adverse effects
Donnelly et al. (118)	NORSE	1 (26 years old)	Case Report	Tocilizumab 300 mg IV. for two times	First dose: 9 weeks after the beginning of treatment Second dose: 12 weeks after the beginning of treatment	Stop seizures after 48 h	No adverse effects
Osminina et al. (119)	CNS disease and DRE associated with LSCS.	1 (2 years 10 months)	Case Report	Tocilizumab 10 mg/kg IV. once in 4 weeks	Start: 16 months after the beginning of symptoms Stop: 26 months after first infusion of Tz.	Reduction of periventricular focus; stop seizures.	No adverse effects
Jaafar et al. (120)	SRSE	1 (8 years old)	Case Report	Tocilizumab, 8 mg/kg/day S.C. divided in two doses 1 week apart	Start: 10 days after admission to hospital	Stops seizure 24 h after	No adverse effects
Cantarín-Extremera et al. (121)	NORSE	2 Pt 1: 1.9 years old Pt 2: 2.7 years old	Case Report	Pt 1 Tocilizumab 4 mg/kg once a week	Start: Day 21 Stop: Day 28	Seizures decrease in frequency, in VEEG critical patterns had disappeared.	No adverse effects
				Pt 2 Tocilizumab 4 mg/kg for 2 times	Start: Day 30 and 40	48–72 h after the first dose, the seizures began to decrease progressively in frequency and intensity, there was global neurological improvement, recovering normality in terms of language, level of consciousness, and motor capacity, but persisting hyperactivity.	No adverse effects
Jun et al. (124)	NORSE	7 [median 25 years old (22–64)]	Prospective	Tocilizumab 4 mg/kg for 2 cycles in 1-week intervals, a monthly dose (8 mg/kg) was added if needed	Start: Median day 25 (6–73)	Resolution of status epilepticus in 6/7 patients 3/6 of the survived patients showed improvement on the mRS	2/7 (2.9%) leukopenia 1/7 (1.4%) diarrhea 1/7 (1.4%) pneumonia 1/7 (1.4%) sepsis

(Continued)

TABLE 3 | Continued

References	Disease	PTS N Age	Study design	Intervention	Timing	Efficacy	Safety
Benucci et al. (122)	Limbic Encephalitis with Anti-CASPR2 Antibodies	1 (64 years old)	Case Report	Tocilizumab 8 mg/kg IV. once a month for 6 months, then 162 mg every week s.c	Start: 2–3 months after admission.	Full seizure control Resolution of behavioral changes and seizures Improvement in mRS	No adverse effects
Vallecoccia et al. (123)	SRSE	1 (34 years old)	Case Report	2 doses of tocilizumab 4 mg/kg at a 1-week interval	Start: day 24	Partial recovery after 7–10 days from the first administration. Resolution of the clinical picture after 1 month (*ketamine and ketogenic diet added)	Sepsis by drug-resistant pathogen

CNS, Central nervous system; DRE: drug-resistant epilepsy; FIRES, Febrile infection-related epilepsy syndrome; LSCS, Linear scleroderma "en coup de sabre;" mRS, modified Rankin scale; NORSE, New-onset refractory status epilepticus; RSE, refractory status epilepticus; SRSE, Super-refractory status epilepticus.

criteria were met: (1) original publication; (2) human studies focusing on RSE and/or DRE; (3) at least one enrolled patient with no age restriction; (4) only papers published in English; (5) only papers published between 1 January 2016 and August 2021.

Exclusion Criteria

We excluded (1) reviews, book chapters, author's replies ad commentaries; (2) animal experiments; (3) all papers published before 2016; (4) all the studies not meeting the inclusion criteria.

Search Strategy and Data Sources

A systematic review of the literature concerning the use of these drugs in patients with epilepsy was conducted in May 2021 and updated in September 2021 on the MEDLINE database (through PubMed). The search terminology was constructed using the name of specific anti-IL-1, anti-IL-6, anti-TNF, anti-CD20, and anti-α4-integrin drugs and the terms "status epilepticus," "epilepsy," and "seizure" with the use of Boolean operators [e.g., "(anakinra AND status epilepticus) OR (anakinra AND seizures)"], ["(tocilizumab AND status epilepticus) OR (tocilizumab AND seizures)"], [(anti-tumor necrosis factor-alpha) OR (anti-TNF)) OR (tumor necrosis factor inhibitor)) OR (Infliximab)) OR (Etanercept)) OR (Adalimumab)) AND ((Epilepsy) OR (seizures))], [((rituximab) OR (anti-CD20)) AND ((Epilepsy) OR (seizures))], [(natalizumab) AND ((Epilepsy) OR (seizures))]. For all searches, the respective Medical Subject Headings (MeSH) and Emtree terms were used, if available.

Study Records

Three review authors (GC, GD, AM) independently screened the titles and abstracts using the previously described inclusion and exclusion criteria. In this first step, the studies considered for potential inclusion were divided into five categories: anti-IL-1, anti-IL-6, anti-TNF agents, anti-CD20, and anti-α4-integrin. In a second step, the same three review authors (GC, DP, AM) evaluated full-text articles and assessed the eligibility for this systematic review. Any disagreement regarding eligibility was resolved through discussion with a third-party member (AO). Data were extracted using a standardized form on Microsoft Excel (Microsoft Corporation, Seattle, USA). The form was designed by GC, and data were extracted by GC, DP, and AM. Any disagreement regarding data extraction was resolved through discussion with a third-party member (AO). The following data were extracted for each study: first author, publication year, number of enrolled patients and their age, study design, specific drugs used, dosage and route of administration (if available), the timing of administration, patients outcomes (decrease in seizure frequency/arrest of seizures or status epilepticus. motor, behavioral and cognitive outcome, adverse events) and the dosage of serum and CSF cytokines. The data obtained from extraction were synthesized through quantitative and qualitative analysis.

Risk of Bias Assessment and Quality of the Evidence

The risk of bias was evaluated using the risk of bias in non-randomized studies of interventions (ROBINS-I) tool (101) for non-randomized studies and the evidence-based medicine (EBM) indications (102) for case series and reports. Each

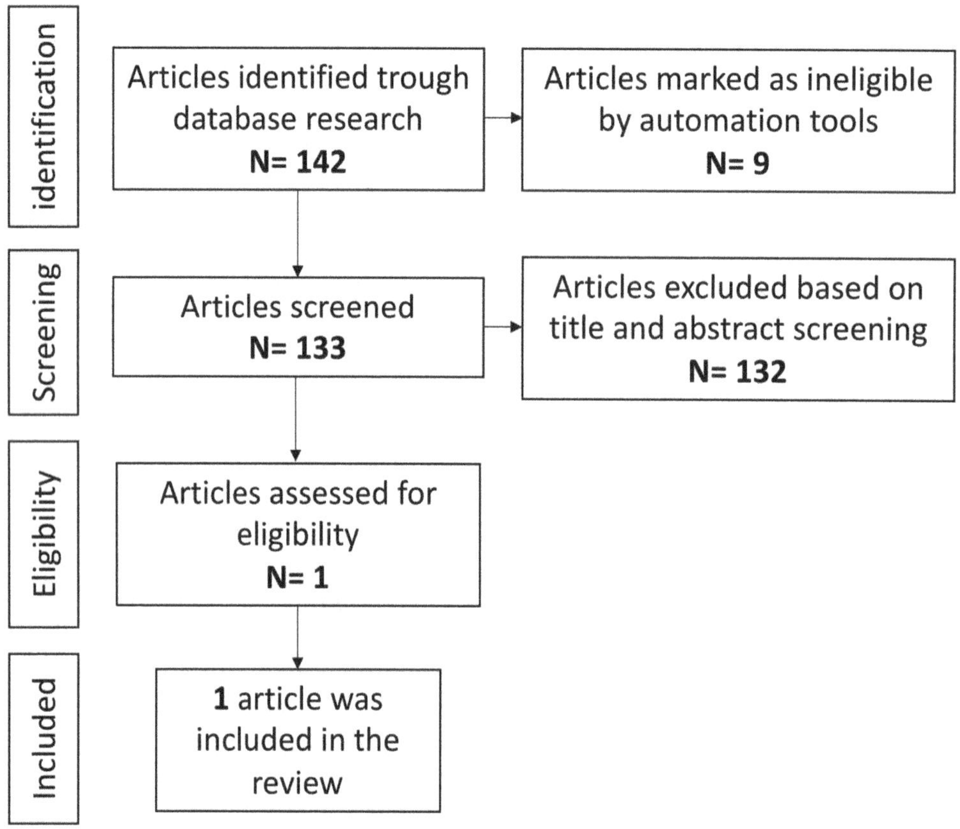

FIGURE 5 | Anti-TNF agents and epilepsy, literature review.

study was assessed by one review author (GC). To estimate the level of evidence reached by this work, the grading of recommendations, assessment, development, and evaluation (GRADE) (103) approach was used. The risk of bias, precision, consistency, directness, and publication bias was analyzed.

Systematic Literature Review: Anti-IL-1 Agents and Epilepsy

Study Selection

Overall, 97 references were identified using the search strategy. After identifying one duplicate and removing 50 articles published before 1 January 2016, the full text of 46 articles was retrieved and evaluated in detail. After a full-text assessment 34 articles were excluded: 10 studies were on animals and 24 were not relevant to the topic of the present review. One paper on multifocal neutrophilic meningoencephalitis (MNM) was excluded as did not directly analyze the effect on the epileptic phenotype (104). Twelve articles were finally included in this review (**Figure 3**), for a total of 37 cases of epilepsy with different etiologies (105–116). All publications were in English, six were from the USA, three were from Europe, one from Asia, and two were international studies, involving different countries. Eleven publications were case reports, while the last was a retrospective observational study.

Results

Among the 37 patients included in this systematic review, the median age was 7 years. Thirty-two patients suffered from FIRES; the other patients suffered from new-onset refractory status epilepticus (NORSE) ($n = 1$), super-refractory status epilepticus (SRSE) ($n = 1$), RE ($n = 1$), encephalopathy with electrical status epilepticus in sleep (ESES) ($n = 1$), and DRE ($n = 1$) (**Tables 1, 2**).

Anakinra was administered with various posologies, ranging from 3 to 20 mg/Kg/day, with a maximum dose of 100 mg SC per administration; canakinumab 300 mg SC was used in one study; no studies were reporting the use of rilonacept. Anti-IL-1 drugs were administrated at least as third-line therapy, after ASM ($n = 37$), corticosteroids ($n = 32$), immunosuppressive agents (sirolimus, $n = 1$), ketogenic diet ($n = 23$), intravenous immunoglobulins ($n = 28$), rituximab ($n = 7$), or plasma exchange ($n = 14$). Two (=2) patients underwent deep brain stimulation and one underwent surgery for DRE. Regarding the timing of administration, anti-IL-1 was started early in 32 cases, with a median delay of 20 days from the onset of seizures. In the remaining five cases, anti-IL-1 treatment was administrated after more than 4 months. Except for five cases in which there weren't improvements (three of them died after drug discontinuation) (105, 110, 114), the use of anti-IL-1 was effective in reducing the seizure burden. Indeed, its use significantly reduced seizures

TABLE 4 | Systematic review of anti-TNF agents in epilepsy.

References	Disease	PTS *N* Age	Study design	Intervention	Timing	Efficacy	Safety
Lagarde et al. (127)	Rasmussen encephalitis.	11 [median 6.5 years (1.5–37)]	Multicenter, open-label, prospective study	Adalimumab 24 mg/m^2 s.c. (maximum 40 mg), every 14 days	Start: Median delay 31 months (range 1–192) after diagnosis	Complete response (>50% seizure frequency decrease) in 5 patients; 3 of these 5 patients had stabilization of functional deficits. One patient showed significant but transitory (6 months) improvement.	One patient discontinued adalimumab due to mild increase of creatine kinase blood levels (normalized after 3 weeks); one patient showed superficial skin infection (not requiring discontinuation of treatment).

(>50%) in 11/15 of the patients described in the cohort by Lai et al. with available clinical data (110), and in 9/12 of the patients described in case reports (**Table 2**). Concerning safety issues, the most frequently reported adverse effect was the development of infections, which have been reported in 11 patients, while four patients experienced drug rash with eosinophilia and systemic symptoms (DRESS) (110, 112). Regarding the cognitive, motor, and behavioral recovery, although in most of the patients presented in case reports (9/12) an improvement was reported, the outcome has been mostly described qualitatively. The study by Lai et al. evidenced that, among the 22 surviving patients, 50% had motor deficit, 77% attention deficit, and more than 50% of the patients had speech, memory, or executive function deficit. In this study, 45% of the surviving patients had mild or moderate disability measured using the pediatric cerebral performance category (PCPC) scale, and 22,7% had a severe disability or vegetative state. Additionally, all the surviving patients in this study have DRE at last follow-up (110). The cytokine serum and CSF levels are reported in 13/37 (35%) and 14/37(37,8%) of the patients, respectively. In the analysis of patients treated with anti-IL drugs, we evidenced some potential biases deriving from missing data, as seizure frequency was not reported for all the included patients (particularly, data are not available for 10/25 patients in the cohort by Lai et al.) (110). Additionally, the lack of use of specific assessment scales did not allow a deeper evaluation of the motor, behavioral and cognitive outcome.

Systematic Literature Review: Anti-IL-6 Agents and Epilepsy

Study Selection

Overall, 32 references were identified using the search strategy. The full text of these 34 articles was retrieved and evaluated in detail, and 25 articles were excluded based on the exclusion criteria. Nine articles were finally included in this review (**Figure 4**), for a total of 16 patients with epilepsy with different etiologies (114, 117–124). Two studies, performed on patients with autoimmune encephalitis and anti-N-methyl-D-aspartate receptor (NMDAR) encephalitis, were excluded as epilepsy was not considered as a specific outcome of the study, although the studies evidenced a global disease activity improvement after treatment with tocilizumab (125, 126). All publications were in English, three from the USA, four from Europe, and two from Asia. Eight publications were case reports, another ($n = 1$), was a prospective study.

Results

Among the 16 patients included in this systematic review, the median age was 23 years. Patients suffered from NORSE ($n = 10$), SRSE ($n = 2$), DRE associated with LSCS ($n = 2$), limbic encephalitis with anti-CASPR2 antibodies ($n = 1$), and FIRES ($n = 1$) (**Table 3**). Tocilizumab was administered in all 16 cases either SC or IV. No other anti-IL-6 was used. Tocilizumab was administered at least as a third-line therapy, after ASM ($n = 16$), corticosteroids ($n = 14$), immunosuppressive agents ($n = 2$), ketogenic diet ($n = 3$), intravenous immunoglobulins ($n = 14$), plasma exchange ($n = 5$), or others (anakinra $n = 1$, electroconvulsive therapy $n = 1$). Tocilizumab was started

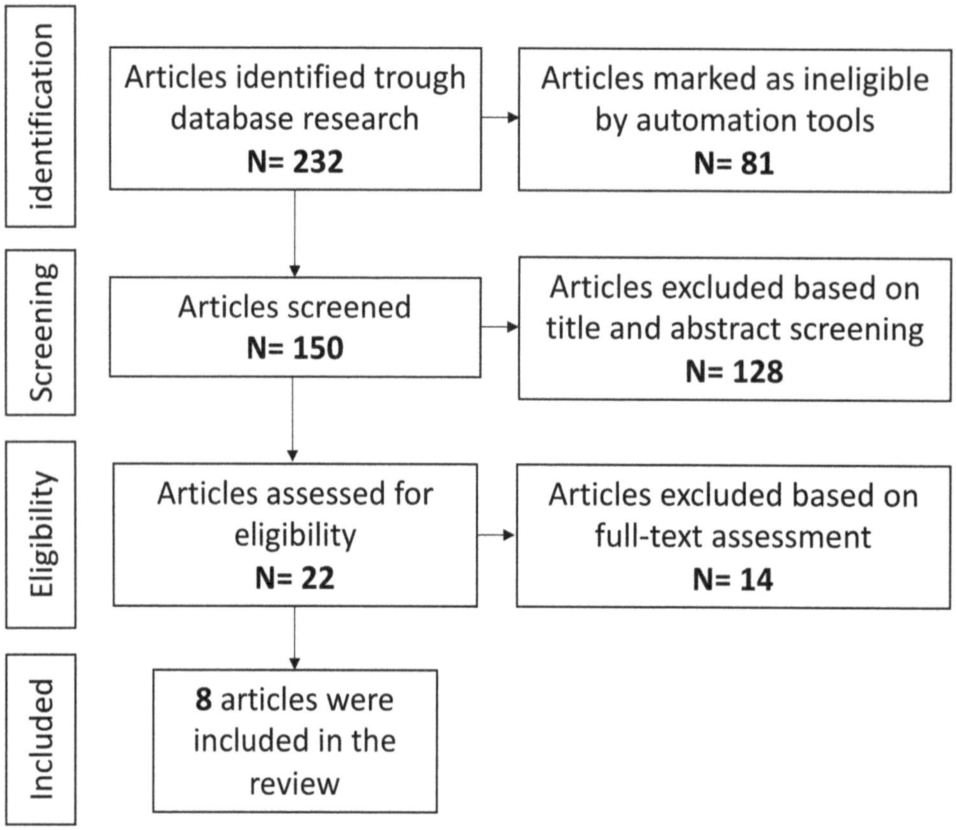

FIGURE 6 | Anti-CD20 agents and epilepsy, literature review.

within the first 6 months of illness in 15 cases (median: 25 days). In only one patient tocilizumab was administered after more than 12 months from the disease onset (**Table 3**). From the available data, it emerges that the use of anti-IL-6 was effective for partial or complete seizure control in most patients [6/7 of the patients described in the cohort study by Jun et al. (124), 9/9 of the patients described in case reports showed reduction or arrest of the seizures]. Concerning safety, although tocilizumab has been well-tolerated by the majority of the patients, our analysis evidenced three cases of infection (one pneumonia and two cases of sepsis), and two patients developed leukopenia (123, 124). The motor, behavioral, and cognitive outcome has been reported mostly with qualitative assessment, showing a reported improvement in seven out of the nine single case reports, with the persistence of behavioral dysregulation (114), mild cognitive impairment, and mild ataxia (118) in two patients. In the study by Jun et al. and the case presented by Benucci et al. the modified Rankin scale (mRS) was used, demonstrating an improvement at follow-up in 4/7 survived patients (122, 124). The dosage of serum and CSF cytokines was available each in 10/16 (62,5%) of the patients. Also in the study of patients treated with tocilizumab, the risk of biases (particularly, missing data) is present, with data being often presented only with qualitative assessment. Additionally, the high rate of therapeutic response in case reports suggests the possibility of a publication bias.

Systematic Literature Review: Anti-TNFα Agents and Epilepsy

Study Selection

Overall a total of 142 references were identified during the initial electronic search, nine of which were marked as not eligible by automation tools because they were not published in English language.

A total of 133 potentially eligible studies were selected. Among these, 132 were excluded (**Figure 5**). One study resulted eligible and was hence included in this review: a multicenter, open-label, prospective study (127).

Results

A total of 11 patients with RE were included in the study (**Table 4**). The median age at first seizure was 6.5 years (range 1.5–37 years). All patients received adalimumab SC (24 mg/m^2 with a maximum of 40 mg) every 14 days. Before adalimumab, patients received treatment with corticosteroids (n = 11), in addition to immunoglobulins (n = 8) and azathioprine (n = 1). The Anti TNF-α agent was started with a median delay of 31 months after the first seizure (range 1 month-16 years). The primary outcome was the decrease of seizures frequency, considering "responders" patients experiencing a decrease in seizure frequency by at least 50%. The secondary outcome measures were neurologic and cognitive outcomes and side

TABLE 5 | Systematic review of anti-CD20 agents in epilepsy.

References	Disease	*N*, (age)	Study design	Intervention	Timing	Efficacy	Safety
Cheli et al. (134)	Anti-LGI1 encephalitis with DRE	1 (54 years old)	Case Report	Rituximab 1,000 mg/day IV, 2 doses 15 days apart then one single dose after 6 months.	Start: 7 weeks after the onset of seizures. Stop: 9 weeks after the onset of seizures.	No further seizures occurred after the treatment. The neuropsychological evaluation resulted within normal range. After 6 months, the patient experienced a cognitive relapse that resolved after the administration of a single dose of Rituximab.	No adverse effects
Kurukumbi et al. (133)	Patient 1: anti-NMDR encephalitis with RSE Patient 2: anti-LGI1 encephalitis with DRE Patient 3: N-type anti-VGCC encephalitis with RSE	3 Pt 1: 32 years Pt 2: 72 years Pt 3: 19 years	Case Series	Pt 1: Rituximab 375 mg/m^2/day IV weekly for 4 weeks, then rituximab 1,000 mg IV every 6 months Pt 2: Rituximab 1,000 mg IV every 6 months Pt 3: Rituximab 1,000 mg IV every 6 months	Pt 1, start: 27 days after the onset of seizures. Pt 2, start: 12 months after diagnosis Pt 3, start: 5 days after the onset of seizures.	Pt 1: resolution of seizures and behavioral disorders, with a return to baseline cognition and personality Pt 2: electrographic and clinical seizure freedom with return of premorbid cognitive function Pt 3: abrogation of seizures and return to baseline functioning	No adverse effects
Sansevere et al. (132)	RE	1 (11 years old)	Case Report	Rituximab 375 mg/m^2 weekly for 4 weeks	Start: 5 days after diagnosis Stop: 33 days after diagnosis	No clinical response. Functional hemispherectomy with right hemisphere deafferentation was performed 3 months after the final dose of rituximab	No adverse effects
Schneider et al. (131)	Anti-NMDAR encephalitis with RSE	1 (22 years old)	Case Report	Rituximab 500 mg IV, followed by a second dose after 6 months and a third after 16 months	Start: not specified Stop: 16 months after the first administration	Complete remission of epileptic seizures and psychotic symptoms	No adverse effects
Jun et al. (124)	NORSE*	6 [median 36 years (22–61)]	Prospective	Rituximab 375 mg/m^2/day IV weekly	Not specified	Persistence of SE despite the treatment. Patients eventually received Tocilizumab	No adverse effects
El Tawil et al. (130)	RE with DRE	1 (61 years old)	Case Report	Rituximab (posology not specified)	Start: 10 years after diagnosis Stop: not specified	Clear and sustained improvement in seizure frequency and severity and patient's disabilities	No adverse effects

(Continued)

TABLE 5 | Continued

References	Disease	*N*, (age)	Study design	Intervention	Timing	Efficacy	Safety
Timarova et al. (129)	RE with RSE	1 (32 years old)	Case Report	Rituximab 375 mg/m^2/day IV weekly (two cycles 22 months apart)	Start: not specified Stop: 22 months after the first administration	Reduction of epileptic seizures with residual 2–3 partial seizures per week. Worsening 18 months after (partial seizures rose to 6 per day). After the second cycle, persistence of one partial seizure per day.	No adverse effects
Byun et al. (128)	AE**	12 [median 32 years (18–68)]	Prospective study	Rituximab 375 mg/m^2/day IV weekly for 4 weeks. The treatment was then repeated every month.	Start: 3–9 weeks after first immunotherapy cycle (with steroid or IVIg).	Remission of seizures in 8/12 patients at 6 months; seizures reduction > 50% in 1/12 patient; no clinical change in 3/12 patients.	Infusion-related reactions (headache, dizziness, chest discomfort) (n = 2); rash with pruritus 24 h after the infusion (n = 1). This patient discontinued the treatment.

AE, autoimmune encephalitis; DRE, drug-resistant epilepsy; IV, intravenous; IVIg, intravenous immunoglobulins; LGI1, leucine rich glioma inactivated 1; NMDAR, N-methyl-D-aspartate receptor; NORSE, New-onset refractory status epilepticus; RE, Rasmussen encephalitis; SRSE, super-refractory status epilepticus; VGCC, voltage-gated calcium channel.

**One patient suffered from anti-NMDAR encephalitis, in the other cases the disease was cryptogenic.*

***AE in these patients was due to anti-NMDAR (n = 8), anti-LGI1 (n = 3), and anti-Ma2/Ta (n = 1).*

effects of the treatment. Although none of the patients became seizure-free, five patients were considered as responders and another one experienced a transitory improvement in frequency of seizures. In three of the five patients, a stabilization of cognitive decline was observed and two patients had improvement of their motor deficiencies. According to the authors, the response to the treatment seemed to occur more likely in slowly progressive forms of RE and patients with concomitant autoimmune diseases (uveitis and juvenile arthritis). None of the responders underwent hemispherectomy, considering the absence of a severe motor and cognitive deficit. On the other hand, three patients experienced a severe progression of the disease, with the requirement of hemispherectomy. Concerning safety, in 1 patient adalimumab was discontinued due to an elevation of creatine kinase levels and another patient showed a superficial skin infection that did not require interruption of the treatment and was successfully controlled with a local antiseptic (127).

Systematic Literature Review: Anti-CD20 Agents and Epilepsy

Study Selection

Overall a total of 232 references were identified during the initial electronic search, 82 of which were marked as not eligible by automation tools because published before 1 January 2016 and/or not in English language. A total of 150 potentially eligible studies were selected. Among these, 128 were excluded for irrelevancy after a screening of the titles and abstracts (**Figure 6**). After a full-text assessment of the remaining 22 studies, eight of them resulted eligible and were therefore included in this review (124, 128–134). Six publications were case reports and two were prospective studies.

Results

A total of 26 patients with different epileptic disorders were included in this review (**Table 5**). The median age of the patients was 32 years (range 11–72). The patients suffered from RE (n = 3) and from AE due to anti-NMDAR (n = 11), anti-LGI1 (n = 5), anti-voltage-gated calcium channels (VGCC) antibodies (n = 1), or onconeural antibodies (anti-Ma2/Ta) (n = 1). Four patients presented a cryptogenic RSE. The posology of rituximab was variable within the different cases and in one case it was not specified (**Table 5**). For all patients, rituximab was started as second-line immunotherapy after the administration of IVIg and steroids. The timing of administration was variable and, given the heterogeneity of the diseases, it is difficult to determine homogeneous timepoints of reference for all the patients. Overall, the treatment with rituximab was effective in abolishing or significantly reducing the burden of seizures in 16/26 patients (61,5%), while in 10/26 patients, the therapy was ineffective. One patient with RE underwent functional hemispherectomy with remission of seizures (132). As discussed in Section Results, the six patients from the cohort of Jun et al. received Tocilizumab with the resolution of status epilepticus (124). Of the three patients in the study of Byun et al. that did not show a clinical change in the course of their disease after the administration of rituximab, one deceased for reasons not related to the therapy itself (128). The two others continued to

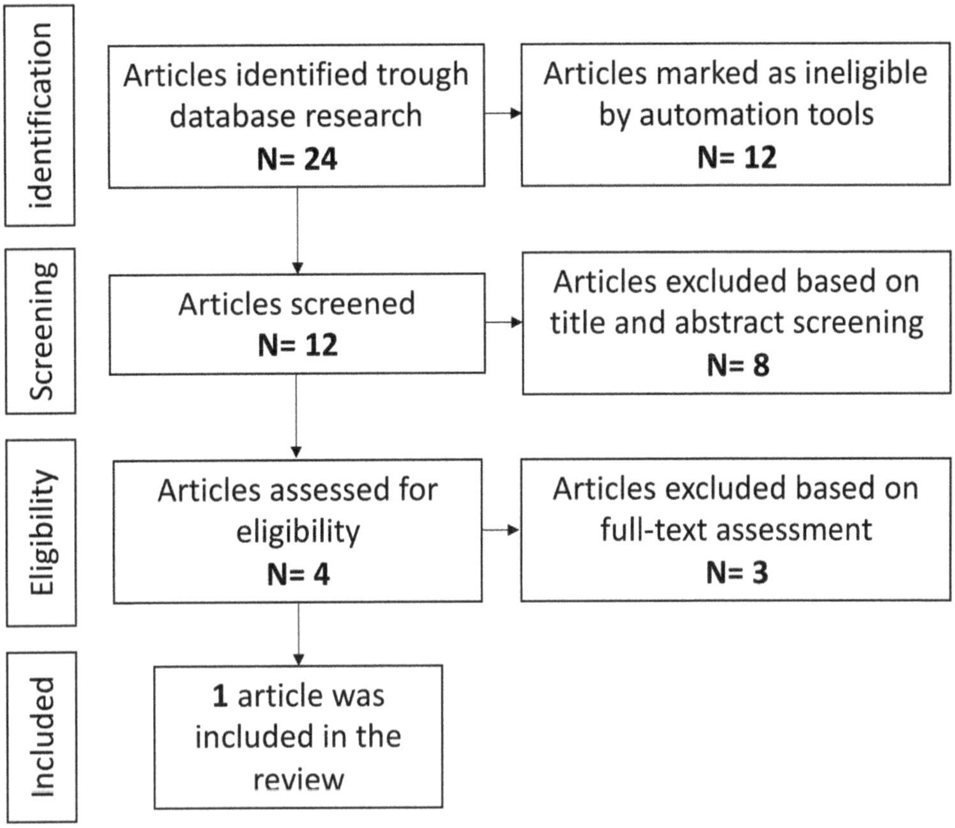

FIGURE 7 | Anti-α4-integrin agents and epilepsy, literature review.

show seizures and there is no mention of additional treatments. Data concerning the behavioral, cognitive, and motor outcomes were available for seven patients (130–134). An improvement was reported in six patients and in five of them the behavioral and cognitive functions were restored to premorbid condition. One patient with RE, albeit improved, showed residual motor and speech dysfunctions (130). In another case, the administration of rituximab resulted ineffective. Finally, only one patient had to discontinue the therapy due to a cutaneous rash associated with pruritus that appeared 24 h after the administration (128). Two other patients experienced mild infusion-related reactions and were able to continue the therapy (126). No adverse effects were reported in the other patients.

Systematic Literature Review: Anti-α4-Integrin Agents and Epilepsy

Study Selection

Overall a total of 24 references were identified during the initial electronic search, 12 of which were marked as not eligible by automation tools because published before 1 January 2016 and/or not in English language. A total of 12 potentially eligible studies were selected. Among these, eight were excluded for irrelevancy after a screening of the titles and abstracts (**Figure 7**). After a full-text assessment of the remaining four studies, three of them resulted ineligible, since the evaluation of seizures frequency and/or severity was not in the outcomes of the studies, or because studies were not concerning patients with RSE or DRE. Therefore, one single study was included in this review, a randomized, placebo-controlled, double-blinded study (phase 2 study OPUS, NCT03283371) (135).

Results

A total of 32 patients with drug-resistant focal epilepsy were included in this review (**Table 6**). The mean age was 42.8 years (±14.56). All patients received natalizumab 300 mg IV every 4 weeks for 24 weeks. The timing of administration was not specified. The primary endpoint of efficacy of the study included was to evaluate the change from baseline in seizure frequency (number of seizures per 28 days) from weeks 8 to 24 of the placebo-controlled period. Overall, the natalizumab-treated group showed a greater reduction in seizure frequency compared to placebo (−14.4%), although the predefined threshold for therapeutic success of 31% relative reduction was not achieved (135). Concerning the secondary endpoints, despite a reduction of ≥50% in seizure frequency from baseline during weeks 8–24 of treatment in 10/32 participants (31.3% compared to 17.6% of the placebo group), none of the participants that received natalizumab remained free from seizures. Reportedly, one patient experienced an inadequate treatment response and withdrew

TABLE 6 | Systematic review of anti-α4-integrin agents in epilepsy.

References	Disease	*N*, (age)	Study design	Intervention	Timing	Efficacy	Safety
French et al. (135)	DRE	32 [mean 42.8 years (±14.56)]	Randomized, placebo-controlled, double-blinded study	Natalizumab 300 mg IV every 4 weeks for 24 weeks	Start: not specified Stop: 24 weeks after the first dose.	Compared to placebo, the natalizumab-treated group showed a greater reduction in seizure frequency from baseline. 10/32 participants showed a reduction of ≥50% from baseline in seizure frequency during weeks 8–24. None of the participants remained free from seizures. One participant experienced an inadequate treatment response (e.g., did not modify ASMs after week 12 of the placebo-controlled period or did not discontinue the treatment after the active run-in period due to lack of efficacy)	24/32 participants experienced adverse effects ranging from mild (15/24), moderate (8/15) and severe (1/32). One participant experienced a serious event (urticaria) and discontinued the treatment.

ASM, anti-seizure medication; DRE, drug-resistant epilepsy; IV, intravenous.

from the treatment (135). Finally, the exploratory endpoints included change from baseline in frequencies of focal to bilateral tonic-clonic seizures and focal seizures. Participants of the natalizumab-treated group showed respectively a decrease of 21.34% and an increase of 6.61% in frequency over placebo. The endpoints of the study did not pertain to the motor, behavioral or cognitive outcome of the participants. Concerning safety, although adverse events were reported in 24/32 participants, ranging from mild (15/24) to moderate (8/15) and severe (1/32), only 2/32 showed events of special interest and only one of these participants discontinued the treatment due to urticaria (135).

Strengths and Limitations

This is the first systematic review exploring the use of anti-cytokine agents and anti-lymphocyte agents in individuals with DRE or RSE. This study has different limitations. Firstly, data on the use of anti-cytokine agents are mostly derived from isolated case reports and case series, with no randomized clinical trials, and the age range of the included patients is considerable. This significantly raises the risk of publication bias, thus favoring the publication of positive reports. Moreover, the administration of concomitant treatments (ASMs, corticosteroids, other immunosuppressive agents) can represent a considerable confounding factor. Therefore, the level of evidence is currently low. However, it is worth highlighting that the administration of anti-IL-1 agents (mainly anakinra) and tocilizumab in patients with severe DRE, such as RSE or FIRES, has shown a reduced seizure burden in most of the described patients, and a good safety profile is usually well-tolerated. Particularly, literature data report that more than 50% of the patients with FIRES respond to anakinra, while tocilizumab has been mostly used in patients with NORSE and SRSE showing partial or complete seizure control in almost all the described cases (**Figure 8**). Therefore, despite the mentioned limitations of this work, literature data suggest considering anti-IL-1 or anti-IL-6 therapeutic approaches in these conditions. Data on the use of adalimumab in patients with RE encourage further studies to assess whether this drug or other TNF-inhibitors could be effective in the treatment of those forms of RE refractory to other immunotherapies, but without the criteria for a surgical approach. Selected patients, like those with slowly progressive forms, may benefit from treatment with Anti TNF-α agents, while less is known regarding their use in other forms of epilepsy since the literature is scarce and studies on animal models are limited. Apart from the effect on seizures, anti-cytokine agents could significantly affect also motor, behavioral, and cognitive recovery, although this outcome has been heterogeneously reported in the different studies, with only four studies analyzing specific scales (110, 122, 124, 127). Notably, the serum and CSF cytokine profile was determined in <50% of the included patients. Although this investigation is not part of routine clinical practice (difficulty of interpretation, limited availability) the increasing knowledge of the involvement of cytokines in DRE and RSE could lead to a more diffuse use of this dosage, to provide a therapeutic strategy targeted on the main mediator involved in the individual patient.

The administration of Rituximab resulted to be effective in the majority of patients with DRE and RSE, with a more conspicuous

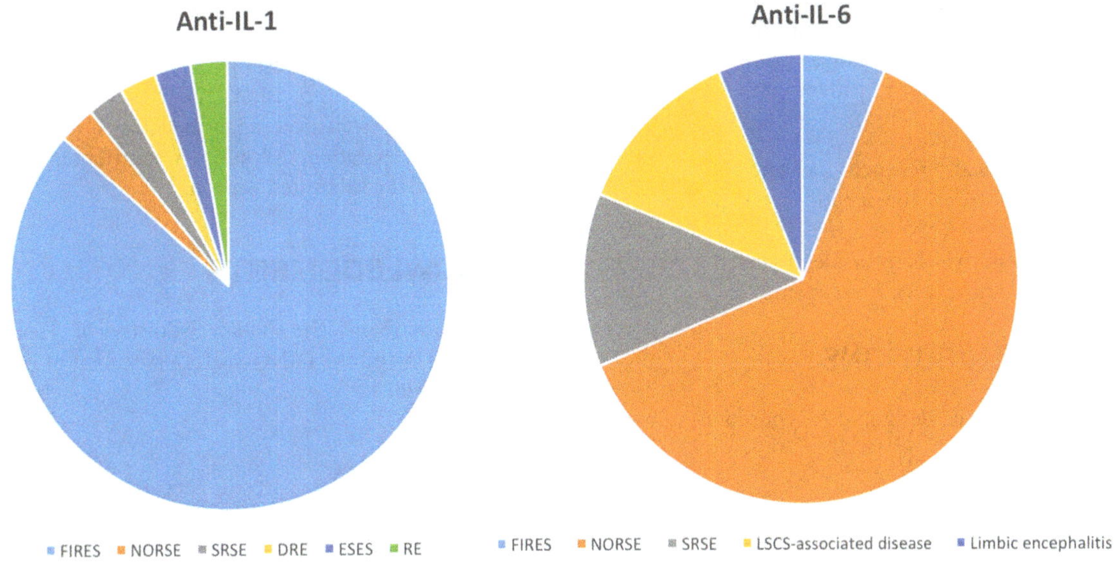

FIGURE 8 | Use of anakinra and tocilizumab in epilepsy, data from the literature.

response in individuals affected by AE-related seizures. Once more, a possible limitation and source of bias comes from the fact that studies concerning the use of Rituximab consit mainly in case reports or case series. This may also be the cause of the considerable heterogeneity in the timing and posology of the treatment that was evidenced. Future studies in this field should prioritize the definition of an appropriate treatment regimen.

Although targeting the leukocyte extravasation to brain parenchyma appeared to be a creditable therapeutic opportunity for patients with intractable epilepsy, the results of a randomized, double-blinded, placebo-controlled study showed that the administration of natalizumab did not significantly change seizure frequency in adults with drug-resistant focal epilepsy (135). Future trials, with a larger sample size, may overcome the limits of this latter study in detecting statistically significant differences.

OTHER INFLAMMATORY TARGETS AND EPILEPSY: FUTURE THERAPEUTIC PERSPECTIVES

Preclinical research is focusing on the identification of novel therapeutic targets for the treatment of neuroinflammation. In this regard, the role of agents targeting the human high-mobility group box-1 (HMGB-1) and chemokines are of particular interest. HMGB-1, a regulator of gene transcription and DNA remodeling/repair (136), mediates inflammatory responses *via* interactions with the receptor for advanced glycation end products (RAGE) and toll-like receptor (TLR) 4. It promotes the release of pro-inflammatory cytokines (e.g., TNF-α and IL-6) and acts as a key initiator of inflammation particularly within the brain (136–138). Anti-HMGB1 mAbs have proven to be effective in different mouse models of epilepsy (138–140), reducing also the chronic inflammatory pathways (upregulation of inflammation-related genes, microglial activation, and neuronal cell death). Chemokines are involved at different levels in CNS homeostasis, and have been implicated in the pathogenesis of different CNS diseases, including epilepsy (26, 141). In animal models of epilepsy, the administration of a CCL2 transcription inhibitor (Bindarit) or a selective antagonist of the CCR2 receptor (RS102895) suppressed the LPS-induced seizure enhancement (142, 143). Additionally, CX3CL1/CX3CR1 and the CC-chemokine receptor CCR5, widely expressed in the CNS microglia, have been implicated in the pathogenesis of epilepsy and represent other potential therapeutic targets (144–147). Overall, these findings, albeit resulting form preclinical experiments, might build the basis for new therapeutic strategies in the upcoming years.

CONCLUDING REMARKS

The involvement of the immune and inflammatory response in the pathogenesis of DRE and RSE are being progressively elucidated, leading to the increasing use of anti-cytokine agents in the treatment of these conditions. The experience with anti-IL-1, anti-IL-6, and anti-TNF drugs in the treatment of epilepsy is still limited and derives mostly from the observation of isolated case reports or small case series. In this work, we performed a systematic review that, despite the low evidence reached, showed promising results regarding the use of anti-cytokine agents in specific patients with DRE and RSE in terms of both efficacy and safety.

Beyond these anti-cytokine agents, there is increasing interest in the use of drugs targeting cells of adaptive immunity. The experience in the use of rituximab in RSE and DRE is fragmentary and there is a lack of a uniform regimen of treatment but this drug resulted to be effective in the major part of patients. Concerning the employment of natalizumab, the experience is limited to a single study that did not evidence a significant advantage in patients with DRE receiving the treatment.

Hopefully, preclinical research advances will allow the identification of new therapeutic strategies targeting neuroinflammation in epilepsy, and the collection of a larger number of clinical data will help in identifying those patients who will benefit from anti-cytokine treatments.

AUTHOR CONTRIBUTIONS

GC, GD, and AM: study design, data collection, statistical analysis, data interpretation, manuscript preparation, and literature search. TF, AO, DP, and AB: study design, data interpretation, and manuscript revision. PS, GM, SS, and RC: study design, supervision, and manuscript revision. AR: data collection, statistical analysis, data interpretation, and manuscript preparation. All authors contributed to the article and approved the submitted version.

ACKNOWLEDGMENTS

The authors thank the Italian Ministry of Health-Ricerca Corrente 2021 and the DINOGMI, Department of Excellence of MIUR 2018–2022.

REFERENCES

1. Behr C, Goltzene MA, Kosmalski G, Hirsch E, Ryvlin P. Epidemiology of epilepsy. *Rev Neurol.* (2016) 172:27–36. doi: 10.1016/j.neurol.2015.11.003
2. Scheffer IE, French J, Hirsch E, Jain S, Mathern GW, Moshé SL, et al. Classification of the epilepsies: New concepts for discussion and debate-Special report of the ILAE Classification Task Force of the Commission for Classification and Terminology. *Epilepsia Open.* (2016) 1:37–44. doi: 10.1002/epi4.5
3. Fisher RS. The new classification of seizures by the International League Against Epilepsy 2017. *Curr Neurol Neurosci Rep.* (2017) 17:48. doi: 10.1007/s11910-017-0758-6
4. Kalilani L, Sun X, Pelgrims B, Noack-Rink M, Villanueva V. The epidemiology of drug-resistant epilepsy: a systematic review and meta-analysis. *Epilepsia.* (2018) 59:2179–93. doi: 10.1111/epi.14596
5. Kwan P, Arzimanoglou A, Berg AT, Brodie MJ, Hauser WA, Mathern G, et al. Definition of drug-resistant epilepsy: consensus proposal by the *ad-hoc* Task Force of the ILAE Commission on Therapeutic Strategies. *Epilepsia.* (2010) 51:1069–77. doi: 10.1111/j.1528-1167.2009.02397.x
6. Téllez-Zenteno JF, Hernández-Ronquillo L, Buckley S, Zahagun R, Rizvi S. A validation of the new definition of drug-resistant epilepsy by the International League Against Epilepsy. *Epilepsia.* (2014) 55:829–34. doi: 10.1111/epi.12633
7. Trinka E, Cock H, Hesdorffer D, Rossetti AO, Scheffer IE, Shinnar S, et al. A definition and classification of status epilepticus–report of the ILAE Task Force on Classification of Status Epilepticus. *Epilepsia.* (2015) 56:1515–23. doi: 10.1111/epi.13121
8. Fisher RS, Acevedo C, Arzimanoglou A, Bogacz A, Cross JH, Elger CE, et al. ILAE official report: a practical clinical definition of epilepsy. *Epilepsia.* (2014) 55:475–82. doi: 10.1111/epi.12550
9. Esposito S, Principi N, Calabresi P, Rigante D. An evolving redefinition of autoimmune encephalitis. *Autoimmun Rev.* (2019) 18:155–63. doi: 10.1016/j.autrev.2018.08.009
10. Orsini A, Foiadelli T, Carli N, Costagliola G, Masini B, Bonuccelli A, et al. Rasmussen's encephalitis: from immune pathogenesis towards targeted-therapy. *Seizure.* (2020) 81:76–83. doi: 10.1016/j.seizure.2020.07.023
11. Hirsch LJ, Gaspard N, van Baalen A, Nabbout R, Demeret S, Loddenkemper T, et al. Proposed consensus definitions for new-onset refractory status epilepticus (NORSE), febrile infection-related epilepsy syndrome (FIRES), and related conditions. *Epilepsia.* (2018) 59:739–44. doi: 10.1111/epi.14016
12. Samanta D, Al Khalili Y. Electrical status epilepticus in sleep. In: *StatPearls.* Treasure Island, FL: StatPearls Publishing (2021).
13. Vossler DG, Bainbridge JL, Boggs JG, Novotny EJ, Loddenkemper T, Faught E. Treatment of refractory convulsive status Ep: a comprehensive review by the American Epilepsy Society Treatments Committee. *Epilepsy Curr.* (2020) 20:245–64. doi: 10.1177/1535759720928269
14. DiSabato DJ, Quan N, Godbout JP. Neuroinflammation: the devil is in the details. *J Neurochem.* (2016) 139(Suppl.2):136–53. doi: 10.1111/jnc.13607
15. Heida JG, Pittman QJ. Causal links between brain cytokines and experimental febrile convulsions in the rat. *Epilepsia.* (2005) 46:1906–13. doi: 10.1111/j.1528-1167.2005.00294.x
16. van Vliet EA, Aronica E, Vezzani A, Ravizza T. Review: neuroinflammatory pathways as treatment targets and biomarker candidates in epilepsy: emerging evidence from preclinical and clinical studies. *Neuropathol Appl Neurobiol.* (2018) 44:91–111. doi: 10.1111/nan.12444
17. Orsini A, Foiadelli T, Costagliola G, Michev A, Consolini R, Vinci F, et al. The role of inflammatory mediators in epilepsy: focus on developmental and epileptic encephalopathies and therapeutic implications. *Epilepsy Res.* (2021) 172:106588. doi: 10.1016/j.eplepsyres.2021.106588
18. Greco A, Rizzo MI, De Virgilio A, Conte M, Gallo A, Attanasio G, et al. Autoimmune epilepsy. *Autoimmun Rev.* (2016) 15:221–5. doi: 10.1016/j.autrev.2015.11.007
19. Nosadini M, Granata T, Matricardi S, Freri A, Ragona F, Papetti L, et al. Relapse risk factors in anti-N-methyl-D-aspartate receptor encephalitis. *Dev Med Child Neurol.* (2019) 61:1101–7. doi: 10.1111/dmcn.14267
20. Prinz M, Jung S, Priller J. Microglia biology: one century of evolving concepts. *Cell.* (2019) 179:292–311. doi: 10.1016/j.cell.2019.08.053
21. Garaschuk O, Verkhratsky A. Physiology of microglia. *Methods Mol Biol.* (2019) 2034:27–40. doi: 10.1007/978-1-4939-9658-2_3
22. Ransohoff RM, Schafer D, Vincent A, Blachère NE, Bar-Or A. Neuroinflammation: ways in which the immune system affects the brain. *Neurotherapeutics.* (2015) 12:896–909. doi: 10.1007/s13311-015-0385-3
23. de Vries EE, van den Munckhof B, Braun KP, van Royen-Kerkhof A, de Jager W, Jansen FE. Inflammatory mediators in human epilepsy: a systematic review and meta-analysis. *Neurosci Biobehav Rev.* (2016) 63:177–90. doi: 10.1016/j.neubiorev.2016.02.007
24. Hulkkonen J, Koskikallio E, Rainesalo S, Keranen T, Hurme M, Peltola J. The balance of inhibitory and excitatory cytokines is differently regulated *in vivo* and *in vitro* among therapy resistant epilepsy patients. *Epilepsy Res.* (2004) 59:199–205. doi: 10.1016/j.eplepsyres.2004.04.007
25. Vitaliti G, Pavone P, Marino S, Saporito MAN, Corsello G, Falsaperla R. Molecular mechanism involved in the pathogenesis of early-onset epileptic encephalopathy. *Front Mol Neurosci.* (2019) 12:118. doi: 10.3389/fnmol.2019.00118
26. Cerri C, Caleo M, Bozzi Y. Chemokines as new inflammatory players in the pathogenesis of epilepsy. *Epilepsy Res.* (2017) 136:77–83. doi: 10.1016/j.eplepsyres.2017.07.016
27. Yazdi AS, Ghoreschi K. The interleukin-1 family. *Adv Exp Med Biol.* (2016) 941:21–9. doi: 10.1007/978-94-024-0921-5_2
28. Zhu L, Liu X, Nemeth DP, DiSabato DJ, Witcher KG, Mckim DB, et al. Interleukin-1 causes CNS inflammatory cytokine expression *via*

endothelia-microglia bi-cellular signaling. *Brain Behav Immun.* (2019) 81:292–304. doi: 10.1016/j.bbi.2019.06.026

29. Lamkanfi M, Dixit VM. Inflammasomes and their roles in health and disease. *Annu Rev Cell Dev Biol.* (2012) 28:137–61. doi: 10.1146/annurev-cellbio-101011-155745
30. Gabay C, Lamacchia C, Palmer G. IL-1 pathways in inflammation and human diseases. *Nat Rev Rheumatol.* (2010) 6:232–41. doi: 10.1038/nrrheum.2010.4
31. Li G, Bauer S, Nowak M, Norwood B, Tackemberg B, Rosenow F, et al. Cytokines and epilepsy. *Seizure.* (2011) 20:249–56. doi: 10.1016/j.seizure.2010.12.005
32. Vezzani A, Viviani B. Neuromodulatory properties of inflammatory cytokines and their impact on neuronal excitability. *Neuropharmacology.* (2015) 96:70–82. doi: 10.1016/j.neuropharm.2014.10.027
33. Jesus AA, Goldbach-Mansky R. IL-1 blockade in autoinflammatory syndromes. *Annu Rev Med.* (2014) 65:223–44. doi: 10.1146/annurev-med-061512-150641
34. Dinarello CA. Treatment of inflammatory diseases with IL-1 blockade. *Curr Otorhinolaryngol Rep.* (2018) 6:1–14. doi: 10.1007/s40136-018-0181-9
35. Cavalli G, Dinarello CA. Anakinra therapy for non-cancer inflammatory diseases. *Front Pharmacol.* (2018) 9:1157. doi: 10.3389/fphar.2018.01157
36. Tanaka T, Narazaki M, Kishimoto T. IL-6 in inflammation, immunity, and disease. *Cold Spring Harb Perspect Biol.* (2014) 6:a016295. doi: 10.1101/cshperspect.a016295
37. Erta M, Quintana A, Hidalgo J. Interleukin-6, a major cytokine in the central nervous system. *Int J Biol Sci.* (2012) 8:1254–66. doi: 10.7150/ijbs.4679
38. Lorigados Pedre L, Morales Chacón LM. Follow-up of peripheral IL-1β and IL-6 and relation with apoptotic death in drug-resistant temporal lobe epilepsy patients submitted to surgery. *Behav Sci.* (2018) 8:21. doi: 10.3390/bs8020021
39. Sheppard M, Laskou F, Stapleton PP, Hadavi S, Dasgupta B. Tocilizumab (Actemra). *Hum Vaccin Immunother.* (2017) 13:1972–88. doi: 10.1080/21645515.2017.1316909
40. Lapides DA, McDonald MM. Inflammatory manifestations of systemic diseases in the central nervous system. *Curr Treat Options Neurol.* (2020) 22:26. doi: 10.1007/s11940-020-00636-2
41. Costagliola G, Cappelli S, Consolini R. Behçet's disease in children: diagnostic and management challenges. *Ther Clin Risk Manag.* (2020) 16:495–507. doi: 10.2147/TCRM.S232660
42. Boyce EG, Rogan EL, Vyas D, Prasad N, Mai Y. Sarilumab: review of a second IL-6 receptor antagonist indicated for the treatment of rheumatoid arthritis. *Ann Pharmacother.* (2018) 52:780–91. doi: 10.1177/1060028018761599
43. Crisafulli S, Isgrò V, La Corte L, Atzeni F, Trifirò G. Potential role of anti-interleukin (IL)-6 drugs in the treatment of COVID-19: rationale, clinical evidence and risks. *BioDrugs.* (2020) 34:415–22. doi: 10.1007/s40259-020-00430-1
44. Lieberman AP, Pitha PM, Shin HS, Shin ML. Production of tumor necrosis factor and other cytokines by astrocytes stimulated with lipopolysaccharide or a neurotropic virus. *Proc Natl Acad Sci USA.* (1989) 86:6348–52. doi: 10.1073/pnas.86.16.6348
45. MacEwan DJ, TNF. receptor subtype signalling: differences and cellular consequences. *Cell Signal.* (2002) 14:477–92. doi: 10.1016/S0898-6568(01)00262-5
46. Vezzani A, Aronica E, Mazarati A, Pittman QJ. Epilepsy and brain inflammation. *Exp Neurol.* (2013) 244:11–21. doi: 10.1016/j.expneurol.2011.09.033
47. Stellwagen D, Beattie EC, Seo JY, Malenka RC. Differential regulation of AMPA receptor and GABA receptor trafficking by tumor necrosis factor-alpha. *J Neurosci.* (2005) 25:3219–28. doi: 10.1523/JNEUROSCI.4486-04.2005
48. Schäfers M, Sorkin L. Effect of cytokines on neuronal excitability. *Neurosci Lett.* (2008) 437:188–93. doi: 10.1016/j.neulet.2008.03.052
49. Mayhan WG. Cellular mechanisms by which tumor necrosis factor-alpha produces disruption of the blood-brain barrier. *Brain Res.* (2002) 927:144–52. doi: 10.1016/S0006-8993(01)03348-0
50. De Simoni MG, Perego C, Ravizza T, Moneta D, Conti M, Marchesi F, et al. Inflammatory cytokines and related genes are induced in the rat hippocampus by limbic status epilepticus. *Eur J Neurosci.* (2000) 12:2623–33. doi: 10.1046/j.1460-9568.2000.00140.x
51. Akassoglou K, Probert L, Kontogeorgos G, Kollias G. Astrocyte-specific but not neuron-specific transmembrane TNF triggers inflammation and degeneration in the central nervous system of transgenic mice. *J Immunol.* (1997) 158:438–45.
52. Turrin NP, Rivest S. Innate immune reaction in response to seizures: implications for the neuropathology associated with epilepsy. *Neurobiol Dis.* (2004) 16:321–34. doi: 10.1016/j.nbd.2004.03.010
53. Yamamoto A, Schindler CK, Murphy BM, Bellver-Estelles C, So NK, Taki W, et al. Evidence of tumor necrosis factor receptor 1 signaling in human temporal lobe epilepsy. *Exp Neurol.* (2006) 202:410–20. doi: 10.1016/j.expneurol.2006.07.003
54. Wallach D, Varfolomeev EE, Malinin NL, Goltsev YV, Kovalenko AV, Boldin MP. Tumor necrosis factor receptor and Fas signaling mechanisms. *Annu Rev Immunol.* (1999) 17:331–67. doi: 10.1146/annurev.immunol.17.1.331
55. Salfeld J, Kaymakcalan Z, Tracey D, Roberts A, Kamen R. Generation of fully human anti-TNF antibody D2E7. *Arthritis Rheum.* (1998) 41:S57.
56. Tracey D, Klareskog L, Sasso EH, Salfeld JG, Tak PP. Tumor necrosis factor antagonist mechanisms of action: a comprehensive review. *Pharmacol Ther.* (2008) 117:244–79. doi: 10.1016/j.pharmthera.2007.10.001
57. van Oosten BW, Barkhof F, Truyen L, Boringa JB, Bertelsmann FW, von Blomberg BM, et al. Increased MRI activity and immune activation in two multiple sclerosis patients treated with the monoclonal anti-tumor necrosis factor antibody cA2. *Neurology.* (1996) 47:1531–4. doi: 10.1212/WNL.47.6.1531
58. The Lenercept Multiple Sclerosis Study Group, The University of British Columbia MS/MRI Analysis Group. TNF neutralization in MS: results of a randomized, placebo-controlled multicenter study. *Neurology.* (1999) 53:457–65. doi: 10.1212/WNL.53.3.457
59. Berrios I, Jun-O'Connell A, Ghiran S, Ionete C. A case of neurosarcoidosis secondary to treatment of etanercept and review of the literature. *BMJ Case Rep.* (2015) 2015:208188. doi: 10.1136/bcr-2014-208188
60. Grau RG. Drug-induced vasculitis: new insights and a changing lineup of suspects. *Curr Rheumatol Rep.* (2015) 17:71. doi: 10.1007/s11926-015-0545-9
61. Gherghel N, Stan A, Stan H. Pearls and Oy-sters: rheumatoid meningitis occurring during treatment with etanercept. *Neurology.* (2018) 91:806–8. doi: 10.1212/WNL.0000000000006397
62. Kastrup O, Diener HC. TNF-antagonist etanercept induced reversible posterior leukoencephalopathy syndrome. *J Neurol.* (2008) 255:452–3. doi: 10.1007/s00415-008-0732-y
63. Yamamoto M, Takahashi H, Wakasugi H, Sukawa Y, Saito M, Suzuki C, et al. Leukoencephalopathy during administration of etanercept for refractory rheumatoid arthritis. *Mod Rheumatol.* (2007) 17:72–4. doi: 10.3109/s10165-006-0530-2
64. Shin IS, Baer AN, Kwon HJ, Papadopoulos EJ, Siegel JN. Guillain-Barré and Miller Fisher syndromes occurring with tumor necrosis factor alpha antagonist therapy. *Arthritis Rheum.* (2006) 54:1429–34. doi: 10.1002/art.21814
65. Yokoyama W, Takada K, Miyasaka N, Kohsaka H. Myelitis and optic neuritis induced by a long course of etanercept in a patient with rheumatoid arthritis. *BMJ Case Rep.* (2014) 2014:bcr-2014-205779. doi: 10.1136/bcr-2014-205779
66. Simsek I, Erdem H, Pay S, Sobaci G, Dinc A. Optic neuritis occurring with anti-tumour necrosis factor alpha therapy. *Ann Rheum Dis.* (2007) 66:1255–8. doi: 10.1136/ard.2006.066787
67. Kameda T, Dobashi H, Kittaka K, Susaki K, Hosomi N, Deguchi K, et al. A case of rheumatoid arthritis complicated by demyelination in both cerebral cortex and spinal cord during etanercept therapy. *Mod Rheumatol.* (2008) 18:399–402. doi: 10.3109/s10165-008-0062-z
68. Sammut L, Wallis D, Holroyd C. Progressive multifocal leukoencephalopathy associated with infliximab. *J R Coll Physicians Edinb.* (2016) 46:163–5. doi: 10.4997/JRCPE.2016.305
69. Mohan N, Edwards ET, Cupps TR, Oliverio PJ, Sandberg G, Crayton H, et al. Demyelination occurring during anti-tumor necrosis factor alpha therapy for inflammatory arthritides. *Arthritis Rheum.* (2001) 44:2862–9. doi: 10.1002/1529-0131(200112)44:12<2862::AID-ART474>3.0.CO;2-W
70. Kemanetzoglou E, Andreadou E, CNS. Demyelination with TNF-α blockers. *Curr Neurol Neurosci Rep.* (2017) 17:36. doi: 10.1007/s11910-017-0742-1

71. Sedger LM, McDermott MF. TNF and TNF-receptors: from mediators of cell death and inflammation to therapeutic giants - past, present and future. *Cytokine Growth Factor Rev.* (2014) 25:453–72. doi: 10.1016/j.cytogfr.2014.07.016
72. Robinson WH, Genovese MC, Moreland LW. Demyelinating and neurologic events reported in association with tumor necrosis factor alpha antagonism: by what mechanisms could tumor necrosis factor alpha antagonists improve rheumatoid arthritis but exacerbate multiple sclerosis? *Arthritis Rheum.* (2001) 44:1977–83. doi: 10.1002/1529-0131(200109)44:9<1977::AID-ART345>3.0.CO;2-6
73. Mausner-Fainberg K, Regev K, Kolb H, Vaknin-Dembinsky A, Karni A. Increased neutralization capacity of TNF-α in sera of relapsing remitting multiple sclerosis patients is not related to soluble TNF-α receptors or anti-TNF-α autoantibody levels. *J Neuroimmunol.* (2015) 286:83–5. doi: 10.1016/j.jneuroim.2015.07.005
74. Arulsamy A, Shaikh MF. Tumor necrosis factor-α, the pathological key to post-traumatic epilepsy: a comprehensive systematic review. *ACS Chem Neurosci.* (2020) 11:1900–8. doi: 10.1021/acschemneuro.0c00301
75. Carson MJ, Doose JM, Melchior B, Schmid CD, Ploix CC. CNS immune privilege: hiding in plain sight. *Immunol Rev.* (2006) 213:48–65. doi: 10.1111/j.1600-065X.2006.00441.x
76. Wilson EH, Weninger W, Hunter CA. Trafficking of immune cells in the central nervous system. *J Clin Invest.* (2010) 120:1368–79. doi: 10.1172/JCI41911
77. Vezzani A, Lang B, Aronica E. Immunity and inflammation in epilepsy. *Cold Spring Harb Perspect Med.* (2015) 6:a022699. doi: 10.1101/cshperspect.a022699
78. Yamanaka G, Morichi S, Takamatsu T, Watanabe Y, Suzuki S, Ishida Y, et al. Links between immune cells from the periphery and the brain in the pathogenesis of epilepsy: a narrative review. *Int J Mol Sci.* (2021) 22:94395. doi: 10.3390/ijms22094395
79. Wiendl H, Bien CG, Bernasconi P, Fleckenstein B, Elger CE, Dichgans J, et al. GluR3 antibodies: prevalence in focal epilepsy but no specificity for Rasmussen's encephalitis. *Neurology.* (2001) 57:1511–4. doi: 10.1212/WNL.57.8.1511
80. Steinman L. Autoimmune disease. *Sci Am.* (1993) 269:106–14. doi: 10.1038/scientificamerican0993-106
81. Zuliani L, Graus F, Giometto B, Bien C, Vincent A. Central nervous system neuronal surface antibody associated syndromes: review and guidelines for recognition. *J Neurol Neurosurg Psychiatry.* (2012) 83:638–45. doi: 10.1136/jnnp-2011-301237
82. Bernal F, Graus F, Pifarré A, Saiz A, Benyahia B, Ribalta T. Immunohistochemical analysis of anti-Hu-associated paraneoplastic encephalomyelitis. *Acta Neuropathol.* (2002) 103:509–15. doi: 10.1007/s00401-001-0498-0
83. Xu D, Robinson AP, Ishii T, Duncan DS, Alden TD, Goings GE, et al. Peripherally derived T regulatory and $\gamma\delta$ T cells have opposing roles in the pathogenesis of intractable pediatric epilepsy. *J Exp Med.* (2018) 215:1169–86. doi: 10.1084/jem.20171285
84. Neumann H, Cavalié A, Jenne DE, Wekerle H. Induction of MHC class I genes in neurons. *Science.* (1995) 269:549–52. doi: 10.1126/science.7624779
85. Alexopoulos H, Biba A, Dalakas MC. Anti-B-cell therapies in autoimmune neurological diseases: rationale and efficacy trials. *Neurotherapeutics.* (2016) 13:20–33. doi: 10.1007/s13311-015-0402-6
86. Pescovitz MD. Rituximab, an anti-cd20 monoclonal antibody: history and mechanism of action. *Am J Transplant.* (2006) 6:859–66. doi: 10.1111/j.1600-6143.2006.01288.x
87. Chisari CG, Sgarlata E, Arena S, Toscano S, Luca M, Patti F. Rituximab for the treatment of multiple sclerosis: a review. *J Neurol.* (2021) 2021:1–25. doi: 10.1007/s00415-020-10362-z
88. Savasta S, Foiadelli T, Vegezzi E, Cortese A, Lozza A, Pichiecchio A, et al. Efficacy of rituximab as third-line therapy in combined central and peripheral demyelination. *Neurol Clin Pract.* (2017) 2017:534–7. doi: 10.1212/CPJ.0000000000000388
89. Nepal G, Shing YK, Yadav JK, Rehrig JH, Ojha R, Huang DY, et al. Efficacy and safety of rituximab in autoimmune encephalitis: a meta-analysis. *Acta Neurol Scand.* (2020) 142:449–59. doi: 10.1111/ane.13291
90. Titulaer MJ, McCracken L, Gabilondo I, Armangué T, Glaser C, Iizuka T, et al. Treatment and prognostic factors for long-term outcome in patients with anti-NMDA receptor encephalitis: an observational cohort study. *Lancet Neurol.* (2013) 12:157–65. doi: 10.1016/S1474-4422(12)70310-1
91. Baroncini D, Spagnolo F, Sarro L, Comi G, Volonte MA. A complex case of anti-GAD antibody-related syndrome treated with Rituximab. *Neurol Sci.* (2013) 34:1847–9. doi: 10.1007/s10072-013-1327-7
92. Foiadelli T, Gastaldi M, Scaranzin S, Franciotta D, Savasta S. Seizures and myelin oligodendrocyte glycoprotein (MOG) antibodies: two paradigmatic cases and a review of the literature. *Mult Scler Relat Disord.* (2020) 41:102011. doi: 10.1016/j.msard.2020.102011
93. Brown JW, Martin PJ, Thorpe JW, Michell AW, Coles AJ, Cox AL, et al. Long-term remission with rituximab in refractory leucine-rich glioma inactivated 1 antibody encephalitis. *J Neuroimmunol.* (2014) 271:66–8. doi: 10.1016/j.jneuroim.2014.03.012
94. Thilo B, Stingele R, Knudsen K, Boor R, Bien CG, Deuschl G, et al. A case of Rasmussen encephalitis treated with rituximab. *Nat Rev Neurol.* (2009) 5:458–62. doi: 10.1038/nrneurol.2009.98
95. Caraballo RH, Reyes G, Lopez Avaria MF, Buompadre MC, Gonzales M, Fortini S, et al. Febrile infection-related epilepsy syndrome: a study of 12 patients. *Seizure.* (2013) 22:553–9. doi: 10.1016/j.seizure.2013.04.005
96. Rudick R, Polman C, Clifford D, Miller D, Steinman L. Natalizumab: bench to bedside and beyond. *J Am Med Assoc Neurol.* (2013) 70:172–82. doi: 10.1001/jamaneurol.2013.598
97. Polman CH, O'Connor PW, Havrdova E, Hutchinson M, Kappos L, Miller DH, et al. A randomized, placebo-controlled trial of natalizumab for relapsing multiple sclerosis. *N Engl J Med.* (2006) 354:899–910. doi: 10.1056/NEJMoa044397
98. Kebir H, Carmant L, Fontaine F, Béland K, Bosoi CM, Sanon NT, et al. Humanized mouse model of Rasmussen's encephalitis supports the immune-mediated hypothesis. *J Clin Invest.* (2018) 128:2000–9. doi: 10.1172/JCI97098
99. Bittner S, Simon OJ, Gobel K, Bien CG, Meuth SG, Wiendl H. Rasmussen encephalitis treated with natalizumab. *Neurology.* (2013) 81:395–7. doi: 10.1212/WNL.0b013e31829c5ceb
100. Page MJ, McKenzie JE, Bossuyt PM, Boutron I, Hoffmann TC, Mulrow CD, et al. The PRISMA 2020 statement: an updated guideline for reporting systematic reviews. *Int J Surg.* (2021) 88:105906. doi: 10.1016/j.ijsu.2021.105906
101. Sterne JA, Hernán MA, Reeves BC, Savović J, Berkman ND, Viswanathan M, et al. ROBINS-I: a tool for assessing risk of bias in non-randomised studies of interventions. *BMJ.* (2016) 355:i4919. doi: 10.1136/bmj.i4919
102. Murad MH, Sultan S, Haffar S, Bazerbachi F. Methodological quality and synthesis of case series and case reports. *BMJ Evid Based Med.* (2018) 23:60–3. doi: 10.1136/bmjebm-2017-110853
103. Goldet G, Howick J. Understanding GRADE: an introduction. *J Evid Based Med.* (2013) 6:50–4. doi: 10.1111/jebm.12018
104. Berger JR, Markowitz C, Merkel PA, Kolster RA, Mourelatos Z. Multifocal neutrophilic meningoencephalitis: a novel disorder responsive to anakinra. *J Neurol.* (2021) 268:2995–9. doi: 10.1007/s00415-021-10431-x
105. Sa M, Singh R, Pujar S, D'Arco F, Desai N, Eltze C, et al. Centromedian thalamic nuclei deep brain stimulation and Anakinra treatment for FIRES - two different outcomes. *Eur J Paediatr Neurol.* (2019) 23:749–54. doi: 10.1016/j.ejpn.2019.08.001
106. Yang JH, Nataraj S, Sattar S. Successful treatment of pediatric FIRES with Anakinra. *Pediatr Neurol.* (2021) 114:60–1. doi: 10.1016/j.pediatrneurol.2020.10.009
107. Kern-Smith E, Chen DF, Koh S, Dutt M. The cat's out of the bag: a rare case of new-onset refractory status epilepticus (NORSE) due to Bartonella henselae. *Seizure.* (2020) 81:241–3. doi: 10.1016/j.seizure.2020.08.006
108. Dilena R, Mauri E, Aronica E, Bernasconi P, Bana C, Cappelletti C, et al. Therapeutic effect of Anakinra in the relapsing chronic phase of febrile infection-related epilepsy syndrome. *Epilepsia Open.* (2019) 4:344–50. doi: 10.1002/epi4.12317
109. Jyonouchi H, Geng L. Resolution of EEG findings and clinical improvement in a patient with encephalopathy and ESES with a combination of immunomodulating agents other than corticosteroids: a case report. *Epilepsy Behav Rep.* (2020) 14:100379. doi: 10.1016/j.ebr.2020.100379

110. Lai YC, Muscal E, Wells E, Shukla N, Eschbach K, Lee KH, et al. Anakinra usage in febrile infection related epilepsy syndrome: an international cohort. *Ann Clin Transl Neurol.* (2020) 7:2467–74. doi: 10.1002/acn3.51229
111. Westbrook C, Subramaniam T, Seagren RM, Tarula E, Co D, Furstenberg-Knauff M, et al. Febrile infection-related epilepsy syndrome treated successfully with Anakinra in a 21-year-old woman. *WMJ.* (2019) 118:135–9.
112. Kenney-Jung DL, Vezzani A, Kahoud RJ, LaFrance-Corey RG, Ho ML, Muskardin TW, et al. Febrile infection-related epilepsy syndrome treated with anakinra. *Ann Neurol.* (2016) 80:939–45. doi: 10.1002/ana.24806
113. DeSena AD, Do T, Schulert GS. Systemic autoinflammation with intractable epilepsy managed with interleukin-1 blockade. *J Neuroinflammation.* (2018) 15:38. doi: 10.1186/s12974-018-1063-2
114. Stredny CM, Case S, Sansevere AJ, Son M, Henderson L, Gorman MP. Interleukin-6 blockade with tocilizumab in anakinra-refractory febrile infection-related epilepsy syndrome (FIRES). (2020) 7:2329048x20979253. doi: 10.1177/2329048X20979253
115. Mochol M, Taubøll E, Sveberg L, Tennøe B, Berg Olsen K, Heuser K, et al. Seizure control after late introduction of anakinra in a patient with adult onset Rasmussen's encephalitis. *Epilepsy Behav Rep.* (2021) 16:100462. doi: 10.1016/j.ebr.2021.100462
116. Choi CH, Ma SH, Ma KK, Leung H, Mok VC. Super-refractory status epilepticus in autoimmune encephalitis treated with interleukin-1 receptor antagonist, anakinra. *Epileptic Disord.* (2021) 23:500–5. doi: 10.1684/epd.2021.1283
117. Magro CM, Halteh P, Olson LC, Kister I, Shapiro L. Linear scleroderma "en coup de sabre" with extensive brain involvement-clinicopathologic correlations and response to anti-interleukin-6 therapy. *Orphanet J Rare Dis.* (2019) 14:110. doi: 10.1186/s13023-019-1015-7
118. Donnelly JP, Kasatwar N, Hafeez S, Seifi A, Gilbert A, Barthol C, et al. Resolution of cryptogenic new onset refractory status epilepticus with tocilizumab. *Epilepsy Behav Rep.* (2021) 15:100431. doi: 10.1016/j.ebr.2021.100431
119. Osminina M, Geppe N, Afonina E. Scleroderma "en coup de sabre" with epilepsy and uveitis successfully treated with tocilizumab. *Reumatol Clin.* (2020) 16:356–8. doi: 10.1016/j.reuma.2018.05.001
120. Jaafar F, Haddad L, Koleilat N, Sharara-Chami R, Shbarou R. Super refractory status epilepticus secondary to anti-GAD antibody encephalitis successfully treated with aggressive immunotherapy. *Epilepsy Behav Rep.* (2020) 14:100396. doi: 10.1016/j.ebr.2020.100396
121. Cantarín-Extremera V, Jiménez-Legido M, Duat-Rodríguez A, García-Fernández M, Ortiz-Cabrera NV, Ruiz-Falcó-Rojas ML, et al. Tocilizumab in pediatric refractory status epilepticus and acute epilepsy: experience in two patients. *J Neuroimmunol.* (2020) 340:577142. doi: 10.1016/j.jneuroim.2019.577142
122. Benucci M, Tramacere L, Infantino M, Manfredi M, Grossi V, Damiani A, et al. Efficacy of tocilizumab in limbic encephalitis with anti-CASPR2 antibodies. *Case Rep Neurol Med.* (2020) 2020:5697670. doi: 10.1155/2020/5697670
123. Vallecoccia MS, Martinotti A, Siddi C, Dominedò C, Cingolani E. Use of unconventional therapies in super-refractory status epilepticus: a case report and literature review. *Clin EEG Neurosci.* (2020) 2020:1550059420975612. doi: 10.1177/1550059420975612
124. Jun JS, Lee ST, Kim R, Chu K, Lee SK. Tocilizumab treatment for new onset refractory status epilepticus. *Ann Neurol.* (2018) 84:940–5. doi: 10.1002/ana.25374
125. Lee WJ, Lee ST, Shin YW, Lee HS, Shin HR, Kim DY, et al. Teratoma removal, steroid, IVIG, rituximab and tocilizumab (T-SIRT) in anti-NMDAR encephalitis. *Neurotherapeutics.* (2020) 18:474–87. doi: 10.1007/s13311-020-00921-7
126. Lee WJ, Lee ST, Moon J, Sunwoo JS, Byun JI, Lim JA, et al. Tocilizumab in autoimmune encephalitis refractory to rituximab: an institutional cohort study. *Neurotherapeutics.* (2016) 13:824–32. doi: 10.1007/s13311-016-0442-6
127. Lagarde S, Villeneuve N, Trébuchon A, Kaphan E, Lepine A, McGonigal A, et al. Anti-tumor necrosis factor alpha therapy (adalimumab) in Rasmussen's encephalitis: an open pilot study. *Epilepsia.* (2016) 57:956–66. doi: 10.1111/epi.13387
128. Byun JI, Lee ST, Jung KH, Sunwoo JS, Moon J, Lim JA, et al. Effect of immunotherapy on seizure outcome in patients with autoimmune encephalitis: a prospective observational registry study. *PLoS ONE.* (2016) 11:e0146455. doi: 10.1371/journal.pone.0146455
129. Timarova G, Lisa I, Kukumberg P. Long-term effect of rituximab in a case with late-onset Rasmussen's encephalitis with anti-ganglioside IgGQ1b and anti-GAD antibodies positivity. *Case Report Neuro Endocrinol Lett.* (2016) 37:179–83.
130. El Tawil S, Morris R, Mullatti N, Nashef L, Rajakulendran S. Adult onset Rasmussen's encephalitis associated with reflex language induced seizures responsive to Rituximab therapy. *Seizure.* (2016) 42:60–2. doi: 10.1016/j.seizure.2016.09.009
131. Schneider R, Brüne M, Breuer TG, Börnke C, Gold R, Juckel G. Early multidisciplinary intensive-care therapy can improve outcome of severe anti-NMDA-receptor encephalitis presenting with extreme delta brush. *Transl Neurosci.* (2019) 10:241–3. doi: 10.1515/tnsci-2019-0039
132. Sansevere AJ, Henderson LA, Stredny CM, Prabhu SP, Shah A, Sundel R, et al. Posterior-onset Rasmussen's encephalitis with ipsilateral cerebellar atrophy and uveitis resistant to rituximab. *Epilepsy Behav Rep.* (2020) 2020:100360. doi: 10.1016/j.ebr.2020.100360
133. Kurukumbi M, Dave RH, Castillo J, Shah T, Lau J. Rituximab for autoimmune encephalitis with epilepsy. *Case Rep Neurol Med.* (2020) 2020:5843089. doi: 10.1155/2020/5843089
134. Cheli M, Dinoto A, Tommasini V, Ajčević M, Stella G, Catalan M, et al. Efficacy of rituximab on seizure control and cognitive symptoms in leucine-rich, glioma-inactivated 1 (LGI1) limbic encephalitis: a high-density electroencephalography case study. *Epileptic Disord.* (2020) 22:678–82. doi: 10.1684/epd.2020.1213
135. French JA, Cole AJ, Faught E, Theodore WH, Vezzani A, Liow K, et al. Safety and efficacy of natalizumab as adjunctive therapy for people with drug-resistant epilepsy: a phase 2 study. *Neurology.* (2021) 97:e1757–e67. doi: 10.1212/WNL.0000000000012766
136. Musumeci D, Roviello GN, Montesarchio D. An overview on HMGB1 inhibitors as potential therapeutic agents in HMGB1-related pathologies. *Pharmacol Ther.* (2014) 141:347–57. doi: 10.1016/j.pharmthera.2013.11.001
137. Wang S, Zhang Y. HMGB1 in inflammation and cancer. *J Hematol Oncol.* (2020) 13:116. doi: 10.1186/s13045-020-00950-x
138. Paudel YN, Shaikh MF, Chakraborti A, Kumari Y, Aledo-Serrano A, Aleksovska K, et al. HMGB1: a common biomarker and potential target for TBI, neuroinflammation, epilepsy, and cognitive dysfunction. *Front Neurosci.* (2018) 12:628. doi: 10.3389/fnins.2018.00628
139. Fu L, Liu K, Wake H, Teshigawara K, Yoshino T, Takahashi H, et al. Therapeutic effects of anti-HMGB1 monoclonal antibody on pilocarpine-induced status epilepticus in mice. *Sci Rep.* (2017) 7:1179. doi: 10.1038/s41598-017-01325-y
140. Zhao J, Wang Y, Xu C, Liu K, Wang Y, Chen L, et al. Therapeutic potential of an anti-high mobility group box-1 monoclonal antibody in epilepsy. *Brain Behav Immun.* (2017) 64:308–19. doi: 10.1016/j.bbi.2017.02.002
141. Cartier L, Hartley O, Dubois-Dauphin M, Krause KH. Chemokine receptors in the central nervous system: role in brain inflammation and neurodegenerative diseases. *Brain Res Rev.* (2005) 48:16–42. doi: 10.1016/j.brainresrev.2004.07.021
142. Foresti ML, Arisi GM, Katki K, Montanez A, Sanchez RM, Shapiro LA. Chemokine CCL2 and its receptor CCR2 are increased in the hippocampus following pilocarpine-induced status epilepticus. *J Neuroinflammation.* (2009) 6:40. doi: 10.1186/1742-2094-6-40
143. Cerri C, Genovesi S, Allegra M, Pistillo F, Püntener U, Guglielmotti A, et al. The chemokine CCL2 mediates the seizure-enhancing effects of systemic inflammation. *J Neurosci.* (2016) 36:3777–88. doi: 10.1523/JNEUROSCI.0451-15.2016
144. Louboutin JP, Strayer DS. Relationship between the chemokine receptor CCR5 and microglia in neurological disorders: consequences of targeting CCR5 on neuroinflammation, neuronal death and regeneration in a model of epilepsy. *CNS Neurol Disord Drug Targets.* (2013) 12:815–29. doi: 10.2174/18715273113126660173
145. Xu Y, Zeng K, Han Y, Wang L, Chen D, Xi Z, et al. Altered expression of CX3CL1 in patients with epilepsy and in a rat model. *Am J Pathol.* (2012) 180:1950–62. doi: 10.1016/j.ajpath.2012.01.024

146. Limatola C, Ransohoff RM. Modulating neurotoxicity through CX3CL1/CX3CR1 signaling. *Front Cell Neurosci.* (2014) 8:229. doi: 10.3389/fncel.2014.00229
147. Pawelec P, Ziemka-Nalecz M, Sypecka J, Zalewska T. The impact of the CX3CL1/CX3CR1 axis in neurological disorders. *Cells.* (2020) 9:2277. doi: 10.3390/cells9102277

23

Case Report of Novel Genetic Variant in KCNT1 Channel and Pharmacological Treatment with Quinidine: Precision Medicine in Refractory Epilepsy

M. C. Kravetz[1], M. S. Viola[1], J. Prenz[2], M. Curi[2], G. F. Bramuglia[1,3] and S. Tenembaum[4]*

[1]Department of Pharmacology, Faculty of Farmacy and Biochemistry, University of Buenos Aires, Buenos Aires City, Argentina, [2]Department of Cardiology, Garrahan Hospital, Buenos Aires City, Argentina, [3]Fundacion Investigar, Buenos Aires City, Argentina, [4]Department of Neurology, Garrahan Hospital, Buenos Aires City, Argentina

Correspondence:
M. C. Kravetz
mariaceciliakravetz@gmail.com

Case introduction: In this work we present a female infant patient with epilepsy of infancy with migrating focal seizures (EIMFS). Although many pharmacological schemes were attempted, she developed an encephalopathy with poor response to antiepileptic drugs and progressive cerebral dysfunction.

Aim: To present the pharmacological response and therapeutic drug monitoring of a paediatric patient with a severe encephalopathy carrying a genetic variant in KCNT1 gene, whose identification led to include quinidine (QND) in the treatment regimen as an antiepileptic drug.

Case report: Patient showed slow rhythmic activity (theta range) over left occipital areas with temporal propagation and oculo-clonic focal seizures and without tonic spasms three months after birth. At the age of 18 months showed severe impairments of motor and intellectual function with poor eye contact. When the patient was 4 years old, a genetic variant in the exon 24 of the KCNT1 gene was found. This led to the diagnosis of EIMFS. Due to antiepileptic treatment failed to control seizures, QND a KCNT1 blocker, was introduced as a therapeutic alternative besides topiramate (200 mg/day) and nitrazepam (2 mg/day). Therapeutic drug monitoring (TDM) of QND plasma levels needed to be implemented to establish individual therapeutic range and avoid toxicity. TDM for dose adjustment was performed to establish the individual therapeutic range of the patient. Seizures were under control with QND levels above 1.5 mcg/ml (65–70 mg/kg q. i.d). In addition, QND levels higher than 4.0 mcg/ml, were related to higher risk of suffering arrhythmia due to prolongation of QT segment. Despite initial intention to withdrawal topiramate completely, QND was no longer effective by itself and failed to maintain seizures control. Due to this necessary interaction between quinidine and topiramate, topiramate was stablished in a maintenance dose of 40 mg/day.

Conclusion: The implementation of Precision Medicine by using tools such as Next Generation Sequencing and TDM led to diagnose and select a targeted therapy for the treatment of a KCNT1-related epilepsy in a patient presented with EIMFS in early infancy and poor response to antiepileptic drugs. QND an old antiarrhythmic drug, due to its activity as KCNT1 channel blocker, associated to topiramate resulted in seizures control. Due to high variability observed in QND levels, TDM and pharmacokinetic characterization allowed to optimize drug regimen to maintain QND concentration between the individual therapeutic range and diminish toxicity.

Keywords: epilepsy, pharmacogenomics, pharmacokinetics, precision medicine, TDM, quinidine, HPLC

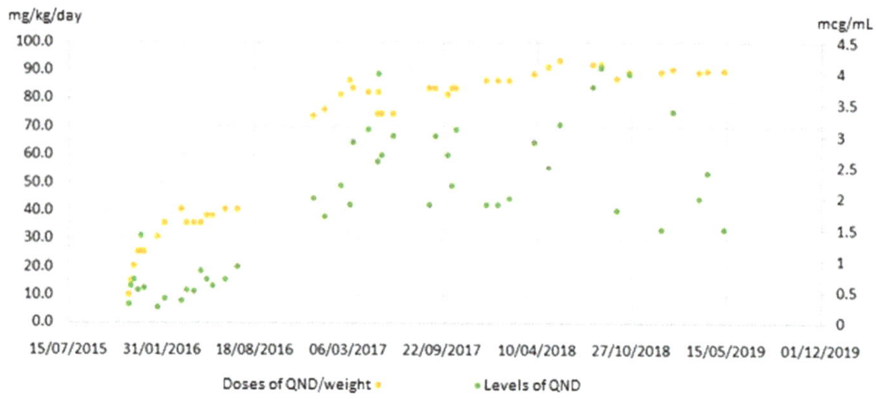

GRAPHICAL ABSTRACT |

INTRODUCTION

Epilepsy of infancy with migrating focal seizures (EIMFS) is a severe encephalopathy affecting children at very early stages. Seizures can begin as early as six months of life, and even a few weeks after delivery. This rare epileptic syndrome is characterized for pharmacological treatment resistance and poor prognosis. Its low prevalence varies from 1/200,000 to 1/1,000,000 habitants depending on of the population studied (Epilepsy of infancy with migrating focal seizures (2020) Epilepsy of infancy with migrating focal seizures | Epilepsy Action).

About etiology, the origin of this complex syndromes of infancy with migrating partial onset is not certain, but it is described the association with pathologic variants of KCNT1, SCN1A, SCN2A, PLCB1, TBC1D24 and CHD2 (International League Against Epilepsy, 2020 Epilepsy of infancy with migrating focal seizures, 2020). Around 70% of patients carries mutations in these and others genes and KCNT1 variants are implied in almost 40% of EIMFS (Lim et al., 2016).

In vitro functional studies have shown that KCNT1 carrying pathogenic variants generate larger currents when compared to wild-type KCNT1 channels, leading to the concept that a gain-of-function mechanism is responsible for epileptogenesis associated with KCNT1 variants (Barcia et al., 2012). Based on the ability to inhibit KCNT1 mutant channels, KCNT1 blockers like quinidine (QND), and old antiarrhythmic drug, and bepridil, have been proposed for the treatment of EIMFS (Milligan et al., 2014). Targeted therapy with QND has been introduced for compassionate use in EIMFS patients, resulting in variable anticonvulsant effect ranging from high pharmacological responses (Fukuoka et al., 2017) to a lack of efficacy or excessive toxicity (Chong et al., 2016; Madaan et al., 2018).

Previous data showed QND produced a concentration-dependent decrease in KCNT1 outward currents (Rizzo et al., 2016; Dilena et al., 2018) and that QND was even more potent in blocking KCNT1 channel carrying previously identified genetic variants, such as R950Q or E893K, in comparison with KCNT1 wild type (Dilena et al., 2018).

In this work we present a female pediatric patient with a severe case of EIMFS. Although many pharmacological schemes were attempted, the patient developed an epileptic syndrome with poor response to antiepileptic drugs and progressive cerebral dysfunction.

The patient had two episodes of apnea during the first week of life and showed poor eye contact, a trend toward a conjugate deviation of the eyes and head to the right or left, with horizontal nystagmus. She was extremely irritable. Three month later the patient was admitted due to three epileptic seizures recorded by electroencephalogram, which indicated slow rhythmic activity (theta range) over left occipital areas with temporal propagation. She presented oculo-clonic focal seizures which she repeated several times during examinations without tonic spasms.

The first year of life the patient received a drug regimen that included phenobarbital, valproic acid 750 mg/day, levetiracetam 600 mg/day, and ketogenic diet. Immunoglobulin therapy was also included because of low serum levels of Ig A and IgG.

As time progressed, the patient demonstrated spastic asymmetric quadriplegia, more prominent on the right, truncal hypotonia with poor head control, and lower-limb pyramidal tract signs. There were no laboratory abnormalities in blood nor CSF, and no sign of skeletal malformation on physical examination.

Electroencephalography during sleep (multiple recordings) demonstrated paroxysmal multifocal discharges with periods of electric attenuation or suppression which were not continuous. Electrographic seizures were also recorded, arising from the left frontal-temporal and right temporal-occipital regions. The clinical presentation and electroencephalographic features resembled an early myoclonic encephalopathy.

When the patient was 18 months old topiramate (TPM) was initiated that was related with a decrease in the frequency of seizures. At two years old (September 2011) seizures could be controlled receiving TPM 7 mg/kg/day, levetiracetam 48 mg/kg/day, and nitrazepam 2 mg/day (ketogenic diet was discontinuated). Nevertheless, electroencephalography during sleep in October 2011 revealed a typical sleep pattern with sleep spindles and vertex waves, in addition to infrequent sharp waves in left occipital region without generalized paroxysms or electric suppression.

A genomic study was performed, and no pathogenic variants were found in Glut1 gene, MCP2, CDKL5, FOXG1. Levetiracetam was finally withdrawn in April 2012 with no seizure recurrence. Due to a clear right-sided hemidystonia, levo-dopa with carbidopa in increasing dose was initiated in May 2012.

A brain MRI was performed at 3 years of age, and revealed subtle signs of cortical atrophy, hypoplastic corpus callosum, T2 and FLAIR high signal abnormalities involving the brain white matter, more prominent in the left hemisphere. Although neurological improvement could be observed, the patient showed a persistent right-sided hemidystonia, increased muscle tone in lower limbs with pyramidal signs and sleep pattern discharges.

AIM

To present the pharmacological response and therapeutic drug monitoring (TDM) of a paediatric patient with a severe encephalopathy refractory to pharmacological treatment, carrying a genetic variant in KCNT1 gene, whose identification by Next Generation Sequencing (NGS) led to include QND as antiepileptic drug.

CASE REPORT

To summarize, the initial years of the patient included epileptic encephalopathy development, cognitive and physical impairment which were part of an undiagnosed syndrome resistant to pharmacological treatment.

On 2013, when the patient was 4 years old, a Whole Exome Sequencing (WES) was performed. The entire exome was captured using reagent that targets coding exons from the consensus coding sequence. Capture enrichment was followed by sequencing on Illumina platform using previously described standard protocols. Illumina sequence analysis was performed using the Human Genome Sequencing Center's integrated Mercury pipeline (Baylor College of Medicine, United States of America). A pathogenic genetic variant associated to EIMFS (Barcia et al., 2012; The ILAE Genetics Commission Blog, 2020 KCNT1 – this is what you need to know, 2020) located in exon 24 (2795 T > C) of the KCNT1 gene (Potassium Sodium-Activated Channel Subfamily T Member 1) was identified.

Due to the remaining nocturnal activity despite many pharmacological schemes, a different approach was implemented.

At that moment new clinical studies showed benefits in using QND in epilepsy (Mikati et al., 2015), due to its activity as KCNT1 blocker. Due to its pharmacological effect and the variant described in the patient, at the age of six years old (in 2015), QND was included as "off label" drug regimen, besides TPM (175 mg/day) and nitrazepam (1.5 mg/day).

Because QND toxicity was well described it was needed to monitor the cardiac function and plasma concentrations. For this aim our laboratory developed and validated HPLC-UV method to quantify QND in human serum. Propranolol was added to the samples as an internal standard, followed by liquid extraction with cyclohexane and evaporation. The chromatography condition included a reversed phase column and a mobile phase consisting of acetonitrile and phosphate buffer (25:75).

Validation parameters studied were specificity (no interferences were found), lineality (0.5–8.0 mcg/ml), repeatability, accuracy (less than 10% CD), sensitivity and stability (in different conditions and time periods). Tests were evaluated according US FDA Guidance for Industry Bioanalytical Method Validation (US FDA Guidance for Industry Bioanalytical Method Validation, 2018).

During QND dose titration, TPM was decreasing the daily doses (initially 175 mg/day) to complete withdrawal, while nitrazepam dose regimen of 2 mg/day was maintained.

TDM was implemented, to establish the individual therapeutic range, as well as electrocardiogram (ECG) studies to assist cardiac follow up. When QND dose was above 50 mg/kg/day in four administrations (achieving a minimum serum level of 1.0 mcg/ml) the therapy started to modify the discharges profile. Only when doses reached 65–70 mg/kg q. i.d (and serum levels were above 1.5 mcg/ml) the patient was seizure free.

According to the original strategy, TPM was almost withdrawn. Surprisingly, QND doses of 65–70 mg/kg which had initially shown therapeutic effectiveness, failed to gain seizures control. Due to this observed synergic effect between TPM and QND, TPM was again indicated. TPM maintenance dose was 2.5 mg/kg/day and then increased to 4.5 mg/kg/day (which achieved levels of 3 mcg/ml and 6 mcg/ml of TPM respectively).

Table 1 shows the variability of QND levels at higher doses compared with lower doses. Initially, when doses increased from 240 to 640 mg/day, QND concentration augmented from 0.6 mcg/ml to 1.0 mcg/ml. But analyzing the same increment in dose (approximately 400 mg/day) with higher doses (from 1,160 to 1,600 mg/day), it resulted in a higher variation of serum levels obtained (1.5–4.1 mcg/ml).

TABLE 1 | Comparison of different variation in lower and higher doses, occurred during patient follow up with TDM. Levels are more disperse in association with doses increment.

Range of doses mg/day	Doses variation (Max–min)	Range of plasma concentration mcg/ml	Plasma concentration variation (Max–min)
240–640	400.0	0.6–1	0.4
1,160–1,600	440.0	1.5–4.1	2.6

TABLE 2 | Serum levels and doses related to QT segment prolongation (Reference <0.46 s). In bold is highlighted those situations where reducing doses was necessary to correct QT segment prolongation.

Date dd/mm/yy	Dose (mg/day)	Plasmatic level (mcg/ml)	QT segment (sec.)
22/03/16	560	0.5	0.48
08/05/17	**1,320**	**4.0**	**0.60**
06/09/17	1,360	3.0	0.46
22/09/17	1,320	2.8	0.52
16/01/18	1,400	1.9	0.46
25/09/18	1,440	1.8	0.52
21/01/19	1,560	3.4	0.50
20/08/19	**1,560**	**5.9**	**0.50**

Values in bold indicate toxicity events.

It is important to mention that the patient received different pharmacological treatment according particular necessities, such as: antimicrobial agents or laxatives, which might affect QND levels. Moreover, changes in TPM doses could contribute to the variability observed. At the beginning of the treatment the increase in QND doses did not correlate with a proportional increase of QND plasma levels. After a reduction in TPM dose regimen below 50 mg/day the increase in QND doses yielded a proportional dose-concentration relationship.

It is also known that QND cardiotoxicity could produce arrhythmia due to prolongation of QT segment. Our patient experienced the risk of suffering this adverse event on several occasions. Nevertheless, we identified two different related patterns (**Table 2**). The first one was observed during the titration period, when QND doses were incremented every 14 days. QT segment values corrected themselves without any medical intervention, once normalized titration could continue. On the other hand, when the levels reached were higher than 4.0 mcg/ml, the prolongation was persistent, and it was mandatory to reduce the doses. To sum up, Graphic 1 shows QND levels achieved during the follow-up, correlated with QND doses.

DISCUSSION

Although pathogenic variants on *KCNT1* are rare in the population, it has been proposed as an important cause of epilepsy with a wide phenotypic spectrum (Barcia et al., 2012). We characterize the genotype, as a pharmacological target, but also a therapeutic drug monitoring strategy to optimize the pharmacological treatment with the potassium channel blocker QND in association with other antiepileptic drugs in a pediatric patient.

KCNT1 encodes the largest potassium channel subunit and is thought to regulate the hyperpolarization that follows repetitive firing. Functional studies have shown that genetic variants in the cytoplasmic C-terminal domain caused constitutive activation of the potassium channel (Milligan et al., 2016), which modify normal neuronal firing and directly led to epileptogenesis.

A KCNT1 variant previously reported as pathogenic (Vanderver et al., 2014; Yang et al., 2014) was identified in the patient. This '*de novo*' variant is highly conserved, and the p.F932I change is, in principle, the most damaging non-synonymous change associated to this variant.

The KCNT1 variant identified in our work is located immediately adjacent to two previously described pathogenic variants (pArg928Cys and pAla934Thr), and therefore was proposed as the underlying disease-causing mechanism in this case. KCNT1 related epilepsies is included in a broader group of potassium channel related epilepsies that may be amendable to channel specific therapies, such as QND.

QND an old antiarrhythmic and antimalarial drug, has emerged as a potential precision therapy for KCNT1-related epilepsy. *In vitro* functional assays have demonstrated that gain of-function effects associated to KCNT-1 gene variants can be reversed by QND. Although previous case reports showed a significant reduction in seizure burden (Bearden et al., 2014; Milligan et al., 2014), subsequent reports demonstrated less favorable results, raising questions about QND effectiveness for treating KCNT1-related epilepsy (Chong et al., 2016; Numis et al., 2018).

In this manuscript we described the pharmacological effects and therapeutic drug monitoring strategy applied after including QND to a patient's drug regimen who carries a KCNT1 variant, receiving also TPM and nitrazepam as pharmacological therapy.

One interesting point to note is that in a previous study, a different pattern of pharmacological response was reported related to the KCNT-1 variant identified. In our work, the less frequent 2795 T > C variant resulted in sustained seizure freedom after quinidine treatment, in agreement with the data showed by Fitzgerald et al. (2019) in a patient treated with QND and receiving TPM and nitrazepam as antiepileptic drugs.

It has been also proposed that the limited efficacy of QND previously reported in KCNT1 patients could be related to the limited bioavailability of QND in the CNS. In this way, it has been shown in healthy volunteers that QND levels in CSF could be lower than in plasma where QND CSF concentration were 16% of unbound serum concentrations (range, 4–37%) (Ochs et al., 1980). Anyway, there is no data available of CSF levels in KCNT1 patients receiving QND to evaluate the CSF/ plasma quinidine concentration relationship and antiepileptic response.

Moreover, the QND dose increment at higher doses resulted in greater variability in QND plasma levels. This phenomenon could in part be explained by the rise in QND free fraction in the range of concentration observed (1.5–4.0 ug/ml), that could be available to be eliminated or re-distributed according to different factors affecting the patient (Ochs et al., 1980). In this sense, the variability observed, justified the QND monitoring of plasma levels with the aim to optimize dose regimen.

In the largest cohort of patient with KCNT1 related epilepsy, that included 43 patients, QND treatment resulted in a >50% reduction in seizure frequency in only 20% of patients receiving this therapy, with sustained seizure freedom occurring rarely (Fitzgerald et al., 2019). In the study mentioned, therapeutic blood levels were not achieved in many patients, with 45% of patients failing to reach a blood level of 2 ug/ml.

There are several potential explanations for this finding, but we can hypothesize that QTc prolongation concern, infrequent use of this drug or lack of knowledge regarding the most appropriate strategies for therapeutic monitoring, could be some of the reasons that prevented reaching higher therapeutic levels.

TDM is a useful tool when allows us to select a goal and to reach a target by developing a pharmacokinetic/ pharmacodynamics (PK/PD) model for a particular patient, but it is useless when there is a lack of skills related to drug monitoring practice, because blood monitoring of a particular drug is very infrequent, or if no pharmacokinetics recommendations are given.

In our study QND drug regimen optimization was performed and a high proportion of QND levels reached the therapeutic target. During the follow-up, intensive therapeutic drug monitoring was accompanied by pharmacokinetics recommendation of QND dose adjustment with a high rate of physician compliance. This strategy allowed to modify QND dose regimen to achieve plasma levels into the individual therapeutic range for this patient.

To highline from our work, the patient got free from seizures receiving QND 70–90 mg/kg q. i.d, TPM 4.5 mg/kg/day and nitrazepam 2.5 mg/day as pharmacological treatment. Due to the fact that QND effectiveness decreased when TPM doses were below 20–30 mg/day during TPM withdrawal, and that QND and TPM does not share the same mechanism of action, we can suggest a potentially synergic effect in this case. Initially, high doses of TPM showed to be ineffective to control seizures in this patient. However low doses of TPM were needed associated to QND to get free from seizures. Although the nature of this interaction needs further studies, QND as monotherapy may not be as effective acting at the KCNT1 receptor level making necessary the association of another antiepileptic drug to maintain the pharmacological response.

From a pharmacokinetic point of view QND is a very potent inhibitor of the efflux transporter P-glycoprotein (PGP), and is involved in the increased bioavailability at the CNS and toxicity of different drugs. It has been shown that TPM is a substrate of PGP, suggesting that up-regulation of MDR-1 gene could affect the TPM brain levels. QND could be acting as a "booster" and might be increasing TPM levels that reach CNS (Sadeque et al., 2000), allowing the use of lower doses of TPM that showed to be effective.

In our experience QND have shown to be affected by other conditions. The patient levels drop off on many occasions neither for changes in doses nor changes in the administration of QND. Levels that were below expected could be associated for example to other pharmacological treatment such as wide spectrum antibiotics which might have affected QND absorption. Laxatives also may have decreased QND absorption because of the increment in bowel motility.

Increasing TPM doses are also suspected of altering serum QND concentrations through several different mechanisms that need to be studied more carefully. According to bibliography, the inhibition of carbonic anhydrase enzyme by TPM (Ruiz Granados et al., 2015) might conduct to metabolic acidosis, producing an increase in urinary pH and QND plasma levels. By the contrary, in our work at higher TPM doses, QND titration was not accompanied by a proportional increase of QND plasma levels until TPM regimen was below 50 mg/day. Anyway, as we mentioned, the fluctuation of QND levels was more significant at higher QND doses, and TDM was successfully applied in order to reach the individual therapeutic range that was defined between 1.5–4.0 ug/ml for this patient.

Considering previous studies and the results presented in this report, we suggest that in patients with KCNT-1 related epilepsy, the inclusion of QND should be accompanied of the analysis of the KCNT-1 genetic variants identified, together with a TDM strategy that allows to characterize the pharmacokinetic of QND, with the aim to reach the individual therapeutic target in order to increase efficacy with minimal side effects.

CONCLUSION

The implementation of Precision Medicine by using tools such as NGS and TDM led to diagnose and select a targeted therapy for the treatment of a KCNT1-related epilepsy in a patient presented with EIMFS in early infancy and poor response to antiepileptic drugs. QND an old antiarrhythmic drug, due to its activity as KCNT1 channel blocker, associated to TPM resulted in seizures control. Due to high variability observed in QND levels, TDM and pharmacokinetic characterization allowed to optimize drug regimen to maintain QND concentration between the individual therapeutic range and diminish toxicity.

AUTHOR CONTRIBUTIONS

All authors listed have made a substantial, direct, and intellectual contribution to the work and approved it for publication.

ACKNOWLEDGMENTS

Pharm. Rodriguez Basso A. G. for assisting HPLC method validation, Bioch. Barrionuevo N.M. and Pharm. Fernández F.A. for technical assistance. Nuñez M and the Institute of Pharmacology at University of Medicine- UBA for equipment backup.

REFERENCES

1. Barcia, G., Fleming, M. R., Deligniere, A., Gazula, V.-R., Brown, M. R., Langouet, M., et al. (2012). De novo gain-of-function KCNT1 channel mutations cause malignant migrating partial seizures of infancy. *Nat. Genet.* 44, 1255–1259. doi:10.1212/NXG.0000000000000036310.1038/ng.2441
2. Bearden, D., Strong, A., Ehnot, J., DiGiovine, M., Dlugos, D., and Goldberg, E. M. (2014). Targeted treatment of migrating partial seizures of infancy with quinidine. *Ann. Neurol.* 76, 457–461. doi:10.1002/ana.24229
3. Chong, P. F., Nakamura, R., Saitsu, H., Matsumoto, N., and Kira, R. (2016). Ineffective quinidine therapy in early onset epileptic encephalopathy withKCNT1mutation. *Ann. Neurol.* 79, 502–503. doi:10.1002/ana.24598
4. Dilena, R., DiFrancesco, J. C., Soldovieri, M. V., Giacobbe, A., Ambrosino, P., Mosca, I., et al. (2018). Early treatment with quinidine in 2 patients with epilepsy of infancy with migrating focal seizures (EIMFS) due to gain-of-function KCNT1 mutations: functional studies, clinical responses, and critical issues for personalized therapy. *Neurotherapeutics* 15 (4), 1112–1126. doi:10.1007/s13311-018-0657-9
5. Epilepsy of infancy with migrating focal seizures (2020). Epilepsy of infancy with migrating focal seizures | Epilepsy Action. Available at: https://www.epilepsy.org.uk/info/syndromes/migrating-partial-epilepsy-in-infancy (Accessed November 30, 2020).
6. Fitzgerald, M. P., Fiannacca, M., Smith, D. M., Gertler, T. S., Gunning, B., Syrbe, S., et al. (2019) Treatment responsiveness in KCNT1-related epilepsy. *Neurotherapeutics* 16, 848–857. doi:10.1007/s13311-019-00739-y
7. Fukuoka, M., Kuki, I., Kawawaki, H., Okazaki, S., Kim, K., Hattori, Y., et al. (2017). Quinidine therapy for West syndrome with KCNTI mutation: a case report. *Brain Development* 39, 80–83. doi:10.1016/j.braindev.2016.08.002
8. International League Against Epilepsy (2020). *Epilepsy of infancy with migrating focal seizures* Available at: https://www.epilepsydiagnosis.org/syndrome/infancy-migrating-focal-genetics.html (Accessed December 20, 2020).
9. Lim, C. X., Ricos, M. G., Dibbens, L. M., and Heron, S. E. (2016). KCNT1mutations in seizure disorders: the phenotypic spectrum and functional effects. *J. Med. Genet.* 53, 217. doi:10.1136/jmedgenet-2015-103508
10. Madaan, P., Jauhari, P., Gupta, A., Chakrabarty, B., and Gulati, S. (2018). A quinidine non responsive novel KCNT1 mutation in an Indian infant with epilepsy of infancy with migrating focal seizures. *Brain Development* 40, 229–232. doi:10.1016/j.braindev.2017.09.008
11. Mikati, M. A., Jiang, Y.-h., Carboni, M., Shashi, V., Petrovski, S., Spillmann, R., et al. (2015). Quinidine in the treatment of KCNT1-positive epilepsies. *Ann. Neurol.* 78, 995–999. doi:10.1002/ana.24520
12. Milligan, C. J., Li, M., Gazina, E. V., Heron, S. E., Nair, U., Trager, C., et al. (2014). KCNT1gain of function in 2 epilepsy phenotypes is reversed by quinidine. *Ann. Neurol.* 75, 581–590. doi:10.1002/ana.24128
13. Milligan, C. X., Ricos, M. G., Dibbens, L. M., and Heron, S. E. (2016). KCNT1mutations in seizure disorders: the phenotypic spectrum and functional effects. *J. Med. Genet.* 53, 217–225. doi:10.1002/ana.2452010. 1136/jmedgenet-2015-103508
14. Numis, A. L., Nair, U., Datta, A. N., Sands, T. T., Oldham, M. S., Patel, A., et al. (2018). Lack of response to quinidine in KCNT1 -related neonatal epilepsy. *Epilepsia* 59 (10), 1889–1898. doi:10.1111/epi.14551
15. Ochs, H. R., Greenblatt, D. J., Lloyd, B. L., Woo, E., Sonntag, M., and Smith, T. W. (1980). Entry of quinidine into cerebrospinal fluid. *Am. Heart J.* 100 (3), 341–346. doi:10.1016/0002-8703(80)90148-9
16. Rizzo, F., Ambrosino, P., Guacci, A., Chetta, M., Marchese, G., Rocco, T., et al. (2016). Characterization of two de novo KCNT1 mutations in children with malignant migrating partial seizures in infancy. *Mol. Cell Neurosci.* 72, 54–63. doi:10.1016/j.mcn.2016.01.004
17. Ruiz Granados, V. J., and Márquez Romero, J. M. (2015). Topiramato en monoterapia o en combinación como causa de acidosis metabólica en adultos con epilepsia. *Rev Neurol* 60, 159–163. doi:10.33588/rn.6004. 2014451
18. Sadeque, A., Wandel, C., He, H., Shah, S., and Wood, A. J. J. (2000). Increased drug delivery to the brain by P-glycoprotein inhibition. *Clin. Pharmacol. Ther.* 68, 231–237. doi:10.1067/mcp.2000.109156
19. The ILAE Genetics Commission Blog (2020). *KCNT1 – this is what you need to know*. Available at: http://epilepsygenetics.net/the-epilepsiome/kcnt1-this-is- what-you-need-to-know/ (Accessed December 29, 2020).
20. US FDA Guidance for Industry Bioanalytical Method Validation (2018). Available at: https://www.fda.gov/files/drugs/published/Bioanalytical-Method-Validation-Guidance-for-Industry.pdf (Accessed on February 25, 2021).
21. Vanderver, A., Simons, C., Schmidt, J. L., Pearl, P. L., Bloom, M., Lavenstein, B., et al. (2014). Identification of a novel de novo p.Phe932Ile KCNT1 mutation in a patient with leukoencephalopathy and severe epilepsy. *Pediatr. Neurol.* 50 (1), 112–114. doi:10.1016/j.pediatrneurol.2013.06.024
22. Yang, Y., Muzny, D. M., Xia, F., Niu, Z., Person, R., Ding, Y., et al. (2014). Molecular findings among patients referred for clinical whole-exome sequencing. *JAMA* 312, 18708–18709. doi:10.1001/jama.2014.14601

24

Case Report: Four Cases of Panayiotopoulos Syndrome Evolving to Juvenile Myoclonic Epilepsy

Hideo Enoki, Shinji Itamura, Shimpei Baba, Tohru Okanishi and Ayataka Fujimoto*

Comprehensive Epilepsy Center, Seirei Hamamatsu General Hospital, Hamamatsu, Japan

***Correspondence:**
Hideo Enoki
enokih.neuropediatr@gmail.com

Panayiotopoulos syndrome (PS) is a self-limited focal epilepsy appearing in childhood. Seizures in PS are self-limiting and do not usually continue into adulthood. Juvenile myoclonic epilepsy (JME) is the most common type of idiopathic generalized epilepsy, developing around puberty and continuing throughout adulthood. We describe four cases of PS in childhood in which JME developed in adolescence. Age at onset ranged from 4 to 8 years for PS, and 11 to 14 years for JME. JME developed after PS subsided, with the interval between last PS seizure and first JME seizure ranging from 1 to 10 years. No link between the two conditions has previously been described. Since PS is considered to show good prognosis and to be self-limiting, long-term observation has been considered unnecessary. No definitive factors were found to predict future evolution to JME in our series, so longer-term follow-up may be warranted for all PS patients.

Keywords: Panayiotopoulos syndrome, juvenile myoclonic epilepsy, self-limited focal epilepsy, idiopathic generalized epilepsy, atypical evolution

INTRODUCTION

Among children, epilepsy syndromes may show changes in the pathological condition within the same patient with development. For example, the age-related evolution of Ohtahara syndrome to West syndrome and Lennox-Gastaut syndrome is well known. In addition to these developmental and epileptic encephalopathies, age-related changes may be observed in other epilepsy syndromes. Whether one causes the other or whether a shared pathology is involved remains unclear. Clarification of the details of age-related evolution could thus contribute to elucidation of the pathophysiology of epilepsies. Here, we report four patients who originally presented with clinical features of Panayiotopoulos syndrome (PS) in childhood and later showed development of juvenile myoclonic epilepsy (JME) in adolescence.

PS is one of the most common self-limited focal epilepsies appearing only in children, with a peak age at onset of 4–5 years old (1, 2). The clinical manifestations of PS are unique. The core symptoms comprise autonomic manifestations, eye deviation, and impairment of consciousness (1). Among these, the most characteristic is the presence of autonomic symptoms, mainly in the form of ictal emesis, and often accompanied by pallor. Ictal non-autonomic symptoms may include clonic convulsions of the face and extremities, often on one side. Seizures typically start during sleep (1, 3). Seizure duration is usually long (4), with almost half lasting >30 min (1–3). Status epilepticus (SE) is usually non-convulsive, with main symptoms in the form of autonomic manifestations. Inter-ictal electroencephalography (EEG) of PS demonstrates significant variability. Occipital spikes represent the main EEG abnormality, but spike discharges may appear anywhere (2).

The prognosis of PS is quite favorable. A quarter of patients with PS experience only a single seizure, and half have two to five seizures (2). Although PS often enters remission within 1–2 years of onset (2–4), evolution to other forms of epilepsy may occur during childhood. A typical example of this evolution is self-limited epilepsy with centrotemporal spikes, formerly called "benign epilepsy with centrotemporal spikes" (BECT). An estimated 13% of patients with PS develop BECT later in childhood (2). BECT is an age-related epilepsy, with remission before 16 years old. Patients with PS, irrespective of whether they develop BECT, thus typically achieve release from epilepsy before reaching adulthood. Textbooks state that the risk of subsequent epilepsy in adult life among patients with a history of PS appears to be no higher than that in the general population (2–4).

JME is the most common type of idiopathic generalized epilepsy, characterized by myoclonic seizures (predominantly in the arms) appearing around puberty. Most patients exhibit generalized tonic-clonic seizures (GTC), and some also experience absence seizures.

Evolution from PS to JME in the same patient does not appear to have been described previously. Similarly, PS has not been reported in the past history of patients with JME. As a result, no link between the two conditions is known. Both syndromes are classed as idiopathic epilepsies, but are classified into totally different syndromes, with PS as a focal epilepsy and JME as a generalized epilepsy. This evolution thus means that the pathological type can change from focal to generalized epileptogenesis with age. In this respect, we have a strong interest in this phenomenon. The present report is the first to describe this rare condition.

PATIENT SELECTION

We conducted a retrospective study of patients with epilepsy who visited Seirei Hamamatsu General Hospital for the first time between January 2004 and December 2014. We collected 1,189, pediatric patients ≤ 15 years old, and identified 56 patients (4.7%) with PS.

The diagnostic criteria for PS we adopted were as follows (2, 4, 5):

- Age at onset between 1 and 14 years;
- Autonomic manifestations, and/or simple motor focal seizures followed or not by impairment of consciousness with or without secondary generalization;
- Functional occipital and extraoccipital spikes alone or combined on interictal EEG, or a normal EEG;
- Normal neurological and mental statuses; and
- Normal results from brain imaging.

The 56 patients we identified were monitored up to July 2020. Ten patients were transferred to another hospital within 1 year due to relocation, etc. Two patients dropped out and were unable to be followed. We then performed long-term observations of 44 patients for 4–13 years (mean, 9.2 years). Of these, 11 patients evolved from PS to other epileptic conditions, comprising 4 cases of JME, 4 cases of epileptic encephalopathy with continuous spikes and waves during sleep (CSWS), 1 case of BECT, 1 case of temporal lobe epilepsy, and 1 case of single unprovoked seizure.

The diagnosis of JME was based on the International League Against Epilepsy (ILAE) classification (6) and recent reviews (7, 8). We encountered four patients who met the diagnostic criteria for PS in childhood and developed JME in adolescence.

CASE PRESENTATION

We conducted retrospective long-term observations for the four patients and analyzed clinical features as summarized in **Table 1**.

Case 1

The patient was a girl who had suffered from six episodes of febrile seizure since 1 year old, one of which lasted for 1 h. We performed EEG four times from 2 to 4 years old, and none revealed epileptic discharges. Developmental history was normal. Her mother had a history of febrile seizure, but all other family members were reportedly free from seizure disorders.

At 5 years and 6 months old, she was transported by ambulance and admitted to our hospital due to impairment of consciousness. Her parents reported sudden vomiting that started during a nap while traveling in a car, and repeating several times. She woke from the nap, and was initially able to speak, but gradually became unconscious. Her eyes then deviated to the right, her complexion became pale, and her limbs became flaccid. When the patient arrived at our hospital 70 min after seizure onset, she was still lethargic, but her eyes were closed without deviation. The emergency room doctor decided that the seizure had already stopped and she was in a state of post-ictal drowsiness. EEG revealed epileptic spikes in the left occipital region, whereas magnetic resonance imaging (MRI) showed no abnormalities. PS was then diagnosed. After observing the course without treatment, the patient experienced another seizure 9 months later. This time, the seizure evolved to left hemiconvulsions with eyes deviating to the left. Medication started with valproic acid (VPA), with later addition of clobazam, but neither achieved resolution of seizures. In total, she experienced nine seizure events equivalent to PS by 7 years and 4 months old, most of which were lengthy seizures lasting >5 min or SE >30 min. The longest seizure lasted 60 min before stopping on intravenous injection of diazepam. Although she experienced no further PS seizures after 7 years old, EEG spike discharges were consistently observed. Medication was continued in accordance with the wishes of the parents until 13 years 6 months old, by which time the EEG abnormalities had disappeared.

At 14 years 6 months old, the patient noticed twitching in the arms, particularly on waking. That same month, she suffered GTC right after waking. EEG showed a 6-Hz wave-and-spike phantom, and results of MRI were normal. Based on the seizure symptomology and laboratory findings, we diagnosed JME. Levetiracetam (LEV) was started, and completely eliminated seizures without adverse effects. The patient is currently 17 years 7 months old and has shown no further symptoms.

Case 2

A 4-year-2-month-old girl was transported by ambulance to our hospital due to a first episode of afebrile convulsions.

TABLE 1 | Clinical information of the 4 cases.

		Case 1	Case 2	Case 3	Case 4
Sex		F	F	M	F
Family history, convulsive disorders		Fs, mother	None	Fs, mother	TLE, sister
Peri- or postnatal disorders		Cesarean section due to pelvic position	None	None	Low birth weight
Past history, convulsive disorders		Febrile SE	None	Fs	Fs
PS	Age at onset	5 y 6 m	4 y 2 m	8 y 6 m	8 y 10 m
	Circadian distribution of sz	Sleep	Sleep	Awake	Awake
	Total no. of sz	9	1	3	6
	No. of prolonged sz (5–30 min)	4	1	1	4
	No. of SE episodes (> 30 min)	4	0	0	1
	EEG discharges	Occipital	Occipital	Occipital	Generalized, frontopolar, OIRDA, FIRDA
	Head MRI	Normal	Normal	Normal	Normal
	AED	VPA, CLB	VPA	VPA	CBZ, LTG
	Age at last sz	7 y 4 m	4 y 2 m	8 y 10 m	10 y 6 m
	Age when AED stopped	13 y 6 m	12 y 6 m	11 y 5 m	12 y 5 m
JME	Age at onset of myoclonic sz	14 y 6 m	14 y 5 m	11 y 8 m	12 y 2 m
	Age at onset of GTC	14 y 6 m	14 y 7 m	12 y 1 m	12 y 7 m
	EEG discharges	Wave-and-spike phantom	Generalized	Generalized	Generalized, PPR
	Head MRI	Normal	Normal	Normal	Normal
	AED	LEV	VPA	VPA	LTG
	Age at last GTC	14 y 6 m	14 y 7 m	12 y 1 m	20 y 3 m
Interval between last PS and first JME sz		7 y 2 m	10 y 3 m	2 y 3 m	1 y 8 m
Reported neurobehavioral disorders*		None	Borderline intellectual function (IQ 72)	None (IQ 110)	None
Present age		17 y 7 m	16 y 7 m	16 y 7 m	20 y 5 m

*sz, seizure/s; SE, status epilepticus; AED, antiepileptic drug; GTC, generalized tonic-clonic seizure; PS, Panayiotopoulos syndrome; JME, juvenile myoclonic epilepsy; Fs, febrile seizure; TLE, temporal lobe epilepsy; OIRDA, occipital intermittent rhythmic delta activity; FIRDA, frontal intermittent rhythmic delta activity; PPR, photoparoxysmal response; VPA, valproic acid; CLB, clobazam; LEV, levetiracetam; CBZ, carbamazepine; LTG, lamotrigine. *Evaluated in adolescence.*

During a nap, she started to vomit and turned pale, and proved unresponsive to her parents' calls. Right upper limb convulsions then began. The whole course of the seizure was about 8 min. No information was available on whether her eyes showed a deviation during the seizure. EEG demonstrated a left occipital spike-and-wave pattern. Results of MRI were normal. Although we advised observation of her condition without medication, VPA was started based on the strong desire of the parents. No subsequent seizures appeared, but left occipital spike-and-wave discharges persisted for a long time (**Figure 1**). VPA was discontinued at 12 years 6 months old, after confirming the disappearance of EEG abnormalities.

Two years later, she suffered myoclonic jerks and a GTC. EEG showed generalized polyspikes and waves. MRI was again performed, but demonstrated no abnormalities. We diagnosed JME and explained the need for medication throughout adulthood. Considering side effects of VPA on women of childbearing potential, we recommended a new-generation antiepileptic, such as LEV or lamotrigine (LTG). However, the patient and her parents opted to use the same drug she had used before. VPA was restarted at a low dose, and achieved total seizure control.

Case 3

An 8-year-old boy suffered from three episodes of afebrile seizure that occurred while awake. Symptoms consisted of repeated vomiting and impairment of consciousness. One of the episodes was accompanied by left upper limb convulsions and deviation of the eyes to the left. Seizure duration ranged from 3 to 10 min. Right occipital spike discharges were confirmed on EEG. Results of MRI were normal. VPA was started after the third seizure, and achieved control of seizures. The drug was discontinued at 11 years old, after confirming complete normalization of EEG findings.

However, after stopping the drug, generalized spike-and-wave discharges appeared on EEG. After a while, he started experiencing myoclonic jerks. In addition, at 12 years 1 month old, he suffered a GTC. VPA was restarted, and effectively stopped the seizures.

Case 4

A 12-year-7-month-old girl was referred to our outpatient clinic due to an episode of GTC. She had a history of focal epilepsy that started at 8 years old. Focal seizures were characterized by initial vomiting, followed by deviation of the eyes and impairment of consciousness without convulsions of the extremities. She

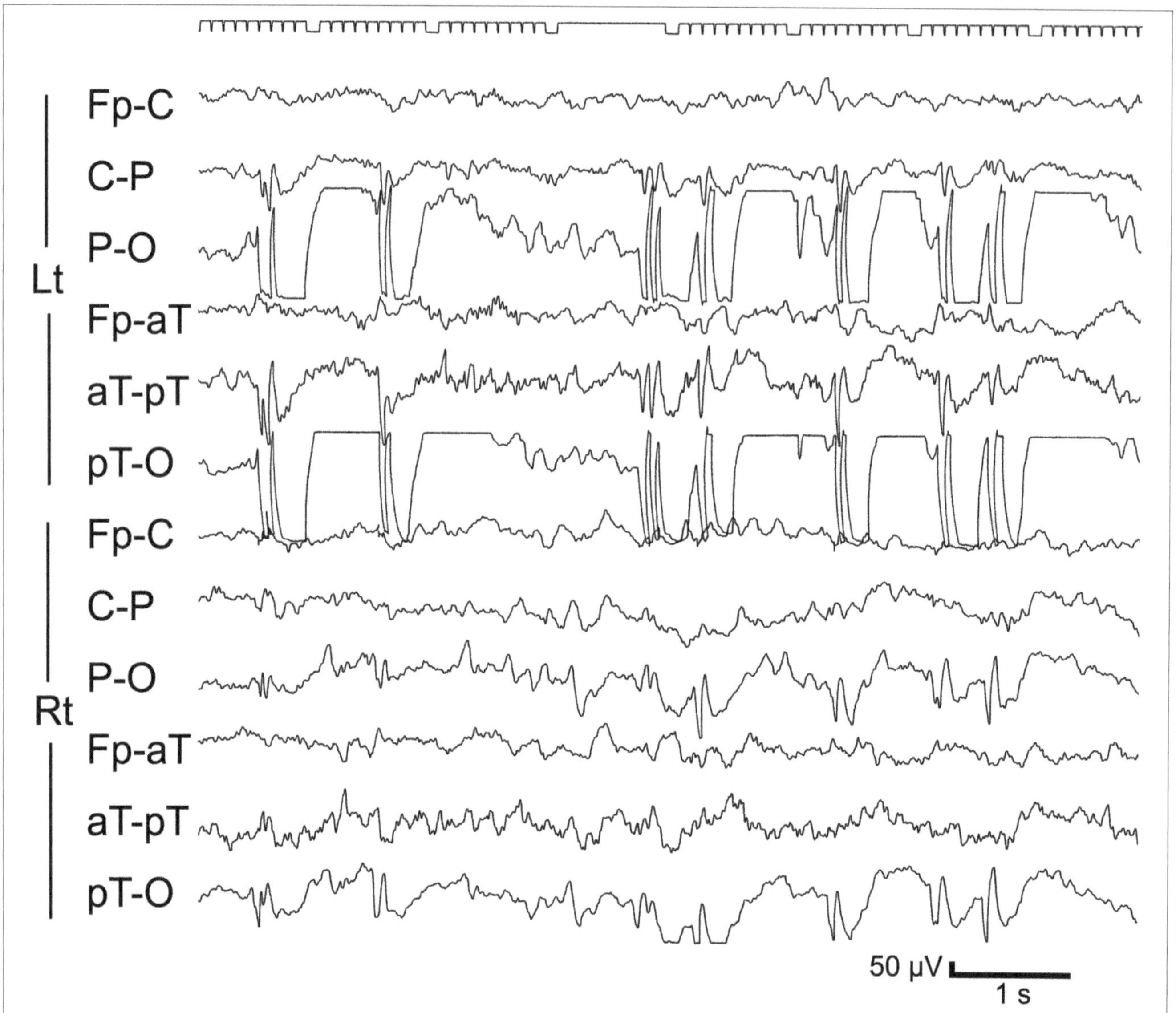

FIGURE 1 | Representative EEG from Case 2 during the PS period. Sleep record at 5 years 9 months old. Upon medication with valproic acid. Frequent spike-and-waves are seen in the left occipital region.

had been administered carbamazepine (CBZ) and LTG. At 12 years 2 months old, she noticed twitching in the arms. She discontinued the medication without medical advice at 12 years 5 months old. GTC subsequently occurred at 12 years 7 months old. EEG revealed frequent generalized polyspike-and-wave discharges (**Figure 2**) and photoparoxysmal responses. LTG effectively improved the EEG abnormalities, but GTCs did not completely cease and appeared triggered by menstruation or a lack of sleep.

DISCUSSION

We have presented here a series of four patients who developed PS in childhood with evolution to JME in adolescent. Although all patients fulfilled the diagnostic criteria for PS, age at onset in Cases 3 and 4 was relatively high (8 years old) and seizures in these patients appeared while awake. As mentioned earlier, peak age at onset is 4–5 years and seizures tend to occur during sleep in PS. Differential diagnosis would thus be important in these cases. Idiopathic etiology, focal seizures while awake, and onset age at 8 years lead to consideration of childhood occipital epilepsy of Gastaut. In that syndrome, the main seizure symptom is visual hallucinations, with frequent complaints of post-ictal headache. No such symptoms were reported in Cases 3 and 4, and EEG in the latter case showed no occipital spikes. A diagnosis of Gastaut-type epilepsy thus could not be given.

Transition of PS to JME has not been reported previously and is clearly rare. The characteristics of such patients thus require investigation. We therefore compared our series with previous PS case studies of large groups. We identified two

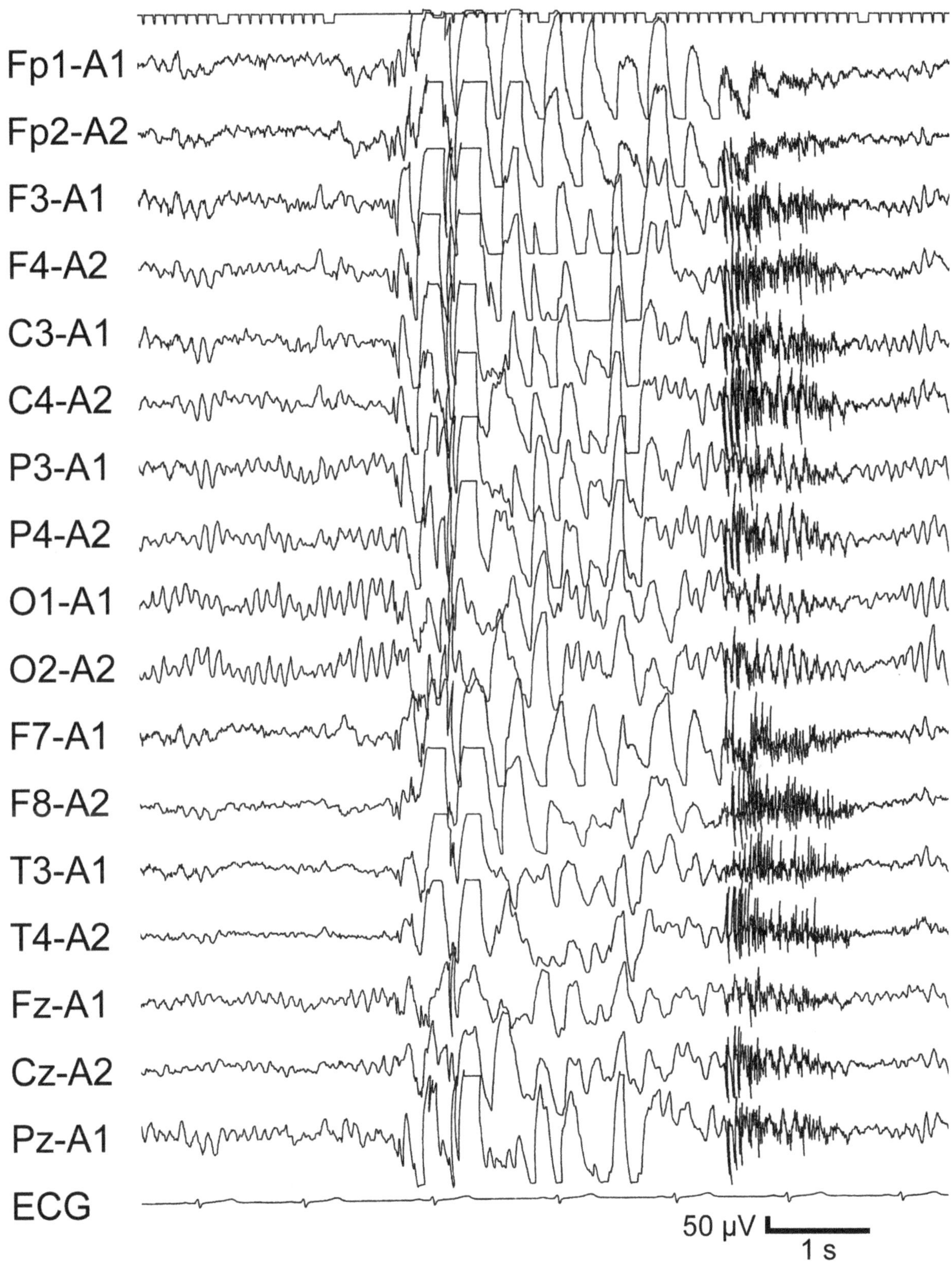

FIGURE 2 | Interictal EEG from Case 4 when JME developed. Awake record at 12 years 7 months old, on no medication. Generalized polyspikes-and-waves are apparent.

TABLE 2 | Comparison with clinical studies of Panayiotopoulos syndrome.

	Caraballo et al. (5)	Specchio et al. (9)	Present series
Number of patients	192	93	4
Sex, %	Girls 44, boys 56	Girls 55.9, boys 44.1	Girls 75, boys 25
Family history, %	Epilepsy 31.3, Fs 13.5	Epilepsy/Fs 45.2	Epilepsy 25, Fs 50
Past history of Fs, %	28.5	6.5	75
Age at onset, y (median)	1.7–12.5 (4.5)	1.1–8.6 (4.1)	4–8 (6.5)
Circadian distribution of sz, %	Sleep 97.4 Awake 30.7	Sleep 69.9 Awake 17.2 Awakening 12.9	Sleep 50 Awake 50
Sz semiology, %			
Ictal emesis	82.3	77.4	100
Eye deviation	88.5	73.1	75*
Impairment of consciousness	78.1	89.2	100
SE, %	36.4	54.8	50
Single sz, %	44.2	33.1	25
Occipital EEG discharges, %	75	76.1	75

*Fs, febrile seizure; sz, seizure/s; SE, status epilepticus. *Details unknown in remaining 25%.*

studies (5, 9), in which the evolution of PS to JME did not appear, and summarized the cases in **Table 2**. We did not perform statistical analyses, because the number of cases in our series was small. However, the frequency of a history of febrile seizures seemed high in our series. No characteristic differences were seen in other factors, such as sex, family history, age at onset, circadian distribution, seizure semiology, SE, single seizure, and EEG findings. Of course, a history of febrile seizure alone cannot determine the prognosis. We were thus unable to identify any factors predicting future evolution.

Aside from JME, evolution from PS to other epilepsy syndromes has been reported in the literature. The representative condition for this situation is BECT (5, 10). This pathology develops after a seizure-free period, or coexists with PS. Other than BECT, the visual seizures of occipital epilepsy might arise in rare cases (3, 4). All these evolutions result in the development of focal seizures.

Aside from these focal seizures, generalized seizures have been described in PS as an atypical evolution in very rare cases, such as absence seizures (5, 11–14), negative myoclonus (5), and myoclonic seizures (13). With these atypical evolutions, worsening of EEG as characterized by diffuse spike-and-wave discharges was shown. As a consequence of the worsening of EEG findings, encephalopathy related to status epilepticus during slow sleep (ESES) or epileptic encephalopathy with continuous spikes and waves during sleep (CSWS) has been reported during the course of PS (5, 15). However, none of our cases showed an EEG pattern consistent with CSWS. Our series appears totally distinguished from the atypical evolutions of PS reported in the literature because our cases demonstrated markedly different findings from EEG.

These atypical evolutions of PS are extremely rare and exceptional. As for the issue of evolution from PS to generalized epilepsy, Caraballo et al. found that 1 of 160 patients with PS developed typical absence seizures and concluded that the absence seizures might have merely been coincidental (11). However, they later found a past history of PS in 3 of 203 patients with childhood absence epilepsy (CAE) (14). This raised the question of whether the relationship between PS and CAE is coincidental, or is a common pathophysiology involved in focal and generalized epilepsy. They hypothesized a close genetic relationship between both epileptic syndromes, while leaving the possibility of mere coexistence. Both CAE and JME are generalized epilepsies. The issue raised by Caraballo et al. in CAE is closely related to the concept of evolution from PS to JME. We speculate that the evolution described here is unlikely to represent coincidence, as the present series collected four cases, not just one. Clarification of this hypothesis will require the accumulation of a larger number of cases in future genetic studies.

From another perspective, the influences of pharmacotherapies should be considered for the atypical evolutions. Kikumoto et al. reported a patient with PS who developed absence and myoclonic seizures due to exacerbation by CBZ (13). However, our cases were unlikely to have involved drug-induced exacerbation. In Cases 1–3, medications had already been discontinued before onset of JME. In the remaining case, myoclonic seizures appeared during treatment with CBZ and LTG, but discontinuation of these agents did not achieve seizure cessation, and GTC appeared during the drug-free period. Neither CBZ nor LTG was thus considered a trigger for JME development in Case 4.

The evolutions of PS previously described in the literature, namely BECT, occipital epilepsy, ESES or CSWS, CAE, and exacerbations due to drugs are all transient pathologies. All are age- or drug-dependent and can remit eventually. However, JME persists throughout adulthood. In that respect, the evolution of PS to JME appears distinct from any previously reported evolutions of PS.

Our series suggests the evolution from self-limited focal epilepsy to JME represents a natural course, rather than an anthropogenic effect such as drug-induced exacerbation. The commonalities between focal epilepsy and JME have also been reported in other epilepsy syndromes, such as idiopathic photosensitive occipital epilepsy (IPOE). IPOE is a focal epilepsy that develops from late childhood to adolescence and has been reported to overlap with JME (16). Both have been suggested to involve a common genetic determinant (16). Our series provides a contribution to the literature on the spectrum of childhood-onset focal epilepsies that may evolve to JME.

In this study, long-term observation revealed that 11 of the 56 PS cases evolved to other epileptic pathologies, including JME. This rate of evolution was surprisingly high. Given that epileptic conditions in these cases were not actually "self-limited" and that the rate of evolution to other conditions was so high, the prognosis of so-called "self-limited epilepsies" needs to be reassessed. Further long-term, observational studies of large groups are thus required.

CONCLUDING REMARKS

Although the background pathology in the evolution cannot yet be clarified from this case series alone, the purpose of this paper was to show the existence of such rare cases and to recommend that clinicians pay attention after PS. Since PS is known to display a good prognosis, the need for long-term observation has not been recognized. In our series, JME appeared even 10 years after the end of PS. We now understand that PS can evolve to a specific epileptic state and definitive factors predicting this future evolution have yet to be identified. Further accumulation of data with long-term follow-up is needed for all PS patients to clarify the pathophysiology of this evolution.

AUTHOR CONTRIBUTIONS

HE and AF contributed to the conceptualization, drafting, and revision of the study. SI, SB, and TO contributed to the acquisition and interpretation of clinical information and EEG data. All authors contributed to the article and approved the submitted version.

REFERENCES

1. Fejerman N. Early-onset benign childhood occipital epilepsy (Panayiotopoulos type). In: Engel J, Pedley T, editors. *Epilepsy: A Comprehensive Textbook*. 2nd ed. Philadelphia, PA: Lippincott Williams & Wilkins (2008). p. 2379–86.
2. Panayiotopoulos CP. Panayiotopoulos syndrome. In: Panayiotopoulos CP, editor. *A Clinical Guide to Epileptic Syndromes and Their Treatment. 2nd ed. Based on the ILAE Classifications and Practice Parameter Guidelines*. London: Springer-Verlag (2010). p. 347–56.
3. Demirbilek V, Bureau M, Çokar Ö, Panayiotopoulos CP. Self-limited focal epilepsies in childhood. In: Bureau MGP, Dravet C, Delgado-Escueta A, Guerrini R, Tassinari CA, Thomas P, et al., editors. *Epileptic Syndromes in Infancy, Childhood and Adlescence*. 6th ed. Montrouge: John Libbey EUROTEXT (2019). p. 219–60.
4. Ferrie C, Caraballo R, Covanis A, Demirbilek V, Dervent A, Kivity S, et al. Panayiotopoulos syndrome: a consensus view. *Dev Med Child Neurol.* (2006) 48:236–40. doi: 10.1017/S0012162206000508
5. Caraballo R, Cersósimo R, Fejerman N. Panayiotopoulos syndrome: a prospective study of 192 patients. *Epilepsia.* (2007) 48:1054–61. doi: 10.1111/j.1528-1167.2007.01085.x
6. Scheffer IE, Berkovic S, Capovilla G, Connolly MB, French J, Guilhoto L, et al. ILAE classification of the epilepsies: position paper of the ILAE Commission for Classification and Terminology. *Epilepsia.* (2017) 58:512–21. doi: 10.1111/epi.13709
7. Baykan B, Wolf P. Juvenile myoclonic epilepsy as a spectrum disorder: a focused review. *Seizure.* (2017) 49:36–41. doi: 10.1016/j.seizure.2017.05.011
8. Wolf P, Yacubian EM, Avanzini G, Sander T, Schmitz B, Wandschneider B, et al. Juvenile myoclonic epilepsy: a system disorder of the brain. *Epilepsy Res.* (2015) 114:2–12. doi: 10.1016/j.eplepsyres.2015.04.008
9. Specchio N, Trivisano M, Di Ciommo V, Cappelletti S, Masciarelli G, Volkov J, et al. Panayiotopoulos syndrome: a clinical, EEG, and neuropsychological study of 93 consecutive patients. *Epilepsia.* (2010) 51:2098–107. doi: 10.1111/j.1528-1167.2010.02639.x
10. Caraballo R, Cersósimo R, Fejerman N. Idiopathic partial epilepsies with rolandic and occipital spikes appearing in the same children. *J Epilepsy.* (1998) 11:261–4 doi: 10.1016/S0896-6974(98)00014-0
11. Caraballo RH, Sologuestua A, Grañana N, Adi JN, Cersósimo RO, Mazza E, et al. Idiopathic occipital and absence epilepsies appearing in the same children. *Pediatr Neurol.* (2004) 30:24–8. doi: 10.1016/S0887-8994(03)00409-0
12. Ferrie CD, Koutroumanidis M, Rowlinson S, Sanders S, Panayiotopoulos CP. Atypical evolution of Panayiotopoulos syndrome: a case report. *Epileptic Disord.* (2002) 4:35–42. Available online at: https://www.jle.com/fr/revues/epd/e-docs/atypical_evolution_of_panayiotopoulos_syndrome_a_case_report_published_with_video_sequences_._110061/article.phtml
13. Kikumoto K, Yoshinaga H, Oka M, Ito M, Endoh F, Akiyama T, et al. EEG and seizure exacerbation induced by carbamazepine in Panayiotopoulos syndrome. *Epileptic Disord.* (2006) 8:53–6. Available online at: https://www.jle.com/download/epd-268134-3365-eeg_and_seizure_exacerbation_induced_by_carbamazepine_in_panayiotopoulos_syndrome-a.pdf
14. Caraballo RH, Fontana E, Darra F, Bongiorni L, Fiorini E, Cersosimo R, et al. Childhood absence epilepsy and electroencephalographic focal abnormalities with or without clinical manifestations. *Seizure.* (2008) 17:617–24. doi: 10.1016/j.seizure.2008.03.009
15. Oguni H, Hirano Y, Nagata S. Encephalopathy related to status epilepticus during slow sleep (ESES) as atypical evolution of Panayiotopoulos syndrome: an EEG and neuropsychological study. *Epileptic Disord.* (2020) 22:67–72. doi: 10.1684/epd.2020.1128
16. Taylor I, Marini C, Johnson MR, Turner S, Berkovic SF, Scheffer IE. Juvenile myoclonic epilepsy and idiopathic photosensitive occipital lobe epilepsy: is there overlap? *Brain.* (2004) 127:1878–86. doi: 10.1093/brain/awh211

25

Case Report: Multisystem Autoimmune and Overlapping GAD65-Antibody-Associated Neurological Disorders with Beneficial Effect of Epilepsy Surgery and Rituximab Treatment

Petia Dimova[1]* *and Krassimir Minkin*[2]

[1] *Epileptology Unit at Epilepsy Surgery Center, Department of Neurosurgery, St. Ivan Rilski University Hospital, Sofia, Bulgaria,*
[2] *Functional and Epilepsy Surgery Center, Department of Neurosurgery, St. Ivan Rilski University Hospital, Sofia, Bulgaria*

Correspondence:
Petia Dimova
psdimova@gmail.com

Glutamic acid decarboxylase (GAD) antibodies are associated with disabling conditions such as stiff person syndrome, temporal lobe epilepsy (TLE), limbic encephalitis, cerebellar ataxia (CA), and ocular movement disorders, which are usually chronic and difficult to treat. GAD-related TLE has poor response to anti-seizure medications and immune therapies, and epilepsy surgery is rarely successful. We report on a 47-year-old female with history of migraine, autoimmune thyroid disease, ankylosing spondylitis, and drug-resistant TLE. A video electroencephalography recorded frequent seizures with temporo-insular semiology, correlating to left temporal epileptiform activity and left mesiotemporal hyperintensity on magnetic resonance imaging. GAD autoimmunity was confirmed by very high GAD antibody titers in serum and cerebrospinal fluid. Steroids, immunoglobulins, and cyclophosphamide had no effect, and selective left amygdalectomy was performed based on very restricted hypermetabolism on positron-emission tomography. After transient seizure freedom, significant epilepsy improvement was observed in spite of memory decline. Transient worsening was noted 1 year later during diabetes mellitus manifestation and 5 years later during presentation of progressive CA, which stabilized on rituximab treatment. We believe this case illustrates the diversity and the frequent overlap of GAD-associated disorders, the need of early and aggressive immunotherapy in severe patients, as well as the possible benefit from epilepsy surgery in some GAD-TLE.

Keywords: autoimmune, GAD, cerebellar, diabetes, epilepsy, insular, temporal, surgery

INTRODUCTION

Glutamic acid decarboxylase antibodies (GAD-Abs; against the enzyme isoform GAD65) are usually associated with chronic conditions, increasingly recognized during the last three decades. Besides type-1 diabetes mellitus (DM1), GAD-Abs have been associated with a number of neurological syndromes, such as stiff-person syndrome (SPS), cerebellar ataxia (CA), limbic encephalitis (LE) and temporal lobe epilepsy (TLE), ocular movement disorder, and myelitis (1–3). Diverse clinical manifestations are thought to be dictated by GAD-Ab specificity, targeting different epitopes in the catalytic domain of the enzyme (1). Nonetheless, because of massive overlap in epitope recognition, presentations with signs and symptoms of several affected systems may be observed (1, 3, 4). Common features of GAD-Ab-associated neurological disorders are frequent comorbidity with other systemic autoimmune diseases, possibility of developing overlap syndromes, and poor to moderate response to immunotherapies. Here, we present a case with refractory TLE, who was historically diagnosed with migraine, autoimmune thyroid disease, and ankylosing spondylitis (AS). A delayed diagnosis of GAD-Ab autoimmunity was established, and DM1 and CA developed 6 and 10 years after the epilepsy onset, respectively. Immunotherapy with steroids, immunoglobulins, and cyclophosphamide had no effect on seizures, while selective amygdalectomy achieved substantial epilepsy improvement. Rituximab treatment led to stabilization of CA and further seizure reduction.

CASE PRESENTATION

A 42-year-old woman presented for presurgical evaluation due to very frequent epileptic seizures. No febrile convulsions or significant medical antecedents in childhood were reported except for rare migraine attacks since puberty. Historically, the patient was operated at the age of 32 for autoimmune Hashitoxicosis (unfortunately, detailed medical documentation is missing) and was on treatment with 100 μg L-thyroxin. At the age of 36, she was diagnosed with HLA-B27-negative AS based on 6-month clinical manifestation of progressive (predominantly low) back and hip pain, 3-plane limitation of lumbar spine mobility, morning stiffness improving with motion, and confirmation by laboratory (elevated C-reactive protein and negative rheumatoid factor) and radiological findings (bilateral sacroiliac joints changes, syndesmophytosis, and enthesitis in neck and lumbar spine on X-ray). Anti-tumor necrosis factor (anti-TNF) therapy with etanercept (ETN) for 2 years led to AS remission and was discontinued due to tuberculosis (TBC) treated with 4-drug regimen for 4 months.

The epilepsy started at the of age 37 with six bilateral tonic-clonic seizures in sleep. A few months later, focal seizures with preserved or impaired awareness started, initially only few per month but later became weekly and in clusters. According to patient description, they did not change over time and occurred in awake state, and were characterized by goosebumps in the back of the neck, left shoulder, and left arm, followed by a cold sensation in the left hemibody, mostly in the upper extremity and shoulder, subsequent unpleasant, strong and sharp smell, "déjà-vu"/"déjà-vécu" experiences, and trembling of both hands, more on the right. Sometimes, because of a feeling of "breathlessness," she tried to breathe more deeply and frequently. Her relatives confirmed that usually she could warn at onset. Afterwards, motion arrest, eye closure, oral automatisms and facial flush were observed. Her right hand became stiff and immobile, while the left hand was squeezing. Postictally she could not speak and respond for minutes. Several anti-seizure drugs (ASDs) had no or minimal efficacy (oxcarbazepine and levetiracetam), and some of them had also marked adverse effects (valproate and carbamazepine). Therefore, the therapy consisted of lamotrigine (LTG) and low-dose clonazepam (CZP). Standard electroencephalograms (EEGs) were reported as showing left temporal epileptic focus, and four brain magnetic resonance imaging (MRI) examinations were interpreted as demonstrating left hippocampal sclerosis (HS). Memory problems appeared 2 years after epilepsy onset and increased 5 months before admission, when seizure frequency reached 30 to 40 per day.

During 3-day video-EEG monitoring, more than 150 seizures were recorded. They lasted 40–60 s and correlated to left temporal ictal change of initial attenuation and subsequent rhythmic epileptiform discharge (**Figure 1A**). In wakefulness, seizures occurred at fairly regular intervals of 3 to 4 per hour (**Figure 1B**). Rapid titration of topiramate and intravenous (IV) phenytoin did not reduce seizure frequency.

Brain MRI demonstrated bilateral mesiotemporal hyperintensity with clear left predominance and enlarged left amygdala (**Figure 2A**). Neuropsychological testing confirmed verbal memory deficit. Based on clinical history, presentation, and results from the examinations performed, we strongly suspected an autoimmune etiology. Serum and cerebrospinal fluid (CSF) autoimmunity testing by ELISA (Oxford University Hospitals Neuroimmunology Laboratory) was negative for anti-Caspr2, anti-NMDAR, anti-AMPAR-1/2, anti-GABA-b, anti-VGCC, anti-VGKC, and anti-LGI1 Ab, but very high anti-GAD-Ab titers of > 50,000 IU/ml (serum) and >10,000 IU/ml were (CSF) detected. Immunotherapy was immediately started with IV methylprednisolone (MPR), and later continued with IV immunoglobulins (IVIG) and cyclophosphamide, with only brief and transient effect despite decreased serum anti-GAD Ab-titers (15,000 IU/ml).

Control brain MRI did not show progression of mesiotemporal abnormalities but fluorodeoxyglucose-positron emission tomography (FDG-PET) revealed very restricted hypermetabolism in the left amygdala correlating to an ictal event during the examination, as reported by the patient (**Figures 2B,C**). Because of lacking efficacy of ASDs and immunotherapy, and after thorough discussions with the patient and relatives on the chances and risks of epilepsy surgery, we performed a very selective left amygdalectomy. Postoperatively, the patient was 3 months seizure-free but later continued to experience shorter focal aware/unaware seizures mostly with behavioral arrest, decreased/absent responsiveness, and milder dyscognitive features but without the initial vegetative/somatosensory and the later motor signs. Seizure frequency stabilized at 3 to 4 per month with no change in ASDs, an outcome corresponding to Engel Class IIIA (5).

One year later, the patient was diagnosed with DM1 that was initially difficult to compensate, and transient increase in seizure frequency of up to 1–2 daily for about 2 months was also noted. Later on, with Insulin Apart 6 UI t.i.d. and Insulin Degludec 16 UI q.d., the condition with regard to both DM1 and TLE (weekly non-disabling

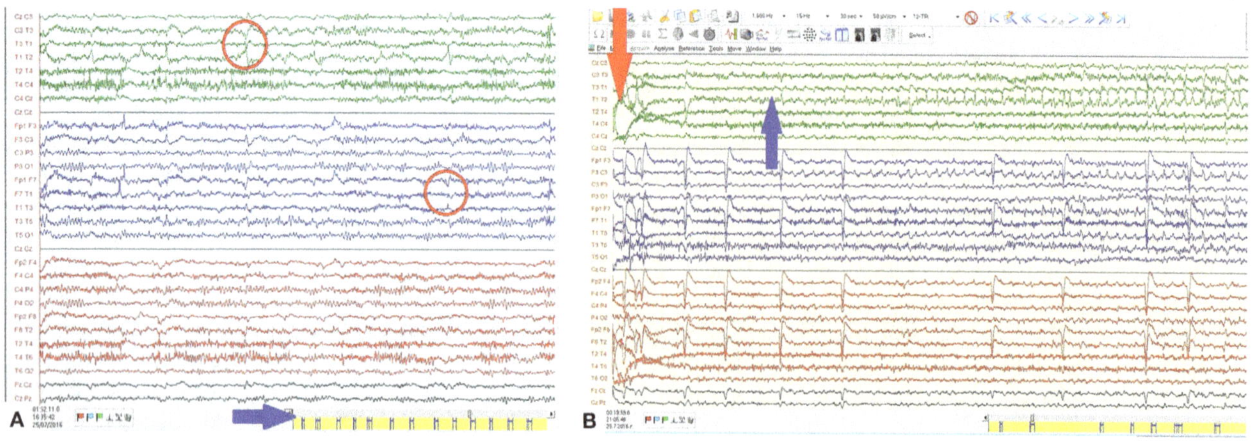

FIGURE 1 | (A) EEG in wakefulness with left temporal sharp- and spike-wave (SW) complexes with maximum and phase reversal on T1-T3 (red arrow). Individual seizures occurring at fairly regular interval and high frequency (blue arrow). **(B)** Ictal EEG epoch from the clinical seizure onset (red arrow) demonstrating the evolution of the left temporal ictal discharge consisting of rhythmic SW with an increasing amplitude and a spread mostly to the central region.

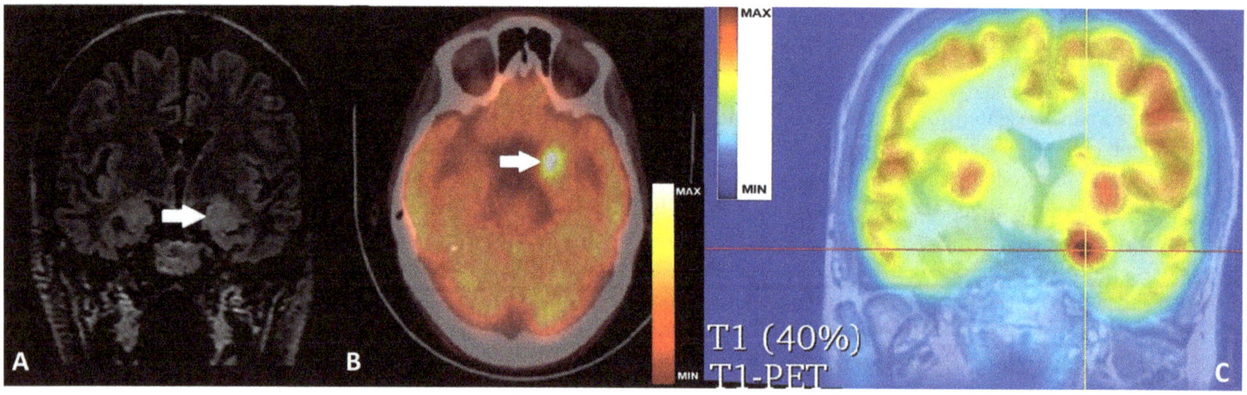

FIGURE 2 | (A) Coronal FLAIR MRI with bi-mesiotemporal hyperintensity, more prominent on the left, with increased volume of left amygdala (white arrow). **(B)** Axial PET-CT scan with hypermetabolic left mesiotemporal spot(white arrow). **(C)** PET-T1 MRI co-registration with clear hyperactivity in the left amygdala (crossed lines' center).

focal seizures) was stable and did not require further treatment adjustments.

Approximately 4 years after the operation, rare episodes of dizziness and falls were reported and interpreted by the patient as probable seizures. They were not recorded on VEEG, but right temporal epileptiform activity was registered, and lacosamide (LCM) was added. The patient continued to report intermittent unsteady gait, diplopia, vertigo, and more frequent falls, related or not to LCM intake. No changes in the neurological exam, MRI, and EEG were found; therefore, these complaints were attributed to LCM and prompted its replacement with brivaracetam without any improvement. Gradually, over the next 5 months, the patient developed a full-blown picture of CA with severe locomotor ataxia, dysdiadochokinesis, dysmetria, nystagmus, and dysarthria. Brain MRI did not reveal obvious signs of cerebellar atrophy but only progress in left HS (**Figure 3**). Paraneoplastic auto-Ab testing was negative for anti-Hu (ANNA-1), anti-Ri (ANNA-2), anti-Yo (PCA-1), anti-PNMA2 (Ma2/Ta), anti-Tr (DNER), anti-amphiphysin, anti-CV-2, anti-Sox-1, anti-ZIC4, anti-recoverin, and anti-titin Ab, but high anti-GAD65 titers of 67 U/ml persisted (positive if $\geq$ 10 U/ml, strong positive $\geq$ 50 U/ml; [10 U/ml $\approx$180 IU/ml]).

Immunotherapy with IV MPR and IVIG had no effect; therefore, rituximab treatment was started. After the first application, marked but transient improvement in CA was noted, and after the second dose, the condition stabilized. Further decrease in seizure frequency to two per month was observed as well, but due to the locomotor and distal limb ataxia at present, the 47-year-old woman is independent and able to fulfill her usual activities at home only. In addition, neuropsychological testing before, 6 months after and most recently, 4.5 years after surgery, demonstrated significant worsening of the memory function from mild short-term verbal memory deficit prior to the selective left amygdalectomy to marked verbal and

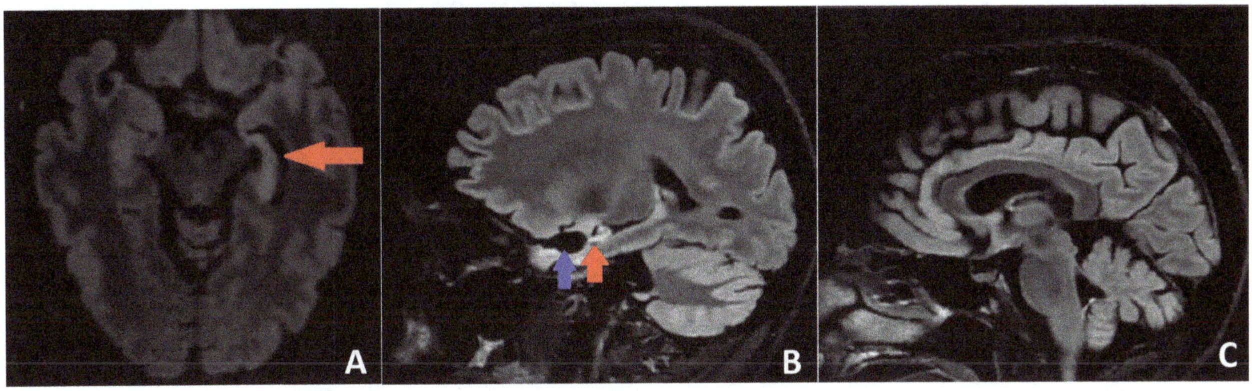

FIGURE 3 | (A) Axial FLAIR MRI with left HS (red arrow). **(B)** Sagittal FLAIR MRI scan demonstrating the postoperative defect (blue arrow) and the left HS (red arrow). **(C)** Sagittal FLAIR MRI without obvious signs of cerebellar and brainstem atrophy.

non-verbal memory decline, favoring continuing underlying bilateral damage, regardless of the stable and even improving epilepsy situation with several EEGs free of left and right temporal epileptiform or slow-wave activity.

The timeline of diseases' onset and course, most important diagnostic workup with relevant results, and therapeutic interventions including doses of the medications are presented in **Figure 4**.

DISCUSSION

After SPS and CA, GAD-TLE is considered the third most common GAD-associated neurological syndrome and one of the most common types of autoimmune epilepsy (3). GAD-Ab association must be suspected in cases with no obvious cause of TLE, and it has been postulated that GAD-Ab need to be found in high serum titers or to be detected in CSF to prove the causal relationship (1, 2, 4, 6, 7). In our case, a very high GAD-Ab titer was found both in serum and CSF, where the recognized abnormal level is >1,000 IU/ml by ELISA (2), and similar to previous reports, the serum level was much higher than that in CSF (7, 8). Although the serum GAD-Ab titer significantly decreased already after the first IV MPR trial, the disease course did not correlate to this Ab-reduction, since very frequent disabling seizures persisted and later on, two other GAD-related conditions (DM1 and CA) developed as well. In our case, the lacking clinical response to the immunomodulatory treatment despite the positive "relative" trend of Ab-decrease confirms important previous observations that without early immunotherapy this autoimmune disorder has a chronic and hard to treat course (9, 10). Obviously, in such difficult cases, GAD-Ab titer changes seem not be an effective indicator of the ongoing inflammation, and the clinical picture with treatment response is the only guide for short- and long-term therapeutic decisions (10).

As in the other GAD-associated neurological syndromes, comorbidity with other autoimmune disorders, such as DM1, could be present in >1/3 of patients with GAD-TLE/LE (11). It was found that usually the epilepsy preceded DM1 in patients with high GAD-Ab titers (12). Our case supports this observation, as TLE developed 6 years before DM1.

An important issue in our case is the possibility of a causal relationship of the autoimmune neurological disorders to the preceding anti-TNF treatment for AS. It is well known that the fundamental change in the treatment of diverse chronic inflammatory diseases brought by anti-TNF drugs increasingly raises many concerns about the safety of those agents because of various adverse events during this targeted biological treatment (13, 14). Our patient suffered from TBC, the most frequent opportunistic infection, after 2-year treatment with ETN, thus exhibiting one of the most frequent anti-TNF therapy complications, as TNFα is critical for localizing and preventing reactivation of latent mycobacterial TBC infection (14).

As to the autoimmunity, up to now, it has been reported that all anti-TNF drugs induce the development of anti-drug Ab, and that the neurological complications related to those agents are demyelinating central and peripheral nervous system diseases (13, 14). Several speculative hypotheses have been proposed to explain the mechanism of the possible relationship between anti-TNF and demyelination, but none is considered unique and adequate; moreover, several factors argue against the true association between anti-TNF therapy and demyelinating disease (14). Based on t available literature data and uncertainties on this issue, we do not consider the GAD-Ab-associated neurological disorders in our case to be related to the anti-TNF treatment, but rather we adopt the view that they are part of a multisystem autoimmune syndrome, especially having in mind the initial manifestation of a (poorly documented) autoimmune thyroid disorder, i.e., Graves' disease alone or in combination with Hashimoto's thyroiditis, as already well-documented (15).

Glutamic acid decarboxylase antibody (GAD-Ab)-associated focal epilepsy seems not to be restricted to the TL and hippocampus; the limbic system is most often affected bilaterally, and insular hypometabolism on PET could serve as an important diagnostic clue (10, 16). In our case, the seizure semiology was in favor of early insular involvement, as ictal onset was with autonomic and somatosensory signs, suggesting generation in the insula or temporo-insular circuit (10, 16–18). Autoimmune

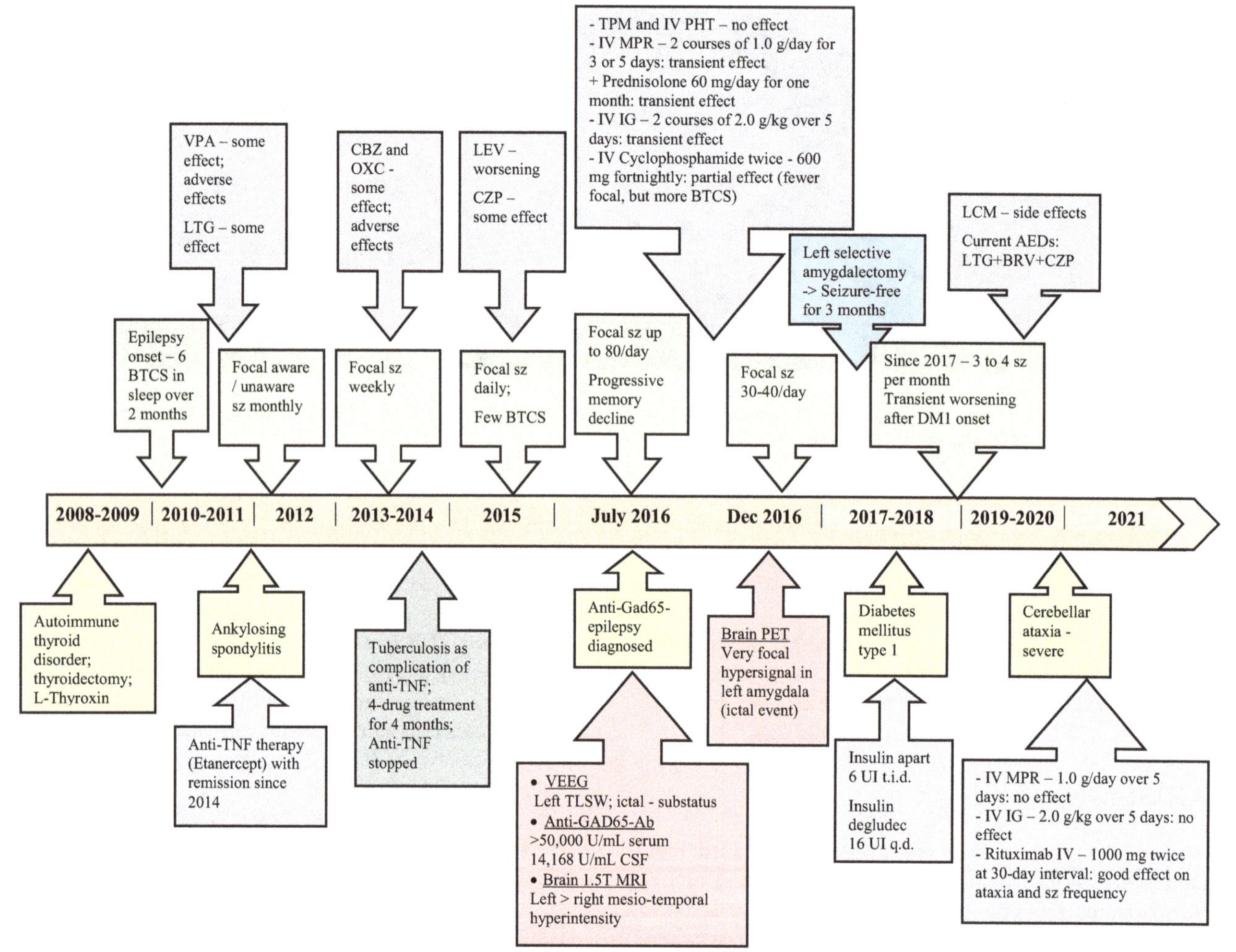

FIGURE 4 | Timeline with diseases' onset and course, the diagnostic work-up, relevant results and therapeutic management.

etiology in seizures with piloerection has been reported in autoimmune TLE (19–23), and to our knowledge there is only one published case of such semiology in GAD-associated temporo-perisylvian epilepsy (23).

Our patient presented for presurgical evaluation 5 years after epilepsy onset with dramatic seizure frequency increase over a few months, concomitantly to progressive memory disturbances, bilaterally hyperintense and swollen mesio-temporal structures, and high GAD-Ab levels. Although one major diagnostic criterion for definite limbic encephalitis is the subacute onset (<3 months) of working memory deficits and seizures (24), we believe that the other findings in our case (bilateral FLAIR-T2 mesio-temporal abnormalities, EEG showing epileptiform and slow-wave activity involving the temporal lobes, and high GAD Ab-titers both in serum and CSF) are sufficient to reasonably exclude alternative causes (24), and to speculate that the condition of our patient could be regarded as an exacerbation of "chronic" LE rather than just worsening of chronic TLE.

In the above cornerstone position article (24), it has been underlined that brain FDG-PET is much more often abnormal than time-matched MRI in cases of autoimmune LE (24–26). Moreover, hypermetabolic PET findings were found to be related to the specific antibody-type, i.e., all patients with Ab against intracellular antigens (such as GAD) showed mesio-temporal PET hyperactivity more frequently than patients with Ab against surface antigens (25). Our patient confirmed that during the PET examination she has had a usual seizure. Therefore, we considered the circumscribed hyperintense area corresponding to the left amygdala as presumable hypermetabolic ictal onset zone, most probably on top of a very active inflammation in the mesiotemporal complex, rather than as possible hypometabolism on the right side.

The surgical outcome in GAD-TLE is worse than in other refractory TLE, as it has been demonstrated by several studies that the majority of operated cases had minimal or no improvement, and that only few became seizure-free (9, 12, 27–29). Moreover, even when selective amygdalohippocampectomy controlled or improved the seizures, in combination with immunotherapy, the long-term performance in verbal and figural memory was worse than with immunomodulation only (27). It is suggested that high seizure recurrence and memory decline over the long run are related to the frequent bilaterality, widespread involvement of the limbic system by GAD-autoimmunity, and structural changes in the third stage of GAD-TLE rather than to the ongoing inflammatory process (2, 16). In our case, despite significant postoperative seizure decrease, HS on MRI and memory problems progressed; therefore, continuing autoimmune activity seems to be of major role, since DM1 and CA manifested as well.

Cerebellar ataxia (CA) is the second most frequent GAD-autoimmune disorder and is often comorbid with DM1 (3, 30–32). Although infrequent, association with epilepsy is possible, including refractory GAD-TLE preceding the CA by up to 15 years (32). Similar to what was already described (32), the full-blown CA in our case was antedated by intermittent episodes of diplopia, vertigo, and ataxia wrongly attributed to new AED. Most likely, the transient episodes represented subtle dysfunctions that in already proven GAD autoimmunity should raise concern about impending CA and prompt evaluation and immunotherapy to increase the chance of improvement (32).

Patients with delayed diagnosis of GAD-associated epilepsy were found to be usually ASD-resistant and not responding to immunotherapy (29). In such difficult cases, "the interplay between AEDs and immunotherapy" (29) is the cornerstone of management, which, in our patient, was further complicated by the subsequent manifestation of DM1 and CA. The treatment approach in every case must be individually oriented, and in this regard, epilepsy surgery cannot be excluded as an option for improvement. We hope that our case could be accepted as an example of complex clinical scenarios, in which tailored and very selective epilepsy surgery might be a useful treatment option to reduce seizure frequency and improve quality of life.

AUTHOR CONTRIBUTIONS

PD participated in patient management, clinical data analysis, and writing of the article. KM participated in patient management and revision of the article. All authors contributed to the article and approved the submitted version.

ACKNOWLEDGMENTS

The authors thank Dr. Tsocho Kmetski, Neurology Clinic, Uni Hospital, Panagyurishte, Bulgaria, for his help in patient management.

REFERENCES

1. Dade M, Berzero G, Izquierdo C, Giry M, Benazra M, Delattre JY, et al. Neurological syndromes asociated with anti-GAD antibodies. *Int J Mol Sci.* (2020) 21:3701. doi: 10.3390/ijms21103701
2. Li X, Guo Q, Zheng Z, Wang X, Liu S. Immune-mediated epilepsy with GAD65 antibodies. *J Neuroimmunol.* (2020) 341:577189. doi: 10.1016/j.jneuroim.2020.577189
3. Tsiortou P, Alexopoulos H, Dalakas MC. GAD antibody-spectrum disorders: progress in clinical phenotypes, immunopathogenesis and therapeutic interventions. *TherAdvNeurolDisord.* (2021) 14:17562864211003486. doi: 10.1177/17562864211003486
4. Saiz A, Blanco Y, Sabater L, González F, Bataller L, Casamitjana R, et al. Spectrum of neurological syndromes associated with glutamic acid decarboxylase antibodies: diagnostic clues for this association. *Brain.* (2008) 131:2553–63. doi: 10.1093/brain/awn183
5. Engel J Jr, Van Ness PC, Rasmussen TB, Ojemann LM. "Outcome with respect to epileptic seizures," In: editor Engel J. *Surgical Treatment of the Epilepsies.* New York, NY: Raven Press. (1993), p. 609–21.
6. Dubey D, Alqallaf A, Hays R, Freeman M, Chen K, Ding K, et al. Neurological autoantibody prevalence in epilepsy of unknown etiology. *JAMA Neurol.* (2017) 74:397–402. doi: 10.1001/jamaneurol.2016.5429
7. Falip M, Carreno M, Miro J, Saiz A, Villanueva V, Quilez A, et al. Prevalence and immunological spectrum of temporal lobe epilepsy with glutamic acid decarboxylase antibodies. *Eur J Neurol.* (2012) 19:827–33. doi: 10.1111/j.1468-1331.2011.03609.x
8. Malter MP, Helmstaedter C, Urbach H, Vincent A, Bien CG. Antibodies to glutamic acid decarboxylase define a form of limbic encephalitis. *Ann Neurol.* (2010) 67:470–8. doi: 10.1002/ana.21917
9. Malter MP, Frisch C, Zeitler H, Surges R, Urbach H, Helmstaedter C, et al. Treatment of immune-mediated temporal lobe epilepsy with GAD antibodies. *Seizure.* (2015) 30:57–63. 05.017 doi: 10.1016/j.seizure.2015.05.017
10. Di Giacomo R, Deleo F, Pastori C, Didato G, Andreetta F, Del Sole A, et al. Predictive value of high titer of GAD65 antibodies in a case of limbic encephalitis. *J Neuroimmunol.* (2019) 337:577063. doi: 10.1016/j.jneuroim.2019.577063
11. Gagnon MM, Savard M. Limbic encephalitis associated with GAD65 antibodies: brief review of the relevant literature. *Can J Neurol Sci.* (2016) 43:486–93. doi: 10.1017/cjn.2016.13
12. Moloney TC, Idris I, Waters P, Howell S, Vincent A, Lang B, et al. Autoantibodies to glutamic acid decarboxylase in patients with epilepsy and their relationship with type 1 diabetes: a pilot study. *J NeurolNeurosurg Psychiatry.* (2016) 87:676–7. doi: 10.1136/jnnp-2015-310512
13. Atzeni F, Nucera V, Gerratana E, Cirillo M, Marino F, Miceli G, et al. Concerns about the safety of anti-TNF agents when treating rheumatic diseases. *Expert Opin Drug Saf.* (2020) 19:695–705. doi: 10.1080/14740338.2020.1763299
14. Kaltsonoudis E, Voulgari PV, Konitsiotis S, Drosos AA. Demyelination and other neurological adverse events after anti-TNF therapy. *Autoimmun Rev.* (2014) 13:54–8. doi: 10.1016/j.autrev.2013.09.002
15. Trummer C, Schwetz V, Aberer F, Pandis M, Lerchbaum E, Pilz S. Rapid changes of thyroid function in a young woman with autoimmune thyroid disease. *Med PrincPract.* (2019) 28:397–400. doi: 10.1159/000499754
16. Falip M, Rodriguez-Bel L, Castañer S, Sala-Padró J, Miro J, Jaraba S, et al. Hippocampus and insula are targets in epileptic patients with glutamic acid decarboxylase antibodies. *Front Neurol.* (2019) 9:1143. doi: 10.3389/fneur.2018.01143
17. Loddenkemper T, Kellinghaus C, Gandjour J, Nair DR, Najm IM, Bingaman W, et al. Localising and lateralising value of ictal piloerection. *J NeurolNeurosurg Psychiatry.* (2004) 75:879–83. doi: 10.1136/jnnp.2003.023333
18. Isnard J, Guénot M, Sindou M, Mauguière F. Clinical manifestations of insular lobe seizures: a stereo-electroencephalographic study. *Epilepsia.* (2004) 45:1079–90. doi: 10.1111/j.0013-9580.2004.68903.x
19. Rocamora R, Becerra JL, Fossas P, Gomez M, Vivanco-Hidalgo RM, Mauri JA, et al. Pilomotor seizures: an autonomic semiology of limbic encephalitis? *Seizure.* (2014) 23:670–3. doi: 10.1016/j.seizure.2014.04.013
20. Wieser S, Kelemen A, Barsi P, Vincent A, Borbely C, Rasonyi G, et al. Pilomotor seizures and status in non-paraneoplastic limbic encephalitis. *Epileptic Disord.* (2005) 7:205-11
21. Baysal-Kirac L, Tuzun E, Erdag E, Ulusoy C, Vanli-Yavuz EN, Ekizoglu E, et al. Neuronal autoantibodies in epilepsy patients with peri-ictal autonomic findings. *J Neurol.* (2016) 263:455–66. doi: 10.1007/s00415-015-8002-2
22. Yang J, Sun Q, Yang G. Pilomotor seizures in a patient with LGI1 encephalitis. *Front Neurol.* (2020) 11:61. doi: 10.3389/fneur.2020.00061
23. Gillinder L, Tjoa L, Mantzioris B, Blum S, Dionisio S. Refractory chronic epilepsy associated with neuronal auto-antibodies: could perisylvian semiology be a clue? *Epileptic Disord.* (2017) 19:439–449. doi: 10.1684/epd.2017.0946

24. Graus F, Titulaer MJ, Balu R, Benseler S, Bien CG, Cellucci T, et al. A clinical approach to diagnosis of autoimmune encephalitis. *Lancet Neurol.* (2016) 15:391–404. doi: 10.1016/S1474-4422(15)00401-9
25. Baumgartner A, Rauer S, Mader I, Meyer PT. Cerebral FDG-PET and MRI findings in autoimmune limbic encephalitis: correlation with autoantibody types. *J Neurol.* (2013) 260:2744–53. doi: 10.1007/s00415-013-7048-2
26. Moreno-Ajona D, Prieto E, Grisanti F, Esparragosa I, Sánchez Orduz L, Gállego Pérez, et al. 18F-FDG-PET imaging patterns in autoimmune encephalitis: impact of image analysis on the results. *Diagnostics (Basel).* (2020) 10:356. doi: 10.3390/diagnostics10060356
27. Hansen N, Widman G, Witt JA, Wagner J, Becker AJ, Elger CE, et al. Seizure control and cognitive improvement *via* immunotherapy in late onset epilepsy patients with paraneoplastic versus GAD65 autoantibody-associated limbic encephalitis. *Epilepsy Behav.* (2016) 65:18–24. doi: 10.1016/j.yebeh.2016.10.016
28. Carreño M, Bien CG, Asadi-Pooya AA, Sperling M, Marusic P, Elisak M, et al. Epilepsy surgery in drug-resistant temporal lobe epilepsy associated with neuronal antibodies. *Epilepsy Res.* (2017) 129:101–5. doi: 10.1016/j.eplepsyres.2016.12.010
29. Mäkelä KM, Hietaharju A, Brander A, Peltola J. Clinical management of epilepsy with glutamic acid decarboxylase antibody positivity: the interplay between immunotherapy and anti-epileptic drugs. *Front Neurol.* (2018) 9:579. doi: 10.3389/fneur.2018.00579
30. Honnorat J, Saiz A, Giometto B, Vincent A, Brieva L, de Andres C, et al. Cerebellar ataxia with anti-glutamic acid decarboxylase antibodies: study of 14 patients. *Arch Neurol.* (2001) 58:225–30. doi: 10.1001/archneur.58.2.225
31. Mitoma H, Hadjivassiliou M, Honnorat J. Guidelines for treatment of immune-mediated cerebellar ataxias. *Cerebellum Ataxias.* (2015) 2:14. doi: 10.1186/s40673-015-0034-y
32. Ariño H, Gresa-Arribas N, Blanco Y, Martínez-Hernández E, Sabater L, Petit-Pedrol M, et al. Cerebellar ataxia and glutamic acid decarboxylase antibodies: immunologic profile and long-term effect of immunotherapy. *JAMA Neurol.* (2014) 71:1009–16. doi: 10.1001/jamaneurol.2014.1011

26

Case Report: Benign Infantile Seizures Temporally Associated with COVID-19

Marcos García-Howard[1], Mercedes Herranz-Aguirre[2], Laura Moreno-Galarraga[3,4], María Urretavizcaya-Martínez[1], Josune Alegría-Echauri[1], Nerea Gorría-Redondo[5], Laura Planas-Serra[6,7], Agatha Schlüter[6,7], Marta Gut[8,9], Aurora Pujol[6,7,10] and Sergio Aguilera-Albesa[3,5]**

[1] Department of Pediatrics, CHN, Navarra Health Service Hospital, Pamplona, Spain, [2] Pediatric Infectious Disease Unit, Department of Pediatrics, CHN, Navarra Health Service Hospital, Pamplona, Spain, [3] NavarraBioMed and IdiSNA, Health Research Institute, Pamplona, Spain, [4] Pediatric Respiratory Medicine, Department of Pediatrics, CHN, Navarra Health Service Hospital, Pamplona, Spain, [5] Pediatric Neurology Unit, Department of Pediatrics, CHN, Navarra Health Service Hospital, Pamplona, Spain, [6] Neurometabolic Diseases Laboratory, Bellvitge Biomedical Research Institute (IDIBELL), Barcelona, Spain, [7] Center for Biomedical Research on Rare Diseases (CIBERER), ISCIII, Madrid, Spain, [8] CNAG-CRG, Centre for Genomic Regulation, Barcelona Institute of Science and Technology, Barcelona, Spain, [9] Universitat Pompeu Fabra (UPF), Barcelona, Spain, [10] Catalan Institution of Research and Advanced Studies (ICREA), Barcelona, Spain

***Correspondence:**
Sergio Aguilera-Albesa
saguilea@navarra.es
Aurora Pujol
apujol@idibell.cat

Background: Non-febrile illness seizures may present in previously healthy children as afebrile seizures associated with minor infections, such as mild gastroenteritis or respiratory tract infections, and are linked to a genetic predisposition. For the novel human coronavirus SARS-CoV-2, causing COVID-19, fever, cough, and gastrointestinal complaints are the most common symptoms in children, and a hyperimmune response may be present. No detailed temporally associated neurological complications have been documented in pediatric case series so far.

Case description: We present the case of a 3-months-old girl with non-febrile repeated seizures in a COVID-19 family setting. The infant started with a mild fever and cough that lasted for 2 days. At day 6 from onset, the girl presented with two focal motor seizures with impaired consciousness and awareness. All investigations ruled out signs of meningo-encephalitis or active epilepsy, including normal electroencephalogram and cerebral magnetic resonance imaging. PCR from nasal and throat swabs was positive for SARS-CoV-2. Remarkably, blood ferritin and D-dimer levels were increased. At day 9, the infant presented another afebrile motor seizure, and levetiracetam dose was modified there was a favorable response within 3 months of the follow-up. Much interest has been raised with regards to host genetic determinants to disease severity and susceptibility to COVID-19. We thus performed whole exome sequencing, revealing a pathogenic frameshift mutation in the PRRT2 gene in both the mother and the infant. The mother had presented two late infantile febrile convulsions with normal outcome afterwards.

Discussion: The hyperimmune response described in adult cases with COVID-19 can be seen in infants, even in the absence of respiratory symptoms. Moreover, COVID-19 may present in infants as non-febrile seizures, triggering early onset seizures in infants with a genetic predisposition. In this pandemic situation, precision medicine using massive sequencing can shed light on underlying molecular mechanisms driving the host response to COVID-19.

Keywords: coronavirus, SARS-CoV-2, COVID-19, pediatric COVID-19, non-febrile seizures, afebrile seizures, PRRT2 mutations, benign familial infantile epilepsy

INTRODUCTION

Non-febrile illness seizures are described as afebrile seizures associated with minor infections in previously healthy children. Seizures occur mainly in infants in the setting of acute infections, such as mild gastroenteritis or respiratory tract infections, without structural correlate or hydro-electrolytic imbalance (1–4). Rotaviruses are frequently found in non-febrile convulsions associated with gastroenteritis, and noroviruses have been recently identified as an emergent pathogen in these cases (1, 5). In infants with non-febrile seizures related to respiratory tract infections, common seasonal viruses, such as influenza, respiratory syncytial virus (RSV), and metapneumovirus, have been pointed out as plausible causative pathogens (3, 4, 6).

Human coronavirus (HCoV) causes respiratory infections with a seasonal pattern in children, and in some cases, extra-pulmonar manifestations have been described. It has been increasingly recognized that HCoV shows some neurotropism due to its capacity to reach the central nervous system after the nasal infection, shown for HCoV-OC43 and HCoV-NL63 (7, 8). Neurological complications of common HCoV infections have been reported, including febrile seizures, convulsions, loss of consciousness, encephalomyelitis, and encephalitis (9). Another HCoV, SARS-CoV, emerged in Guandong province, southern China, in 2002, and it spread to many countries and caused severe lower respiratory tract infection with an overall case-fatality rate of 10%. The SARS-CoV was associated with milder disease in children compared to adults, with some case series reporting febrile seizures in 10% of a total sample of 41 children (10–12). Fortunately, no human SARS-CoV infections have been identified since July 2003 (8).

In December 2019, a novel HCoV (SARS-CoV-2) was reported from Wuhan city, Hubei province, China, and it rapidly spread worldwide causing a pandemic outbreak by March 2020, producing a respiratory disease called COVID-19. Initial case series have shown that children present milder clinical symptoms than adults and that most pediatric cases were infected in family clusters. Fever, cough, respiratory distress, myalgia, and gastrointestinal complaints are the most common symptoms (13–18), but no detailed neurological complications have been documented in pediatric case series so far.

In this article, we describe the case of a 3-months-old girl with non-febrile repeated seizures in a COVID-19 family setting. Whole exome sequencing was applied and revealed an underlying genetic pathogenic variant that may cause the clinical presentation.

CASE PRESENTATION

A previously healthy, with uneventful pregnancy and delivery, 3-months-old girl was admitted to the pediatric emergency department early morning on April 1 after her mother reported two episodes of convulsions without fever. During the night, the mother, who was a nurse, reported a first episode of clonic movements of the face with tonic posture of extremities and trismus, without consciousness, lasting 3 min approximately. Few hours later, the infant presented with a second episode, described as staring gaze, clonic movements of the face and right extremities, and repeating sucking movements of the mouth, lasting <5 min. At admission, vital constants were normal; physical and neurological examination showed mild hypotonia and drowsiness without focal deficits. The mother informed us that, on March 27–28, the infant had presented with a low fever of <38.1°C, rhinorrhea, cough, and diarrhea with subsequent improvement. No fever was documented the 3 days before these convulsions. Interestingly, the mother referred herself as having persistent symptoms of anosmia and dysgeusia since March 23, and showed no signs of fever or respiratory symptoms since.

At admission, patient blood tests did not show any abnormalities except for a high ferritin value (385 μg/L; normal values 10–204). PCRs of nasopharyngeal and throat swabs tested positive for SARS-CoV-2. Additional testing for other viruses was negative, including HCoV-NL63, HCoV-OC43, HCoV-229E, RSV, rhinovirus, metapneumovirus, influenza, adenovirus, bocavirus, and enterovirus. Chest x-ray and brain CT scans did not reveal abnormalities; the CSF analysis for cells, glucose, and protein was normal. PCRs for herpes virus family (HSV-1, HSV-2, and VZV) and enterovirus in CSF were negative. Bacteria cultures in blood, urine, and CSF were also negative.

During hospitalization, three interictal electroencephalograms (EEG) and a cerebral 1.5T MRI showed normal results. Levetiracetam was started the 1st day as prophylactic antiepileptic treatment (28 mg/Kg/day), but the infant presented with another afebrile seizure on April 4, consisting of upright tonic eye deviation, clonic movements of face muscles, and tonic posture of four limbs in extension, lasting 90 s. The seizure was recorded by the mother and was checked by pediatric neurologists. Pre-dosing blood levels of levetiracetam were within therapeutic range (15 mcg/mL; normal values 10–40). Hydroxychloroquine was then started on April 4, as compassionate use due to the persistence of seizures in a COVID-19 setting, at a dosage of 6.5 mg/Kg/day for 5 days with excellent tolerance. Blood test controls revealed a sustained decrease of ferritin values, with a late increase of D-dimer levels. Unfortunately, D-dimer control was not possible due to technical procedures. The rest of the lab tests were within normal limits. Following discharge, the patient was followed as an outpatient, and she presented with normal neurological development and an absence of seizures. A timeline of clinical course, lab test, and investigations is summarized in **Figure 1**. Informed and written consent to publish clinical details was obtained from the parents. Additionally, during hospitalization, the patient and her mother were included in a collaborative study of genomic medicine for identifying genetic variants causing hyperimmunity due to SARS-CoV-2 infection. The local ethics committee approved the study. Whole exome sequencing was performed, and prioritized genes were analyzed. No pathogenic variants of susceptibility genes for hyperimmunity were found, but both the infant and the mother carried a loss-of-function variant in the PRRT2 gene (NM_145239.3), c.649dupC (p.Arg217fs), at the heterozygous state. This frameshift variant has been recurrently described in ClinVar as pathogenic. It is associated with benign familial infantile convulsions (OMIM 605751), but it is also allelic to infantile convulsions and choreoathetosis (OMIM 602066) (19). A revision of maternal family history revealed that the mother could have had two convulsions during late infancy, related to mild infections and fever, with normal development afterwards.

DISCUSSION

SARS-CoV-2 infection in children is being increasingly recognized. However, detailed clinical data are still lacking and individual cases, such as the one presented, can shed some light to comprehend the complex systemic manifestations of this disease in the youngest.

A review of the Chinese Center for Disease Control and Prevention on February 24 has shown than <1% of the COVID-19 cases were in children younger than 10 years of age (20). In Wuhan Children's Hospital, China, 1,391 children were tested through February, and a total of 171 (12.3%) were positive for SARS-CoV-2 infection, with a median age of 6.7 years. Of these, 65% presented pneumonia and three required invasive mechanical ventilation. Only 18% of the positive children were infants younger than 1 year of age, and no cases were reported with neurological features. In Spain, by March 16, 41 of the 4,695 confirmed cases (0.8%) in the Madrid region were children younger than 18 years, and 60% of the pediatric cases required hospitalization (21). In a systematic review of SARS-CoV-2 infection in children, Castagnoli et al. found, by April 22, 444 participants younger than 10 years of age, but no details about clinical symptoms were revealed (22).

Our infant presented with afebrile seizures during the course of COVID-19, some of them with focal semiology, and these were

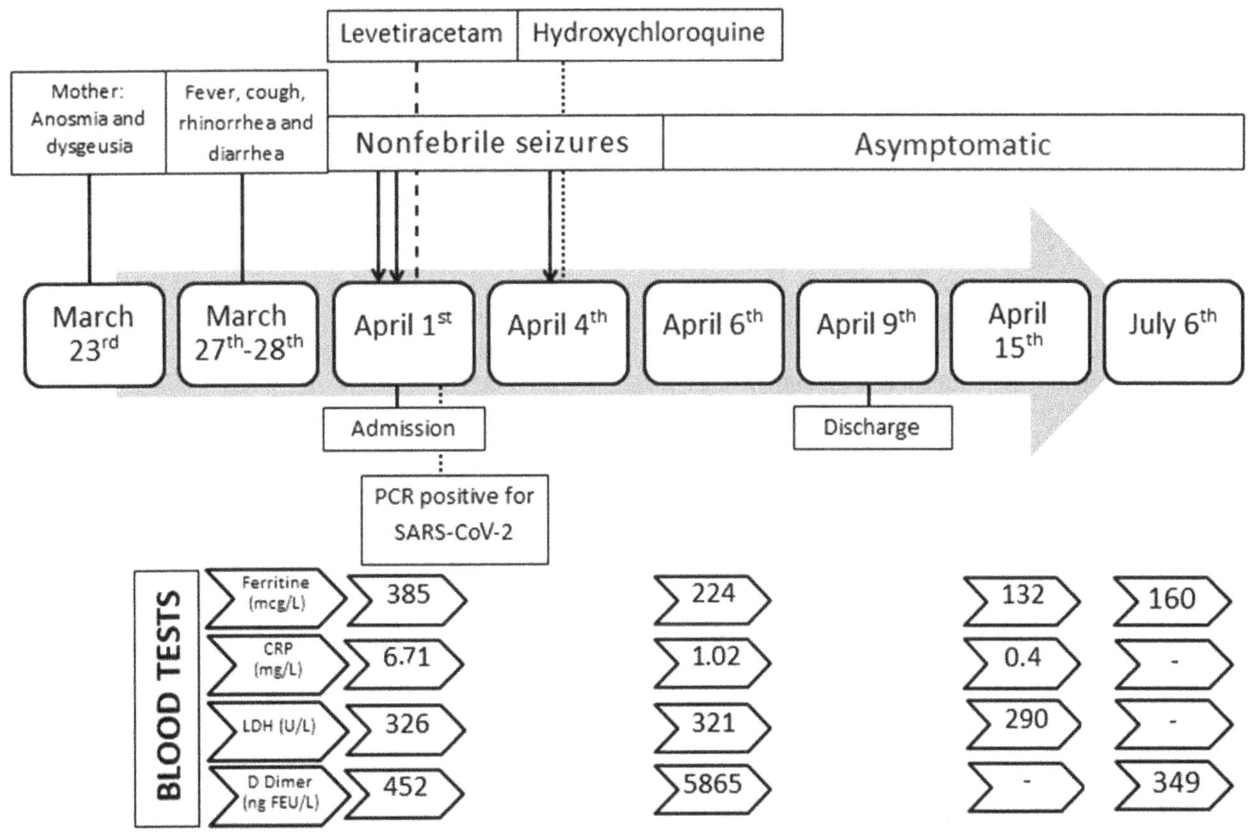

FIGURE 1 | Timeline course of the patient's COVID-19 disease.

not associated with signs of encephalitis, structural damage, or other concomitant infection. The clinical picture is compatible with the definition of non-febrile illness seizures, which occur in association with an acute infection the week before or 3 days after the seizure, although without presenting with fever on the day of the seizure (3, 23).

Besides respiratory symptoms, HCoV infections may present with febrile seizures in susceptible infants (9–12). Very recently, a febrile convulsion in a 2-years-old girl with COVID-19 was reported (15). However, several studies have suggested that non-febrile illness seizures are a different seizure category from febrile seizures or unprovoked seizures. Non-febrile illness seizures may share some genetic predisposition in a similar manner as febrile seizures or epilepsy, and, as with febrile seizures, the prognosis is favorable in most cases (3).

This pandemic has sparked an interest in genomic medicine to elucidate host determinants of phenotype severity (24, 25). We thus performed whole exome sequencing as described (26) and uncovered the genetic predisposition of the infant to develop afebrile seizures due to a well-known recurrent pathogenic PRRT2 mutation associated with benign familial infantile convulsions (OMIM 605751) and infantile convulsions and choreoathetosis (OMIM 602066) (19). In the mother, the phenotype is benign and self-limited, without movement disorders. Nonetheless, a long-term follow-up is required to detect the possible development of dyskinesias in the infant.

Regarding other investigations in this case, ferritin levels were increased at admission, on day 6 since symptoms onset, and they progressively decreased over time. D-dimers were within normal limits at admission but increased during hospitalization. These findings resemble the hyperimmune response found is adult COVID-19 severe cases, a major driver of adverse outcome (27, 28). Same findings are being reported in severe COVID-19 in children (8), and, during the SARS-CoV epidemic of 2002, some patients presented with decreased lymphocyte count and increased levels of LDH and D-dimers.

Therapeutic strategies and evidence-based protocols for COVID-19 treatment in children are still lacking. On April 4, we thus decided to treat our infant with hydroxychloroquine since this drug is renowned for its antiviral and immunomodulating properties (29), and it has been previously used in young infants (30–33). Preliminary results of hydroxychloroquine on adults COVID-19 clinical trials suggested that 600 mg daily may decrease viral load in nasal swabs (34), but further studies has raised concerns about its use during hospitalization (35). On July 4, the WHO International Steering Committee discontinued clinical trials for hydroxychloroquine in hospitalized patients (www.who.int/news-room).

One limitation of this case is related to the storing of the biological samples. PCR of SARS-CoV-2 in CSF was not available at that moment, and the sample was not stored. Moreover, hyperimmune response in younger children is an uncommon phenomenon and warrants further research in samples of the patients. We would like to encourage pediatricians to collect and store biological samples of patients with COVID-19 for further analysis, as it would be useful for future research.

ETHICS STATEMENT

The studies involving human participants were reviewed and approved by Complejo Hospitalario de Navarra. Written informed consent to participate in this study was provided by the participants' legal guardian/next of kin. Written informed consent was obtained from the minor(s)' legal guardian/next of kin for the publication of any potentially identifiable images or data included in this article.

AUTHOR CONTRIBUTIONS

SA-A and MH-A conceived and designed the manuscript. MG-H wrote the first draft. LM-G, MU-M, JA-E, and NG-R provided data acquisition, clinical details of the patient, and reviewed the literature. LP-S, AS, and MG generated and analyzed the exomes using the CNAG pipeline. AP provided funding and interpreted the variants in its clinical context. SA-A wrote the final manuscript. AP and SA-A added and refined discussion and final conclusions. All authors reviewed and approved the final version as submitted, and agreed to be accountable for all aspects of the work.

ACKNOWLEDGMENTS

The authors would like to thank the patient's family for their cooperation and for consenting to the publication of this manuscript. They will also like to thank the enormous effort done by all our hospital and Spanish health workers in the fight against the current COVID-19 pandemic.

REFERENCES

1. Uemura N, Okumura A, Negoro T, Watanabe K. Clinical features of benign convulsions with mild gastroenteritis. *Brain Dev.* (2002) 24:745–9. doi: 10.1016/S0387-7604(02)00097-9
2. Durá-Travé T, Yoldi-Petri ME, Molins-Castiella T, Souto-Hernández S, Aguilera-Albesa S. Infantile convulsions with mild gastroenteritis: epidemiological and clinical characteristics and outcome. *Rev Neurol.* (2010) 5:12–8. doi: 10.33588/rn.5101.2010018
3. Zhang T, Ma J, Gan X, Xiao N. Are afebrile seizures associated with minor infections a single seizure category? A hospital-based prospective cohort study on outcomes of first afebrile seizure in early childhood. *Epilepsia.* (2014) 55:1001–8. doi: 10.1111/epi.12651
4. Conejo Moreno D, Rodríguez Fernández C, Ruíz Ayúcar de la Vega I, Ortiz Madinaveitia S, Hedrera Fernández A, Maldonado Ruiz. E, et al. Para-infectious seizures: a retrospective multicentre study. *An Pediatr.* (2016) 85:300–4. doi: 10.1016/j.anpede.2016.01.012
5. Ma X, Luan S, Zhao Y, Lv X, Zhang R. Clinical characteristics and follow-up of benign convulsions with mild gastroenteritis among children. *Medicine.* (2019) 98:e14082. doi: 10.1097/MD.0000000000014082
6. Cha T, Choi YJ, Oh JW, Kim CR, Park DW, Seol IJ, et al. Respiratory syncytial virus-associated seizures in Korean children, 2011–2016. *Korean J Pediatr.* (2019) 62:131–7. doi: 10.3345/kjp.2018.07066

7. St-Jean JR, Jacomy H, Desforges M, Vabret A, Freymuth F, Talbot PJ. Human respiratory coronavirus OC43: genetic stability and neuroinvasion. *J Virol.* (2004) 78:8824–34. doi: 10.1128/JVI.78.16.8824-8834.2004
8. Zimmermann P, Curtis N. Coronavirus infections in children including COVID-19: an overview of the epidemiology, clinical features, diagnosis, treatment and prevention options in children. *Pediatr Infect Dis J.* (2020) 39:355–68. doi: 10.1097/INF.0000000000002660
9. Bohmwald K, Gálvez NMS, Ríos M, Kalergis AM. Neurologic alterations due to respiratory virus infections. *Front Cell Neurosci.* (2018) 12:386. doi: 10.3389/fncel.2018.00386
10. Hon KL, Leung CW, Cheng WT, Chan PK, Chu WC, Kwan YW, et al. Clinical presentations and outcome of severe acute respiratory syndrome in children. *Lancet.* (2003) 361:1701–3. doi: 10.1016/S0140-6736(03)13364-8
11. Chiu WK, Cheung PC, Ng KL, Ip PL, Sugunan VK, Luk DC, et al. Severe acute respiratory syndrome in children: experience in a regional hospital in Hong Kong. *Pediatr Crit Care Med.* (2003) 4:279–83. doi: 10.1097/01.PCC.0000077079.42302.81
12. Bitnun A, Allen U, Heurter H, King SM, Opavsky MA, Ford-Jones EL, et al. Children hospitalized with severe acute respiratory syndrome-related illness in Toronto. *Pediatrics.* (2003) 112:e261. doi: 10.1542/peds.112.4.e261
13. Chan JF, Yuan S, Kok KH, To KK, Chu H, Yang J, et al. A familial cluster of pneumonia associated with the 2019 novel coronavirus indicating person-to-person transmission: a study of a family cluster. *Lancet.* (2020) 395:514–23. doi: 10.1016/S0140-6736(20)30154-9
14. Zhu N, Zhang D, Wang W, Li X, Yang B, Song J, et al. A novel coronavirus from patients with pneumonia in China, 2019. *N Engl J Med.* (2020) 382:727–33. doi: 10.1056/NEJMoa2001017
15. Tan YP, Tan BY, Pan J, Wu J, Zeng SZ, Wei HY. Epidemiologic and clinical characteristics of 10 children with coronavirus disease 2019 in Changsha, China. *J Clin Virol.* (2020) 127:104353. doi: 10.1016/j.jcv.2020.104353
16. Shen KL, Yang YH, Jiang RM, Wang TY, Zhao DC, Jiang Y, et al. Updated diagnosis, treatment and prevention of COVID-19 in children: experts' consensus statement (condensed version of the second edition). *World J Pediatr.* (2020) 16:232–9. doi: 10.1007/s12519-020-00362-4
17. Dong Y, Mo X, Hu Y, Qi X, Jiang F, Jiang Z, et al. Epidemiological characteristics of 2143 pediatric patients with 2019 coronavirus disease in China. *Pediatrics.* (2020) 58:712–3. doi: 10.1016/j.jemermed.2020.04.006
18. CDC COVID-19 response team. Coronavirus disease 2019 in children—United States, February 12-April 2, 2020. *MMWR Morb Mortal Wkly Rep.* (2020) 69:422–6. doi: 10.15585/mmwr.mm6914e4
19. Heron SE, Grinton BE, Kivity S, Afawi Z, Zuberi SM, Hughes JN, et al. PRRT2 mutations cause benign familial infantile epilepsy and infantile convulsions with choreoathetosis syndrome. *Am J Hum Genet.* (2012) 90:152–60. doi: 10.1016/j.ajhg.2011.12.003
20. Wu Z, McGoogan JM. Characteristics of and important lessons from the coronavirus disease 2019 (COVID-19) outbreak in China: summary of a report of 72 314 cases from the Chinese Center for Disease Control and Prevention. *JAMA.* (2020). doi: 10.1001/jama.2020.2648. [Epub ahead of print].
21. Tagarro A, Epalza C, Santos M, Sanz-Santaeufemia FJ, Otheo E, Moraleda C, et al. Screening and severity of coronavirus disease 2019 (COVID-19) in children in Madrid, Spain. *JAMA Pediatr.* (2020) e201346. doi: 10.1001/jamapediatrics.2020.1346. [Epub ahead of print].
22. Castagnoli R, Votto M, Licari A, Brambilla I, Bruno R, Perlini S, et al. Severe Acute Respiratory Syndrome Coronavirus 2 (SARS-CoV-2) infection in children and adolescents. A systematic review. *JAMA Pediatr.* (2020). doi: 10.1001/jamapediatrics.2020.1467. [Epub ahead of print].
23. Zerr DM, Blume HK, Berg AT, Del Beccaro MA, Gospe SM Jr, Allpress AL, et al. Non-febrile illness seizures: a unique seizure category? *Epilepsia.* (2005) 46:952–5. doi: 10.1111/j.1528-1167.2005.65204.x
24. Casanova JL, Su HC. A global effort to define the human genetics of protective immunity to SARS-CoV-2 infection. *Cell.* (2020) 181:1194–1199. doi: 10.1016/j.cell.2020.05.016
25. The COVID-19 Host Genetics Initiative. The COVID-19 Host Genetics Initiative, a global initiative to elucidate the role of host genetic factors in susceptibility and severity of the SARS-CoV-2 virus pandemic. *Eur J Human Genet.* (2020) 28:715–8. doi: 10.1038/s41431-020-0636-6
26. Pant DC, Dorboz I, Schluter A, Fourcade S, Launay N, Joya J, et al. Loss of the sphingolipid desaturase DEGS1 causes hypomyelinating leukodystrophy. *J Clin Invest.* (2019) 129:1240–56. doi: 10.1172/JCI123959
27. Qin C, Zhou L, Hu Z, Zhang S, Yang S, Tao Y, et al. Dysregulation of immune response in patients with COVID-19 in Wuhan, China. *Clin Infect Dis.* (2020) ciaa248. doi: 10.2139/ssrn.3541136. [Epub ahead of print].
28. Mehta P, McAuley DF, Brown M, Sanchez E, Tattersall RS, Manson JJ, et al. COVID-19: consider cytokine storm syndromes and immunosuppression. *Lancet.* (2020) 395:1033–4. doi: 10.1016/S0140-6736(20)30628-0
29. Sturrock BR, Chevassut TJ. Chloroquine and COVID-19—a potential game changer? *Clin Med.* (2020) 20:278–1. doi: 10.7861/clinmed.2020-0129
30. White NJ. The treatment of malaria. *N Engl J Med.* (1996) 335:800–6. doi: 10.1056/NEJM199609123351107
31. Colson P, Rolain JM, Raoult D. Chloroquine for the 2019 novel coronavirus SARS-CoV-2. *Int J Antimicrob Agents.* (2020) 55:105923. doi: 10.1016/j.ijantimicag.2020.105923
32. Vincent MJ, Bergeron E, Benjannet S, Erickson BR, Rollin PE, Ksiazek TG, et al. Chloroquine is a potent inhibitor of SARS coronavirus infection and spread. *Virol J.* (2005) 2:69. doi: 10.1186/1743-422X-2-69
33. Yao X, Ye F, Zhang M, Cui C, Huang B, Niu P, et al. *In vitro* antiviral activity and projection of optimized dosing design of hydroxychloroquine for the treatment of Severe Acute Respiratory Syndrome Coronavirus 2 (SARS-CoV-2). *Clin Infect Dis.* (2020) ciaa237. doi: 10.1093/cid/ciaa237. [Epub ahead of print].
34. Gautret P, Lagier JC, Parola P, Hoang VT, Meddeb L, Mailhe M, et al. Hydroxychloroquine and azithromycin as a treatment of COVID-19: results of an open-label non-randomized clinical trial. *Int J Antimicrob Agents.* (2020) 105949. doi: 10.1016/j.ijantimicag.2020.105949. [Epub ahead of print].
35. Alexander PE, Debono VB, Mammen MJ, Iorio A, Aryal K, Berg D, et al. COVID-19 coronavirus research has overall low methodological quality thus far: case in point for chloroquine/hydroxychloroquine. *J Clin Epidemiol.* (2020) 123:120–6. doi: 10.1016/j.jclinepi.2020.04.016

27

Three Cases of Hemiconvulsion-Hemiplegia-Epilepsy Syndrome with Focal Cortical Dysplasia Type IIId

Shinji Itamura [1], Tohru Okanishi [1], Yoshifumi Arai [2], Mitsuyo Nishimura [3], Shimpei Baba [1], Naoki Ichikawa [4], Yoshimichi Hirayama [5], Naoko Ishihara [6], Takuya Hiraide [7], Hidetoshi Ishigaki [7], Tokiko Fukuda [7], Yoshiro Otsuki [2], Hideo Enoki [1] and Ayataka Fujimoto [4]*

[1] Department of Child Neurology, Seirei-Hamamatsu General Hospital, Shizuoka, Japan, [2] Department of Pathology, Seirei-Hamamatsu General Hospital, Shizuoka, Japan, [3] Department of Clinical Laboratory, Seirei-Hamamatsu General Hospital, Shizuoka, Japan, [4] Epilepsy Center, Seirei-Hamamatsu General Hospital, Shizuoka, Japan, [5] Department of Pediatrics, Naha City Hospital, Okinawa, Japan, [6] Department of Pediatrics, Fujita Health University School of Medicine, Toyoake, Japan, [7] Department of Pediatrics, Hamamatsu University School of Medicine, Hamamatsu, Japan

***Correspondence:**
Tohru Okanishi
t.okanishi@sis.seirei.or.jp;
okanishipediatrics@gmail.com

Hemiconvulsion-hemiplegia-epilepsy syndrome (HHES) is a subset of acute encephalopathy characterized by infantile-onset with acute hemiconvulsive febrile status and subsequent unilateral cerebral atrophy and hemiparesis. In the chronic phase, patients with HHES develop epilepsy, typically displayed as intractable focal seizures. The patients are often intractable with antiepileptic drugs and need surgical treatment. Although viral encephalitis and genetic abnormalities are presumed to be the underlying etiology, the pathogenesis remains mostly unknown. We describe three cases of successful functional hemispherotomy for intractable epilepsy in HHES. Patients developed acute asymmetrical convulsive status following viral infections during the ages of 17–30 months. Their seizures were intractable with antiepileptic drugs and required hemispherotomy. On the basis of the pathological findings, all cases were diagnosed as focal cortical dysplasia (FCD) type IIId. The epileptogenic mild cortical malformations may be the cause of HHES.

Keywords: hemiconvulsion-hemiplegia-epilepsy syndrome, hemispherotomy, focal cortical dysplasia, cortical malformation, intractable epilepsy, epilepsy surgery, pathology, histopathology

INTRODUCTION

Hemiconvulsion-hemiplegia-epilepsy syndrome (HHES) is a rare condition first described by Gastaut et al. in 1960 (1) that starts with virus infection-associated acute encephalopathy in the unilateral hemisphere. This condition is characterized by prolonged febrile status of hemiconvulsion (asymmetrical convulsion) in the acute phase, and development of hemiparesis/hemiplegia and intractable epilepsy in the chronic phase. Hemispheric cytotoxic edema occurs in the acute phase and is presented as reduced diffusivity in brain magnetic resonance imaging (MRI), including diffusion-weighted imaging (DWI). The affected hemisphere evolves into atrophy in the chronic phase. Only a few pathologic investigations have been reported; therefore, the pathogenesis of HHES has not yet been determined (2–5).

Focal cortical dysplasia (FCD) is an epileptogenic cortical tissue frequently seen in the resected cortices of patients who have undergone epilepsy surgery. In the 2011 International League Against Epilepsy (ILAE) classification, FCD was classified into type I: dyslamination and disrupted organization of tissue architecture with morphologically normal neurons and glial cells; type II:

presence of dysplastic, megalocytic neurons mixed with normal neurons; and type III: adjacent to another principal lesion. Type IIId is diagnosed in association with epileptogenic lesions acquired early in life (6).

We herein report three cases of HHES with FCD type IIId in the affected cortices.

CASE PRESENTATION

We summarized the clinical information of the three cases in **Table 1**.

Case 1

An 18-month-old boy with a healthy clinical history presented with left-sided status of clonic convulsion lasting over 30 min following fever. Enterovirus was isolated from his pharyngeal secretion on the day of admission. Three days following onset, brain DWI showed reduced diffusivity on subcortical white matter in the right hemisphere. He was diagnosed with viral infection associated-acute encephalopathy and treated with methylprednisolone pulse therapy, high dose immunoglobulin and continuous intravenous midazolam. After the acute phase of the encephalopathy, he presented with left hemiparesis. Left side dominant-tonic spasms recurred 3 months following onset. Despite treatment with clobazam, lamotrigine, topiramate, carbamazepine, and levetiracetam, the seizures continued to occur daily.

He was referred to our epilepsy center at the age of 39 months. He had left hemiparesis and could only speak a few words. His developmental quotient (DQ) was 46 on the Kinder Infant Development Scale. Long-term video-electroencephalogram (EEG) monitoring revealed that the left side dominant-tonic spasms (10/day) coincided with ictal changes of diffuse spike bursts followed by biphasic or triphasic diffuse slow waves, and that the myoclonic seizures (>30/day) coincided with diffuse polyspikes and waves. Brain MRI revealed right cerebral atrophy and hypoperfusion with arterial spin labeling (ASL). At the age of 41 months, he underwent right hemispherotomy. He was free from any seizures up to the last follow-up at 10 months after

TABLE 1 | Clinical information and pathological findings in the 3 cases.

	Case 1	Case 2	Case 3
Age at onset of acute encephalopathy	18 mo	28 mo	17 mo
Side of affected hemisphere	Right	Right	Left
Type of convulsive status at onset	Left-sided clonic seizures	Left-sided clonic seizures	Right-sided clonic seizures
Causative virus	Enterovirus	Influenza type A	Human herpesvirus 6
DWI findings in the acute phase (d of onset)	Subcortical high intensities diffusely in the right hemisphere (3d)	Cortical and subcortical high intensities diffusely in the right hemisphere (5d)	Cortical and subcortical high intensities diffusely in the left TPO (3d)
Treatment for acute encephalopathy	mPSL, IV	mPSL, IV, mannitol, PB, MDZ	mPSL, MDZ
Antiepileptic drugs before surgery	CLB, LTG, TPM, CBZ, LEV	PB, VPA, CLB, PER, LTG, LEV	VPA, CLB, LTG, PER, TPM, LEV
MRI findings in the chronic phase	Diffuse atrophy and hypoperfusion in the right hemisphere	Diffuse atrophy and hypoperfusion in the right hemisphere	Diffuse atrophy in the left hemisphere
Development quotient before surgery (age)	46 (39 mo)	31 (56 mo)	34 (56 mo)
Motor disability before surgery	Left hemiparesis	Left hemiparesis	No paresis
Seizure types before surgery (frequency)	1: Left side dominant-tonic spasms (10/d); 2: Myoclonic seizures (>30/d)	Left side dominant-tonic spasms (2–5/d)	1: Focal impaired awareness seizures with foci in left F, O; 2: Asymmetrical tonic seizure secondary to seizure 1
Ictal EEG findings	1: Diffuse spike burst followed by polyphasic slow waves; 2: Diffuse polyspikes and waves	Diffuse attenuation in the right hemisphere	1: Frequent spikes and theta burst in left F or O; 2: Fast wave -> spike burst in left hemisphere
Age at epilepsy surgery	41 mo	59 mo	60 mo
Type of epilepsy surgery	Right hemispherotomy	Right hemispherotomy	Left subtotal hemispherotomy
Seizure outcomes of the surgery (follow-up period)	Seizure free (10 mo)	Seizure free (11 mo)	Seizure free (10 mo)
Pathology			
Neocortex	Excessive neuronal cells and glial cells in white matter (FCD type IIId) in temporal lobe	Excessive neuronal cells and glial cells in white matter (FCD type IIId) in temporal lobe	Excessive neuronal cells and glial cells in white matter (FCD type IIId), immature-like in temporal lobe
Amygdala	No change	No change	Immature-like neurons
Hippocampus	No change	No change	Gliosis

y, year(s); mo, month(s); d, day(s); mPSL, methylprednisolone; IV, immunoglobline; MDZ, midazolam; CLB, clobazam; LTG, lamotrigine; TPM, topiramate; CBZ, carbamazepine; LEV, levetiracetum; PB, phenobarbital; VPA, valproic acid; PER, perampanel; F, frontal lobe; T, temporal lobe; O, occipital lobe; FCD, focal cortical dysplasia.

the surgery. The left hemiparesis transiently worsened after the surgery and then recovered to the presurgical level. His attention and cognitive function improved.

The histopathological examination with hematoxylin-eosin staining revealed an excessive number of neurons and glial cells in the white matter with intact cortical architecture and absence of aberrant cells, corresponding to FCD type IIId, on the right tip of the temporal lobe (**Supplementary Figures 1A,B, 2A**). No changes were observed in the right amygdala and hippocampus.

Case 2

A 28-month-old boy with a healthy clinical history presented with left-sided status of clonic convulsions lasting >30 min with fever. His pharynx was positive for the antigen of influenza virus type A. Brain DWI showed reduced diffusivity in the cortex and subcortical white matter in the right hemisphere, at 5 days after the occurrence (**Figure 1A**). He was treated with methylprednisolone pulse therapy and high dose immunoglobulin, mannitol, phenobarbital, and continuous intravenous midazolam. After encephalopathy onset, he presented with left hemiparesis, and suffered from left side dominant- or symmetrical tonic spasms. Although he was treated with phenobarbital, valproic acid, clobazam, perampanel, lamotrigine, and levetiracetam, seizures continued to occur daily.

He was referred to our epilepsy center at the age of 56 months. DQ was 31 on the Kyoto Scale of Psychological Development and he presented with left hemiparesis. Long-term video-EEG revealed left side dominant-tonic spasms and ictal attenuation in the right hemisphere with a frequency of 2–5/day. Brain MRI revealed right hemispheric atrophy and right hemispheric hypoperfusion with ASL (**Figures 1B,C**). At the age of 59 months, he underwent right hemispherotomy. He was free from any seizures up to 11 months after the surgery. The left hemiparesis worsened transiently after the surgery and then recovered to the presurgical level.

The histopathological examination with hematoxylin-eosin staining revealed an excessive number of neurons and glia cells in the white matter with intact cortical architecture and absence of aberrant cells, corresponding to FCD type IIId, in the cerebral tissues of the tip of the right temporal lobe (**Supplementary Figures 1C,D**) and adjacent to the right hippocampus. No changes were observed in the right amygdala and hippocampus.

Case 3

A 17-month-old boy with a healthy clinical history presented with left-sided status of clonic convulsion lasting 60 min. Human herpesvirus 6 was isolated from his pharynx. He was treated with methylprednisolone pulse therapy and continuous intravenous midazolam. Three days following onset, cortical-subcortical restricted diffusivity was observed on the left temporo-parieto-occipital lobes in brain DWI. Following the acute phase, he continuously developed focal seizures accompanied by impaired consciousness and cyanosis. Despite treatment with valproic acid, clobazam, lamotrigine, perampanel, topiramate, and levetiracetam, daily focal seizures accompanied by mouthing, grimacing or expressions of fear continued to occur. Two months following onset, brain MRI revealed left hemispheric atrophy.

He was referred to our epilepsy center at the age of 56 months. He was not paralyzed but was barely able to speak. DQ was 34 on the Kyoto Scale of Psychological Development. Long-term video-EEG monitoring revealed that the focal impaired awareness seizures coincided with ictal EEG activities from the left frontal and occipital areas, which sometimes evolved into asymmetrical tonic seizures (extensions of left extremities and flexion of right extremities). Left hemispheric atrophy was observed in brain MRI. At the age of 60 months, he underwent left subtotal hemispherotomy (hemispherotomy sparing the pyramidal tract). He was free from seizures up to the last follow-up 10 months after surgery.

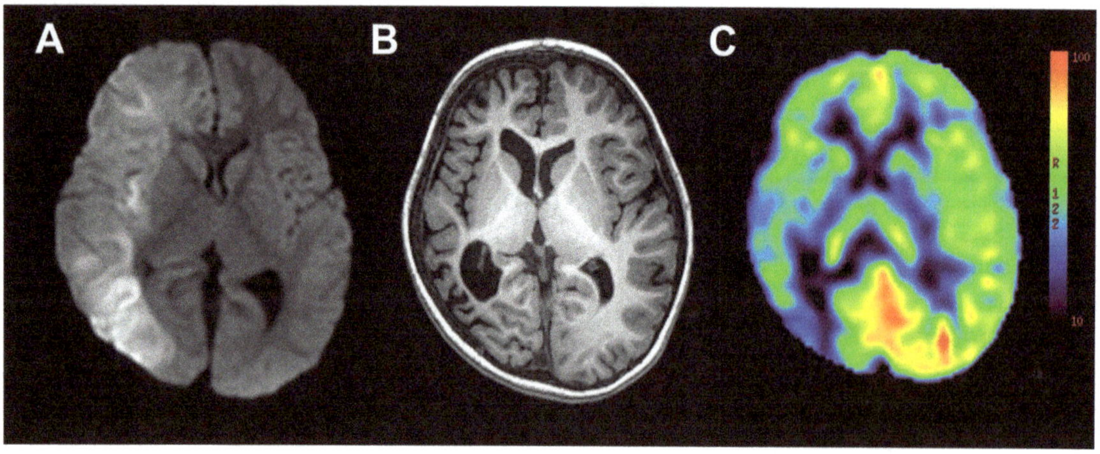

FIGURE 1 | Representative magnetic resonance images from case 2. **(A)** Diffusion weighted imaging at day 5 following onset of left-sided convulsion revealed high signals in subcortical areas in the right hemisphere. **(B)** T1-weighted imaging 2 years following onset revealed right hemispheric atrophy. **(C)** Arterial spin labeling at the same time revealed hypoperfusion in the right hemisphere.

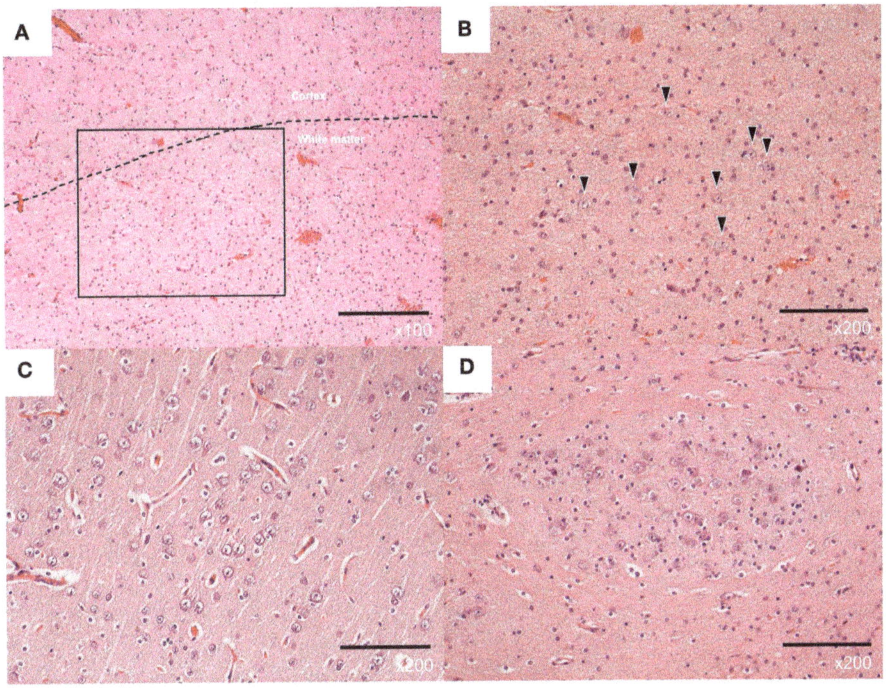

FIGURE 2 | Representative pathological findings with hematoxylin-eosin staining of the left lateral temporal lobe **(A–C)** and left amygdala **(D)** from case 3. **(A)** Normal architecture of cortical and subcortical white matter (×100). **(B)** Excessive number of neurons in the white matter (×200, arrowheads). **(C)** Neurons with increased nuclear/cytoplasmic ratio in the cortex (×200). **(D)** Clustered immature neurons (×200).

The histopathological examination with hematoxylin-eosin staining revealed immature-like neurons with large nuclei in the cerebral cortex of the tip of the left temporal lobe (**Supplementary Figure 2B**). An excessive number of neurons and glial cells was observed in the white matter of the same region, corresponding to FCD type IIId (**Figures 2A–C**). Clustering of immature-like neurons was observed in the left amygdala (**Figure 2D**) and gliosis was observed in the right hippocampus.

Procedures of Hemispherotomy

We performed the hemispherotomies using a standard peri-insula approach, which disconnected the association and commissural fibers in one hemisphere and interrupted the radiation fibers. Medial temporal structures, including the hippocampus and amygdala, were resected, along with the circular sulcus, except in case 3. In case 3, we performed posterior quadrant disconnection, with frontal lobe disconnection preserving the pyramidal tract to secure fine finger motor movement, such as pincer movement.

DISCUSSION

We reported 3 cases of HHES following virus infection associated-acute encephalopathy. Patients suffered from intractable seizures in chronic periods, which were completely resolved by functional hemispherotomy. The histopathological examinations revealed FCD type IIId in the cortices of all cases. One case presented additional aberrant neurons in the neocortex and amygdala.

Some etiologies have been described as the cause of HHES. Viral infections, including human herpesvirus 7, varicella zoster virus, and other viruses, have been reported as the trigger of HHES (7, 8). Genetic background has also been reported. Mutations in *SCN1A* and *CACNA1A*, the causative genes of Dravet syndrome or febrile seizures and familial paralytic migraine headache, respectively, have been reported in HHES patients. The excessive epileptic excitability of the cortex conferred by these mutations may also contribute to the development of HHES (9, 10). However, why the excitation and damage occur only in unilateral hemisphere remains unexplained.

There are only a few reports of pathological investigations regarding HHES. Mori reported neuropathological studies of 17 HHES patients who underwent hemispherectomy (2, 3). One patient had polymicrogyria in the left sylvian fissure and another presented non-specific findings of diffuse cortical scarring in the laminae and demyelination of the white substance. Auvin et al. (4) reported post-mortem specimens without any cell death in the cerebrum as a result of prolonged seizures. The last report was the biopsy case of the right temporal cortex in a patient with HHES in need of decompressive craniectomy. The histopathological examination revealed reduced granular cells in diffuse spongiosis and edema without cell necrosis in the cortical tissue (5). Thus, previous reports indicate no specific pathological findings, other than the case of polymicrogyria.

On the other hand, all our cases showed FCD type IIId. FCD type IIId is observed in the cortical tissues in resective surgical cases of intractable epilepsy and Rasmussen encephalitis, and the aberrant structure has the potential to induce seizures (11, 12).

Our cases indicate that the fever associated with the viral infections triggered the seizures in the hemisphere with FCD type IIId and induced epileptic excitotoxicity. Epileptic excitotoxicity during infant to early childhood can result in cytotoxic edema as observed by DWI and secondary atrophic changes (13). The mild cortical malformation and additional episodes of neuroexcitation may be one of the main causes of HHES. The lack of reporting of these findings in the previous study might be due to the recent establishment of the classification and lack of recognition.

Hemispheric cortical malformation with epileptic excitability has been reported to be caused by somatic mutations related to cortical dysplasia in the affected hemisphere (14). Our cases suggest that somatic mutations related to FCD might increase the susceptibility of developing virus infection associated-acute encephalopathy in the unilateral hemisphere that result in hemispheric involvement. More genetic investigations and pathological cases are necessary to clarify the correlation between mild cortical malformation and emergence of HHES.

In conclusion, we reported 3 cases of HHES likely caused by FCD type IIId in the affected hemisphere.

AUTHOR CONTRIBUTIONS

SI, TO, HE, and AF contributed to conceptualizing, drafting, and revising the study. YA and YO contributed to analyzing and interpreting the pathological examinations. MN, SI, TO, and SB contributed to the interpretation of EEG data. SI, TO, SB, NIc, YH, NIs, TH, HI, and TF contributed to acquiring and the interpreting the clinical information and MRI data.

ACKNOWLEDGMENTS

We are thankful Dr. Akiyoshi Kakita who gave us the comments that the pathological findings in case 1 and 2 remain a matter of debate. This report is not supported by any funding.

REFERENCES

1. Gastaut H, Poirier F, Payan H, Salamon G, Toga M, Vigouroux M. H.H.E. syndrome; hemiconvulsions, hemiplegia, epilepsy. *Epilepsia.* (1960) 1:418–47. doi: 10.1111/j.1528-1157.1959.tb04278.x
2. Mori Y. Anatomopathology and pathogeny of the hemiconvulsion-hemiplegia-epilepsy syndrome. Part II. *J Neurology Sci.* (1978) 22:17–28.
3. Mori Y. Anatomopathology and pathogeny of the hemiconvulsion-hemiplegia-epilepsy syndrome. Part I. *J Neurology Sci.* (1979) 23:1–22.
4. Auvin S, Devisme L, Maurage CA, Soto-Ares G, Cuisset JM, Leclerc F, et al. Neuropathological and MRI findings in an acute presentation of hemiconvulsion-hemiplegia: a report with pathophysiological implications. *Seizure.* (2007) 16:371–6. doi: 10.1016/j.seizure.2007.01.009
5. Berhouma M, Chekili R, Brini I, Kchir N, Jemel H, Bousnina S, et al. Decompressive hemicraniectomy in a space-occupying presentation of hemiconvulsion-hemiplegia-epilepsy syndrome. *Clin Neurol Neurosurg.* (2007) 109:914–7. doi: 10.1016/j.clineuro.2007.07.027
6. Blümcke I, Thom M, Aronica E, Armstrong DD, Vinters HV, Palmini A, et al. The clinico-pathological spectrum of Focal Cortical Dysplasias: a consensus classification proposed by an *ad hoc* Task Force of the ILAE diagnostic methods commission. *Epilepsia.* (2011) 52:158–74. doi: 10.1111/j.1528-1167.2010.02777.x
7. Kawada J, Kimura H, Yoshikawa T, Ihira M, Okumura A, Morishima T, et al. Hemiconvulsion-hemiplegia syndrome and primary human herpesvirus 7 infection. *Brain Dev.* (2004) 26:412–4. doi: 10.1016/j.braindev.2003.12.003
8. Wakamoto H, Ohta M, Nakano N. Hypercytokinemia in hemiconvulsions-hemiplegia syndrome associated with dual infection with varicella zoster and Epstein-Barr viruses. *Neuropediatrics.* (2002) 33:262–5. doi: 10.1055/s-2002-36736
9. Sakakibara T, Nakagawa E, Saito Y, Sakuma H, Komaki H, Sugai K, et al. Hemiconvulsion-hemiplegia syndrome in a patient with severe myoclonic epilepsy in infancy. *Epilepsia.* (2009) 50:2158–62. doi: 10.1111/j.1528-1167.2009.02175.x
10. Yamazaki S, Ikeno K, Abe T, Tohyama J, Adachi Y. Hemiconvulsion-hemiplegia-epilepsy syndrome associated with CACNA1A S218L mutation. *Pediatr Neurol.* (2011) 45:193–6. doi: 10.1016/j.pediatrneurol.2011.04.010
11. Garganis K, Kokkinos V, Zountsas B. Surgical outcome in neocortical resections of type IIId focal cortical dysplasia with accompanying medial temporal pathology. *Epilepsy Behav Case Rep.* (2012) 1:29–31. doi: 10.1016/j.ebcr.2012.11.002
12. Wang D, Blümcke I, Gui Q, Zhou W, Zuo H, Lin J, et al. Clinico-pathological investigations of Rasmussen encephalitis suggest multifocal disease progression and associated focal cortical dysplasia. *Epileptic Disord.* (2013) 1:32–43. doi: 10.1684/epd.2013.0555
13. Takanashi J, Oba H, Barkovich AJ, Tada H, Tanabe Y, Yamanouchi H, et al. Diffusion MRI abnormalities after prolonged febrile seizures with encephalopathy. *Neurology.* (2006) 66:1304–9. doi: 10.1212/01.wnl.0000210487.36667.a5
14. Lee JH, Huynh M, Silhavy JL, Kim S, Dixon-Salazar T, Heiberg A, et al. *De novo* somatic mutations in components of the PI3K-AKT3-mTOR pathway cause hemimegalencephaly. *Nat Genet.* (2012) 44:941–5. doi: 10.1038/ng.2329

28

KCNQ2-Related Neonatal Epilepsy Treated with Vitamin B6: A Report of Two Cases and Literature Review

Greta Amore[1], Ambra Butera[1], Giulia Spoto[1], Giulia Valentini[1], Maria Concetta Saia[1], Vincenzo Salpietro[2,3,4], Francesco Calì[5], Gabriella Di Rosa[1] and Antonio Gennaro Nicotera[1]*

[1] Department of Human Pathology of the Adult and Developmental Age "Gaetano Barresi", Unit of Child Neurology and Psychiatry, University of Messina, Messina, Italy, [2] Department of Neuromuscular Disorders, Institute of Neurology, University College London, London, United Kingdom, [3] Pediatric Neurology and Muscular Diseases Unit, Scientific Institute for Research, Hospitalization and Healthcare (IRCCS) Istituto Giannina Gaslini, Genoa, Italy, [4] Department of Neurosciences, Rehabilitation, Ophthalmology, Genetics, Maternal and Child Health, University of Genoa, Genoa, Italy, [5] Oasi Research Institute-Scientific Institute for Research, Hospitalization and Healthcare (IRCCS), Troina, Italy

***Correspondence:**
Vincenzo Salpietro
v.salpietro@ucl.ac.uk

Potassium Voltage-Gated Channel Subfamily Q Member 2 (KCNQ2) gene has been initially associated with "Benign familial neonatal epilepsy" (BFNE). Amounting evidence arising by next-generation sequencing techniques have led to the definition of new phenotypes, such as neonatal epileptic encephalopathy (NEE), expanding the spectrum of KCNQ2-related epilepsies. Pyridoxine (PN) dependent epilepsies (PDE) are a heterogeneous group of autosomal recessive disorders associated with neonatal-onset seizures responsive to treatment with vitamin B6 (VitB6). Few cases of neonatal seizures due to KCNQ2 pathogenic variants have been reported as successfully responding to VitB6. We reported two cases of KCNQ2-related neonatal epilepsies involving a 5-year-old male with a paternally inherited heterozygous mutation (*c.1639C>T*; p.Arg547Trp), and a 10-year-old female with a *de novo* heterozygous mutation (*c.740C>T*; p.Ser247Leu). Both children benefited from VitB6 treatment. Although the mechanisms explaining the efficacy of VitB6 in such patients remain unclear, this treatment option in neonatal-onset seizures is easily taken into account in Neonatal Intensive Care Units (NICUs). Further studies should be conducted to better define clinical guidelines and treatment protocols.

Keywords: KCNQ2, neonatal epilepsy, vitamin B6, pyridoxine, pyridoxal 5 phosphate, pyridoxine-dependent epilepsy (PDE), pyridoxine-responsive epilepsy

INTRODUCTION

Potassium Voltage-Gated Channel Subfamily Q Member 2 (KCNQ2) gene, first described by Singh et al. (1), is located on chromosome 20q13.3 and encodes for the voltage-gated potassium channel subunit Kv7.2. It has been traditionally related to "Benign familial neonatal epilepsy" (BFNE). This clinical entity often occurs within the first 2 weeks of life and is characterized by tonic/clonic early-onset seizures with apneic episodes and autonomic manifestations. Generally, it presents a self-limiting course for weeks/months with a regular neurodevelopmental outcome (2–4).

Amounting evidence arising from innovative genetic testing, and particularly next-generation sequencing (NGS) techniques, has revealed that different pathogenic variants of the same gene are responsible for several epileptic phenotypes; in particular, KCNQ2-related neonatal epileptic encephalopathy (NEE) contributed to expanding the spectrum of KCNQ2-related epilepsies (5). This is a severe phenotype, with an onset during the first days of life of intractable seizures (usually focal tonic), variably evolving into seizure freedom or a worsening/relapsing of the epileptic attacks over time, and an inevitable, though variable, adverse neurodevelopmental outcome (4–6). The electroencephalogram (EEG) may show a burst-suppression pattern or multifocal epileptiform abnormalities with background attenuation. This phenotype is mostly due to *de novo* missense variants of KCNQ2 causing a dominant-negative effect leading to a loss or a reduction of the M-current (a slow activating non-inactivating potassium current modulating the resting membrane potential) and less commonly to a gain of function effect, but not to a loss of function (haplo-insufficiency) (4, 7–9).

First described by Hunt et al. (10), pyridoxine (PN) dependent epilepsies (PDE) are a heterogeneous group of autosomal recessive disorders associated with neonatal-onset seizures not well-controlled with anti-epileptic drugs (AEDs) but responsive to large daily doses of vitamin B6 (VitB6) (11). PDE are caused by inborn errors of PN metabolism, usually due to pathogenic variants of ALDH7A1 gene (antiquitin). ALDH7A1 encodes for the alpha-aminoadipic semialdehyde (a-AASA) dehydrogenase, a key enzyme in the lysine metabolism, eventually implicated in the activation of VitB6 (12). Moreover, pyridoxamine5'-phosphate oxidase (PNPO) and pyridoxal 5′-phosphate binding protein (PLPBP) genes [both involved in the homeostasis of the active form of PN, namely pyridoxal 5′-phosphate (PLP)], have recently been related to variants of PDE more responsive to PLP than PN (13, 14).

The phenotypic spectrum associated with ALDHE mutation include: (1) Classic PDE-ALDH7A1 (with a dramatic early onset of prolonged or recurrent seizures of different types); (2) Atypical PDE-ALDH7A1 (including a late-onset, or seizures initially responding only to AEDs and eventually controllable only with PN/PLP several months later, or folic acid-responsive seizures, anyhow associated with variable degree of neurocognitive outcomes) (15). Clinical diagnosis is based on the demonstration of seizures ceasing after PN treatment, even after the elimination of all AEDs, and re-occurrence after its withdrawal (11, 16).

In addition to genetic testing, elevated levels of a-AASA in plasma and urine, and of pipecolic acid in plasma, urine and cerebrospinal fluid (CSF), as well as a high plasma-to-CSF PLP ratio, can be suggestive for VitB6 disorders (17, 18). However, a clear interpretation of these results is complicated; in fact, to date, no studies on CSF PLP levels in healthy newborns or infants are available, hence reference ranges derive from neurologically abnormal children undergoing CSF metabolite measurement for diagnostic workup (18).

Interestingly, PN and PLP have been proven to be effective in several early-onset seizures, not meeting the diagnosis of PDE, but instead falling within the category of "Pyridoxine-responsive epilepsy" (PRE) (19).

In this regard, they have been increasingly used in the clinical practice as add-on treatments in early-onset epilepsies, and it should be noted that few reports are today available specifically on KCNQ2-related neonatal epilepsies trialed with VitB6 (either in its inactive or active form) with variable outcomes (**Table 1**). Herein, we reported two new cases of KCNQ2-related neonatal epilepsy who benefited from VitB6 treatment.

CASE REPORTS

Case 1

A 6-year-old Caucasian boy was born at term by eutocic vaginal delivery from an uneventful pregnancy. Birth weight was 2,870 gr. Perinatal period was unremarkable and physical examination at birth normal. He was the second child of healthy related parents with common ancestors. The patient's family history was positive for epilepsy both in the maternal and paternal line; in particular, the father was diagnosed with a KCNQ2-related-epilepsy treated with Valproate (VPA) and Phenobarbital (Pb). It is to note that the father referred this data only at the end of our patient's genetic investigation.

On the second day of life, the patient presented clonic seizures at the limbs. The episodes resolved spontaneously. On the fourth day, he was hospitalized for the re-occurrence of seizures associated with perioral cyanosis. An electroencephalogram (EEG) showed polyspike wave complexes. Given the persistence of continuous clonic seizures, associated with perioral cyanosis, revolving eyes and buccal automatisms (sucking), midazolam by continuous intravenous infusion and intravenous boluses of Pb were administered. Brain magnetic resonance imaging (MRI) was normal. On the 10th day of life, oral Pb treatment was started, with seizure control for almost 3 months. Meanwhile, metabolic tests and the sequencing of KCNQ2 gene were performed.

At 3 months of life, recurrent convulsive seizures/status epilepticus occurred; thus, VPA was started at 10 mg/kg/bid, with subsequent titration up to 30 mg/kg/bid with transient remission of seizures. About a month later, focal clonic seizures at the limbs appeared, mainly with deviation of the eyes and cyanosis, lasting 60 s. An EEG showed "slight abnormalities of electrical brain activity in the left posterior areas." Further brain MRI scans were normal. Given the age of the patient and the partial response to stabilized treatment with VPA (100 mg/bid) and intravenous Pb (7.5 mg/bid), we decided to start PN supplementation as an intramuscular formulation of the vitamin B complex, containing 100 mg/day of PN. Seizure cessation and disappearance of the EEG abnormalities were gained after few days of treatment. Maintenance treatment was carried on, in agreement with the patient's parents (who were hesitant about PN withdrawal, as initially planned), with an oral formulation of multivitamin B complex at a very low dosage of 5 ml/day, equivalent to 0.45 mg of PN, with a seizure-free interval of about a month. In the meanwhile, a Developmental Quotient (DQ) of 70 was measured by using the Brunet-Lezine developmental scale, detecting a neurodevelopmental delay. The next month, in concomitance to an infectious episode, he presented with a further epileptic seizure characterized by clonic movements of the limbs, revolving eyes, perioral cyanosis, lasting about 60 s and resolving spontaneously. Antiepileptic treatment was unchanged. No further seizures occurred thereafter, either during infectious episodes.

TABLE 1 | Patients described in the literature who carry a KCNQ2 mutation and have been trialed with vitamin B6.

References	Patient	Phenotype	Mutation	Sex	Perinatal and early history	Seizure onset	Seizure features	AEDs administered (response)	Type of vitamin B6/Response	EEG	Neuroimaging	Seizure and clinical outcome	Additional information
Our patients	1	Pyridoxine responsive epilepsy	c.1639C>Tp.Arg547Trp Paternally inherited heterozygous mutation	M	Normal	2 d	Clonic szs, perioral cyanosis, revolving eyes and buccal automatisms	MDL (acutely effective) PB, VPA (partially effective)	PN i.m.100 mg/d (later switched to oral maintenance therapy)/ Successful electro-clinical response	Initial EEG: Abnormal After PN initiation: Normal	MRI (4 d and 4 mo): Normal	Sz-free after PN start Today (6 ys): still sz-free; global DD; mild autism-like features	ALDH7A1 sequencing: negative. No further genetic testing was performed
	2	Pyridoxine responsive epilepsy	c.740C>Tp.Ser247Leu *De novo* heterozygous mutation in exon 5	F	Normal	2 d	Myoclonic szs with rolling eye movements	PB (acutely ineffective), Several AEDS at onset (ineffective), VGB, FA (in addition to PLP—effective), CBZ (maintenance therapy)	PN/ Unsuccessful PLP (start at 36 d, p.o. 500 mg/d in 4–6 doses)/Immediate sz control up to 18 mo	Initial EEG: Abnormal After PN initiation: Abnormal	MRI (2 d): Normal	Sz-freedom for 18 mo (after PLP start at 36 d) Today (10 ys): discrete sz-control	ALDH7A1 and PNPO sequencing: normal
Millichap et al. (20)	3	EOEE	c.1009G>A p.Ala337Thr	NR	NR	5 mo	NR	LEV, CBZ, CLB, CLZ, F_B, PB, VPA (NR) EZO (szs began to decrease by the second week on 13 mg/kg/d)	PN/ Unsuccessful	Initial EEG: Abnormal After EZO initiation: Normal	NR	Sz decrease after EZO initiation Abnormal development	Sz proved refractory to multiple AEDs and PN as well
Sands et al. (21)	4–5 (twins)	BFNE	c.1057C>G p.Arg353Gl	F	Born at 34 wks	2 d	Focal asymmetric tonic posturing, associated with apnea and desaturation	PB i.v. 40 mg/kg, CLN p.o., DZP i.v. (NR) CBZ p.o. 10 mg/kg/day (effective)	PN i.v.100 mg/ Unsuccessful	EEG (patient 4): Normal EEG (patient 5): Abnormal	MRI: Normal	Both sz-free off meds at 16 ys Normal development	Family history positive for neonatal szs
Mulkey et al. (22)	6	NEE	c.601C>T p.R201C	NR	Normal	1 d	Exaggerated and sustained startle reaction to touch	EZO, VGB, CLZ, FA (NR)	PN, PLP/ NR	Initial and 1 mo EEG: Abnormal	MRI (1 wk and 3 mo): Abnormal	Sz outcome NR Profound DD Died at 13 mo for cardio-pulmonary arrest	Early neurologic exam: Abnormal
	7	NEE	c.601C>T p.R201C	NR	Normal	1 d	Exaggerated and sustained startle reaction to noise/touch, apnea Infantile spasms at 4 mo	EZO, VGB, PB, VPA, PHT, FA, TPM, LEV, ZNS, LOC, CBZ, STM, KD, CBD enriched cannabis (NR)	PN, PLP/ NR	Initial and 1 mo EEG: Abnormal	MRI (1 wk): Abnormal	Sz outcome NR Profound DD	Early neurologic exam: Abnormal
	8	NEE	c.601C>T p.R201C	NR	Normal	2 d	Stiffening events	VGB, PB, TPM, ACTH, KD, LEV, CLZ, FA (NR)	PN, PLP/NR	Initial and 1 mo EEG: Abnormal	MRI (1 wk): Normal MRI (1 y): Signal anomalies	Sz outcome NR Profound DD	Early neurologic exam: Abnormal
	9	NEE	c.601C>T p.R201C	NR	Born at term: bradycardia prior to delivery via caesarian section	1 d	Exaggerated startle response, apnea	EZO, VGB, CBZ, CLZ, PB, FA, PHT (NR)	PLP/NR	Initial and 1 mo EEG: Abnormal	MRI (2 and 4 mo): Abnormal	Sz outcome NR Profound DD Deceased	Early neurologic exam: Abnormal
	10	NEE	c.602G>A p.R201H	NR	Normal	1 d	Myoclonic spontaneous movements, exaggerated startle to noise/ touch Infantile Spasms at 2 months	VGB, CBZ, ZNS, PB, FA (NR)	PLP/NR	3 mo: Abnormal	MRI (3 mo): Abnormal	Sz outcome NR Profound DD	Early neurologic exam: Abnormal
Sharawat et al. (23)	11	NEE	c.835G >A p.Gly279Ser Likely pathogenic heterozygous Missense variant in exon 6	M	Normal	7 d	Repeated szs with up-rolling of eyeballs, generalized stiffening of body and cry	PB (sz-free for 3 months in combination with PN) CBZ 20 mg/kg/d (sz-free within a week)	PN started at 15 mg/kg/d, later increased to 50 mg/kg/d/Partial response	Initial EEG: Abnormal Repeat EEG: Normal	MRI (28 d): Normal	Sz-free at 3 mo (after PN start) 5 mo: re-occurrence of 1–2 sz/mo 1 y: re-occurrence of 8–10 sz/d Sz-free at last follow-up and mild global DD	Partial and temporary response to PN. Sz-freedom achieved with CBZ and PN together
Spagnoli et al. (24)	12	NEE	c.913_915del p.Phe305del *De novo*	M	Born full-term Apgar Score 3/10 Urgent cesarean section (cardio-tocographic abnormalities)	10 hs	10 hs: versive tonic spasms, ± flushing and desaturation ± focal clonic components	PB, PHT, LEV, MDL (ineffective) CBZ (sz-free)	PN, PLP/ Unsuccessful	Initial EEG: Abnormal After plural AEDS (9 mo): Abnormal	MRI (1 d): Minor abnormalities	Sz-free at 9 mo (after CBZ start) Severe DD; Spastic-dystonic tetraplegia	The patient was trialed with FA as well, unsuccessfully
Vilan et al. (25)	13	BFNE	c.1076C>A p.Thr359Lys Maternally inherited	F	Normal	1 d	Tonic with cyanosis	PB, CZP, PHT, VPA (NR) Lidocaine (partially effective)	PN/ Unsuccessful	Ictal aEEG: Abnormal Interictal: Normal	MRI: Normal	Sz-free at 1.5 mo Recurrence of frequent Sz after 4 years; Mild ID, ADHD (13 y)	Pyridoxine was administered to 8 infants without any beneficial effect. All infants needed ≥2 AEDs to control their szs

(Continued)

TABLE 1 | Continued

References	Patient	Phenotype	Mutation	Sex	Perinatal and early history	Seizure onset	Seizure features	AEDs administered (response)	Type of vitamin B6/Response	EEG	Neuroimaging	Seizure and clinical outcome	Additional information
	14	NR	c.1955dupC p.Pro652fs *De novo*	M	Normal	2 d	Tonic with cyanosis	PB, MDL, CZP (NR) Lidocaine (partially effective)	PN/Unsuccessful	Ictal aEEG: Abnormal Interictal: Normal	MRI: Normal	Sz-free at 21 d Recurrence of 2 Sz at 4 ys. Mild delay in MD (5 ys)	
	15	NR	c.1065C>G p.Asp355Glu *De novo*	M	Normal	2 d	Tonic with cyanosis	PB, MDL (NR) Lidocaine (acutely effective) PHT (effective)	PN/Unsuccessful	Ictal aEEG: Abnormal Interictal: Normal	MRI: Normal	Sz-free at 12 d Normal outcome (2 ys)	
	16	NR	c.2296delC p.Leu766fs *De novo*	M	Normal	3 d	Tonic with cyanosis	PB, MDL (NR) Lidocaine (partially effective)	PN/Unsuccessful	Ictal aEEG: Normal Interictal: Discontinuous normal voltage	MRI: Normal	Sz-free at 14 d Further outcome: NR	
	17	NR	c.1527delA p.Glu509fs *De novo*	M	Normal	24 d	Tonic with cyanosis	PB (not effective)	PN/Unsuccessful	Ictal aEEG: Abnormal Interictal: Normal	MRI: Normal	Sz-free at 14 d Further outcome: NR	
	18	NEE	c.830C>T p.Thr277Ile *De novo*	M	Normal	2 d	Tonic with cyanosis followed by focal clonic activity	PB, MDL, CZP, TPM (NR) LEV and lidocaine (acutely effective) VPA (effective)	PN/Unsuccessful	Ictal aEEG: Abnormal Interictal: Discontinuous normal voltage	MRI: Normal	Sz-free at 1.5 mo Non-verbal, autistic features, delay in MD (3 ys)	
	19	NR	c.1657C>T p.Arg553Trp *De novo*	F	Normal	1 d	Tonic with cyanosis followed by focal clonic activity	PB, LEV, MDL (NR) CBZ (effective)	PN/Unsuccessful	Ictal aEEG: Abnormal Interictal: Normal	MRI: Normal	Sz-free at 15 d Normal outcome (16 mo)	
	20	NEE	c.901G>A p.Gly301Ser *De novo*	F	Normal	1 d	Tonic with cyanosis	PB, MDL, LEV (NR) Lidocaine (acutely effective) CBZ (effective)	PN/Unsuccessful	Ictal aEEG: Abnormal Interictal: Normal	MRI: Signal anomalies	Sz-free at 15 d	
Pisano et al. (26)	21–32	NEE	12 patients were trialed with adequate dose of pyridoxine, 7 received pyridoxal-phosphate. At the onset, all patients showed axial hypotonia. During follow-up, cognitive impairment										
Klotz et al. (27)	33	NEE	c.1023G>C p.Gln341His *De novo*	F	Born at term but SGA	7–8 d	Tonic with cyanosis.	PB, LEV (partially effective, in combination with PN)	PN trial: 30 mg/kg over 3 d/ No immediate effect on sz frequency or EEG Consequent PLP trial: 30 mg/kg/Improvement of sz frequency shortly after its start (in combination with PB and LEV)	Initial EEG: Abnormal Last EEG (date NR): Abnormal	MRI: Normal	Sz reduction (once-twice every few wks) Neuro-cognitive sequelae: abnormal MD and DD	No detected mutations in ALDH7A1 or PNPO After PLP discontinuation: re-occurrence of 20 szs/d After PLP reintroduction seizures resolved Further switch to PN: no change in seizure frequency
Reid et al. (18)	34	NEE?	c.629G>A p.Arg210His *De novo*	F	Born at 38 wks + 6 by spontaneous labor, after an uneventful pregnancy	4 d	Episodes of choking and cyanosis, associated with stiffening after which she became floppy; "cycling" movements of arms; desaturation	PB, LZP (not effective) PHT, CBZ (partially effective in combination with PN)	PN, PLP/Successful 2 mo: sz control after 6 d of 0.25 mg of PN (oral drops), at a time when she was also receiving 6.7 mg/kg/day of PHT and 11 mg/kg/day of CBZ	9 d: Abnormal 7 ys: Abnormal	MRI (28 d); Minor abnormalities	Sz outcome at 7 years: szs presenting only during intercurrent illness 7 y: DD with minimal expressive language	No mutations detected in ALDH7A1 or PNPO
Allen et al. (3)	35	BFNE	c.419_430dupp.Val143_Arg144insGlnTyrPheVal Maternally inherited (affected mother)	F	Normal	4 d	Clonic and tonic szs. Clusters multiple/day or days sz-free. Minor cyanosis subsequently, mainly tonic. Multiple/day, then weeks and months sz–free	LEV (some response, required dose increases) Other drugs used but ineffective: PB, MDZ, LZP	PLP (used acutely)/ NR	Initial EEG: Abnormal 3.5 mo: Normal	MRI (3 wks): Normal	Sz outcome: sporadic breakthrough minor szs Normal developmental outcome (1 y)	
Mefford et al. (16)	36	Pyridoxine-dependent epilepsy?	1.5 Mb terminal deletion of the long arm of chromosome 20	M	Precipitous after a 36 week pregnancy complicated by frequent Braxton-Hicks contractions.	2 wks	Reddening and tonic stiffening of arms, lasting approximately 1 min Initially sporadic but, by 8 wks of age, occurring 4–6/day	PB 15 mg/day (partial response)	PN 100 mg/d, later increased to 200 mg/d and eventually reduced to 150 mg/d/ Good electroclinical response (so that PB was discontinued at 11 months)	Initial EEG: Abnormal 5 ys: Abnormal	First MRI: Minor abnormalities MRI (11 mo): Normal	Sz-free (7 ys) ID and delay in MD	Sequencing of the ALDH7A1 gene did not detect mutations

(Continued)

TABLE 1 | Continued

References	Patient	Phenotype	Mutation	Sex	Perinatal and early history	Seizure onset	Seizure features	AEDs administered (response)	Type of vitamin B6/Response	EEG	Neuroimaging	Seizure and clinical outcome	Additional information
Weckhuysen et al. (5)	37	NEE	c.613A>G p.Ile205Val	M	During the last 2 months of pregnancy rhythmical jerking similar to szs Subsequent normal perinatal and early development	2 d	Generalized tonic with clonic components, lip smacking, back arching, and apnoea. Multiple szs daily	VGB (initially reduced szs and normalized EEG with 7 wks sz freedom) MDZ (partially effective) PB, FA, betamethasone, VPA (all ineffective) TPM, VGB (effective in combination with PN)	PN/The combination of TPM, VGB, and PN controlled szs	7 d: Abnormal 9 mo: Normal	CT scan (2 d) and MRI (11 d and 3.5 ys): Signal anomalies	Status epilepticus at 3 mo; Sz -free from 9 mo until 8 ys ID and delay in MD	
Borgatti et al. (28)	38	BFNE, epileptic encephalopathy and profound mental retardation?	c.1620G>A p.K526N Maternally inherited (Affected mother and two younger sisters)	F	Born at 40 wks by cesarean section due to podalic presentation	3 d	Clonic szs. Subsequently right sided clonic and tonic-clonic szs with oro-alimentary automatism	ACTH (partially effective) PB, VGB, benzodiazepines, PHT, VPA, CZP, immune-globulin (ineffective)	PN/NR	Initial ictal EEG: Abnormal Last EEG (date NR): Abnormal	MRI (around 4 mo): Abnormal	Not achieved complete sz control. Many polymorphic szs/d Severe spastic tetraparesis and profound ID	
Dedek et al. (29)	39	BNFE	p.Ser247Trp	M	Born by cesarean section due to prolonged delivery period and symptoms of fetal distress	3 d	Left or right head deviation, and upper and lower limb involvement	ACTH (effective) PB, PHT,VGB (ineffective)	PN /Unsuccessful	8 d: Normal 2.5 ys: Abnormal	CT (7 d): Normal MRI (41 d): Normal	Sz-free (szs stopped at 13 wks) Immediate improvement of EEG after ACTH initiation DD (2 ys and 5 mo)	
Martin et al. (30)	40	NEE (Ohtahara syndrome)	c.827C>T p.T276I	M	Born at 41 wks by emergency cesarean section due to failure to progress	1 d	Cyanotic episodes, then more obvious szs; tonic spasms	TPM, DZP, and NZP (fits initially continued, but at 5 months were less severe, ceasing by 17 months) CZP, VGB, FA (ineffective)	PLP/ Unsuccessful	1 d: Abnormal 4 ys: Abnormal	MRI: Abnormal	Sz-free Severe DD (4 ys)	
Numis et al. (31)	41	NEE	c.1734 G>Cp.Met578Ile	NR	Born at 34 wks. Lack of visual fixation, decreased spontaneous movements, and axial hypotonia	4 d	Tonic head, conjugate eye, mouth deviation, unilateral tonic abduction of the limbs. Apnoea and desaturation	CBZ (effective—sz free within 2 wks) PB, LEV, TPM, VGB, CLB, CZP, KD, FA (ineffective)	PN, PLP/ Unsuccessful	Interictal and Ictal EEG: Abnormal	MRI (20 and 33 d): Abnormal	Sz-free DD and delay in MD	
Saitsu et al. (32)	42	NEE (Ohtahara syndrome)	c.1010C>G p.A337G	M	NR	7 d	Tonic szs, vomiting. Complex partial szs since age 5	High dose PB (sz-free and burst-suppression disappeared) ZNS (ineffective)	PN/ Unsuccessful	Initial EEG: Abnormal	NR	Sz-free after high dose PB DD and delay in MD	
	43	NEE (Ohtahara syndrome)	c.341C>T p.T114I	F	NR	0 d	Tremor of the upper extremities then generalized convulsions with cyanosis Complex partial szs since age 5	ZNS (sz free) CZP, PHT (ineffective)	PN/ Unsuccessful	Initial EEG: Abnormal	NR	Sz-free after ZNS Profound DD and abnormal MD	
	44	NEE (Ohtahara syndrome)	c.794C>T p.A265V	M	NR	1 d	Apnoeic spell, then tonic spasms with right opsoclonus like movement.	ZNS, VPA, CZP, CBZ (ineffective)	PN/ Unsuccessful	Initial EEG: Abnormal	NR	Intractable szs DD Myoclonus at the bilateral upper extremities	
Kato et al. (7)	45	NEE (Ohtahara syndrome)	c.650C>Ap.Thr217Asn *De novo*	F	NR	0 d	At onset: Pale face for tens of seconds 1 d: Eye deviation to left followed by tonic szs (0.5–1/h)	High dose PB (sz-free) ZNS (ineffective)	PLP/ Unsuccessful	1 d: Abnormal	MRI (2 d, 1 and 6 mo): Signal anomalies MRI (2 ys): Normal	Sz-free after high dose of PB Profound DD and abnormal MD	
	46	NEE?	c.794C>T p.Ala265Val *De novo*	M	NR	2 d	At onset: Facial flushing and eye fixation 3 d: Tonic szs (daily)	DZP, MDL, high-dose PB (partially effective) VPA (ineffective) CBZ (successful)	PLP/ Unsuccessful	5 d:Abnormal	MRI (7 mo and 2 y): Abnormal	Sz-free after CBZ. No szs since 16 mo Moderate DD and abnormal MD	
	47	NEE (Ohtahara syndrome)	c.794C>T p.Ala265Val *De novo*	M	NR	2 d	At onset: No cry, poor suck, stiffening, and arching with eye rolling 5 d: left-sided szs	PB, CLB, MDZ, VGB (ineffective)	PLP/ Unsuccessful	5 d:Abnormal	MRI (0 mo): Normal	Intractable szs DD and abnormal MD Died at 3 mo	

(Continued)

TABLE 1 | Continued

References	Patient	Phenotype	Mutation	Sex	Perinatal and early history	Seizure onset	Seizure features	AEDs administered (response)	Type of vitamin B6/Response	EEG	Neuroimaging	Seizure and clinical outcome	Additional information
	48	NEE (Ohtahara syndrome)	c.854C>A p.Pro285His Maternally inherited	F	NR	0 d	At onset: poor feeding followed irritability with hypoxia and tonic szs (1–4/d).	VPA (sz-free) PB (ineffective)	PLP/ Unsuccessful	12 d:Abnormal	MRI (12 d and 3 mo): Signal anomalies	Sz-free after VPA (since 3 mo) DQ 35. Moderate DD and abnormal MD	
	49	NEE (Ohtahara syndrome)	c.881C>T p.Ala294Val *De novo* Domain in protein: Transmembrane domain (S4)	M	NR	1 w	Convulsion-like movements followed by asymmetric tonic szs	TPM (sz-free) ZNS, VPA (partially effective) CZP, PB (ineffective)	PLP/ Unsuccessful	<1 mo: Abnormal 3 mo: Abnormal	MRI (3 mo and 9 mo): Abnormal	Sz-free since 6 mo Profound DD and abnormal MD	
	50	NEE (Ohtahara syndrome)	c.997C>Tp.Arg333Trp *De novo* C-terminal region	M	NR	2 d	Tonic szs followed by partial ones (eyes rolling up)	ZNS (almost sz-free) VPA, lidocaine (partially effective) DZP, PB, PHT (partially effective)	PLP/ Unsuccessful	42 d:Abnormal	NR	Sz-free. Only one sz in 10 ys. Severe DD	
	51	NEE (Ohtahara syndrome)	c.1689C>Gp.Asp563Glu C-terminal region	F	NR	1 d	Poor feeding with cyanosis, followed by tonic szs, facial clonic sz, and generalized tonic-clonic convulsions	CBZ and CZP (sz-free) PHT, PB (partially effective) VPA, NZP (ineffective)	PLP/ Unsuccessful	4 d: Abnormal	CT (0 m): Normal	No szs since 10 y, but relapsed at 24 ys after a y of drug withdrawal Moderate DD with autistic features	
Milh et al. (6)	52–57	Six patients described that have been treated with vitamin B_6 during the first month of life. Responses to each AED not stated											

NR, not reported; BFNE, Benign familial neonatal epilepsy; EIEE, early infantile epileptic encephalopathy; EOEE, early onset epileptic encephalopathy; NEE, neonatal epileptic encephalopathy; F, female; M, male; IV, intravenous; P.O., per os; S, second(s); Mn, minute(s); H(s), hour(s); D, day/s; Wk(s), week(s); Mo, month(s); Y(s), year(s); CBZ, carbamazepine; CLB, clobazam; CF, calcium folinate; CLZ, clonazepam; EZO, ezogabine; FA, folinic acid; FLB, felbamate; KD, ketogenic diet; LEV, levetiracetam; LOC, lacosamide; LZP, lorazepam; MDL, midazolam; NZP, nitrazepam; PB, phenobarbital; PHT, phenytoin; PN, pyridoxine; PLP, pyridoxal 5′ phosphate; TPM, topiramate; STM, sulthiame; VB6, vitamin B6; VGB, Vigabatrin; VPA, valproic acid; ZNS, zonisamide; Sz(s), seizure(s); DD, developmental delay; ID, intellectual disability; MD, motor development.

Throughout the following years, VPA first, and Pb later, were discontinued. Today the child is seizure-free and takes daily multivitamin B complex, also containing PN. Despite the global neurodevelopmental delay, he is able to walk alone, jump and climb; his expressive language is limited to simple and short phrases and characterized by dyslalia, whereas the comprehension is adequate. The child presents mild autism-like features (such as self-stimulatory, repetitive and stereotyped behaviors, and relational difficulties). He has also gained sphincteric control.

Direct sequencing of the KCNQ2 (NM_172107.4; NP_742105.1) gene demonstrated a paternally inherited heterozygous mutation (c.1639C>T; p.Arg547Trp), leading to the replacement of Arginine with Tryptophan at position 547 of the protein and involving a conserved amino-acid of the protein predicted to have functional consequences on the protein (**Figure 1**). This variant had already been reported in the literature by Zara et al. (2) (as causative of a BFNE in a female patient with a maternal inheritance) and Lindy et al. (33) (no clinical data available). *In silico* analysis performed with bioinformatic tools predicted that mutation has a potential strong damaging effect on the structure/function of the KCNQ2 protein. ACMG standard criteria for assessment of pathogenicity of variants (Varsome) (34) should be considered as "Pathogenic" (**Table 2**).

In the case of our patient, ALDH7A1 sequencing was later reported to be negative, and no further genetic testing was performed. This data prevented us the possibility to explain his positive response to PN and his clinical phenotype (that, despite the clinical continuum existing between BFNE and NEE, seems closer to the NEE phenotype), in which a possible role of other genes on his impaired neurodevelopment cannot be ruled out.

Case 2

A 10-year-old Caucasian female was born at term by eutocic vaginal delivery from an uneventful pregnancy. Birth weight was 3,400 gr. Prenatal and perinatal history was unremarkable. On the second day of life, the baby showed myoclonic seizures associated with sudden loss of muscle tone and rolling eye movements. The patient started treatment with Pb, without effects. The EEG showed a suppression-burst pattern. Brain MRI and routine metabolic investigations resulted to be normal. At day 36 of life, after unsuccessful therapeutic attempts with Pb and VPA, and the start of PN administration, she was admitted to the NICU without considerable response. Herein, she was started on oral PLP therapy (up to a dose of 500 mg/day divided in 4–6 administrations), achieving immediate seizure control. An extended metabolic workup was performed highlighting an elevation of pipecolic acid both in serum and urine, albeit the sequencing of ALDH7A1 and PNPO genes was normal. Given the good clinical response to PLP and the poor neurodevelopment performance (no achievement of motor milestones, marked muscular hypotonia, and visual disturbances), she received a diagnosis of "Focal epilepsy with pyridoxal phosphate-responsive seizures and global neurodevelopmental delay."

Feature key	Position(s)	Description	Mutation	Graphical view
Topological domain	1 – 91	Cytoplasmic		
Transmembrane	92 – 112	Helical; Segment S1		
Topological domain	113 – 122	Extracellular		
Transmembrane	123 – 143	Helical; Segment S2		
Topological domain	144 – 166	Cytoplasmic		
Transmembrane	167 – 187	Helical; Segment S3		
Topological domain	188 – 195	Extracellular		
Transmembrane	196 – 218	Helical; Voltage-sensor; Segment S4		
Topological domain	219 – 231	Cytoplasmic		
Transmembrane	232 – 252	Helical; Segment S5	c.740C>T (p.S247L)	
Topological domain	253 – 264	Extracellular		
Intramembrane	265 – 285	Pore-forming; Segment H5		
Topological domain	286 – 291	Extracellular		
Transmembrane	292 – 312	Helical; Segment S6		
Topological domain	313 – 872	Cytoplasmic	c.1639C>T (p.R547W)	

FIGURE 1 | Functional domain position of p.R547W and p.S247L amino acid changes of KCNQ2 protein (adapted from https://www.uniprot.org). The figure shows the KCNQ2 functional domain position of the variants found in our two cases (p.R547W and p.S247L). *In silico* analysis (**Table 2**) predicted that the two mutations have potential strong damaging effect on the structure/function of the KCNQ2 protein.

TABLE 2 | *In silico* prediction of the KCNQ2 missense mutations*.

NM_172107.4 (NP_742105.1) (GRCh38)	c.1639C>T (p.R547W)	c.740C>T (p.S247L)
PolyPhen2 prediction: B (benign), P (possibly damaging), D (probably damaging)	D	Variable: P;P;B;B;B;B
SIFT prediction	Damaging	Damaging
LRT prediction	Deleterious	Neutral
MutationTaster prediction	Disease causing	Disease causing
MutationAssessor prediction	Medium impact	High impact
FATHMM	Damaging	Damaging
fathmm-MKL	Damaging	Damaging
M-CAP	Damaging	Damaging
CADD [the larger the score the more likely the SNP is damaging (PHRED-like)]	27.2	25.9
MetaSVM	Damaging	Damaging
MetaLR	Damaging	Damaging
PhyloP 20way the larger the score, the more conserved the site (max 1.199000)	−0.409000	0.982000
PhyloP 100way the larger the score, the more conserved the site (max 10.003000)	0.097000	6,62,8000
GERP RS the larger the score, the more conserved the site (max 6.17).	−1.15	3.25
1000 Genomes	No data	No data
gnomAD	No data	No data
Interpro domain	Potassium channel, voltage dependent, KCNQ, C-terminal	Ion transport domain
ClinVar interpretation	Pathogenic/Likely_pathogenic	Pathogenic/Likely_pathogenic
ACMG classification (Varsome**)	Pathogenic	Pathogenic

**Data from HGMD professional database [www.hgmd.cf.ac.uk; (35)].*
***Kopanos et al. (34).*

After 18 months of seizure-free interval, epileptic tonic spasms occurred, both during sleep and wakefulness. The EEG showed multifocal epileptic discharges.

Low CSF folic acid levels were revealed; hence, folic acid was started (7.5 mg/bid, later increased at 7.5 mg/tid), in add-on to her previous therapy, with benefits in terms of number and intensity of epileptic seizures.

Despite the overall discrete seizure control, subsequent interictal EEG recordings showed marked diffuse abnormalities up to a *quasi*-periodic epileptiform pattern. The patient showed severe global neurodevelopmental delay at the follow-up.

Further genetic testing was performed. Array-CGH was not informative. Whereas, trios NGS (epilepsy panel) revealed a *de novo* heterozygous mutation in Exon 5 of the KCNQ2 gene (NM_172107.4; NP_742105.1): c.740C>T/(p.Ser247Leu), affecting a highly conserved aminoacidic region and predicted to be deleterious *in silico* programs (**Figure 1**). However, using the standard procedures for assessment of pathogenicity of variants (ACMG criteria—Varsome) (34), should be considered as "Pathogenic" (**Table 2**). This variant has already been reported in the literature and related to early-onset epileptic phenotypes with a variable degree of neurocognitive impairment (36–41). However, none of these reports shows evidence of VitB6 supplementation. Our patient was maintained on Vigabatrin, PLP, and Folic acid for several years. By the age of 10 years, given the occurrence of severe behavioral and sleep disorders, PN, Folic acid, and Vigabatrin were withdrawn, and maintenance therapy with carbamazepine, in add-on to Lorazepam and Promazine, was started.

To date, the child failed to achieve trunk control, independent standing or walking. She shows axial hypotonia and limbs hypertonia. Language is limited to vocalizations and she presents severe intellectual disability. In addition, behavioral disturbances are evident, with aggressive manifestations and sleep disorders. She displays a good clinical control, with occurrence of rare seizures (one episode/1–2 years).

DISCUSSION

Herein, we reported two cases of KCNQ2-related epilepsy, a 5-year-old male with a paternally inherited heterozygous mutation (c.1639C>T; p.Arg547Trp), and a 10-year-old female with a *de novo* heterozygous mutation (c.740C>T; p.Ser247Leu), who benefited from PN treatment.

The first patient presented with neonatal epilepsy with an onset during the first week of life, which was later ascribed to a KCNQ2 pathogenic variant paternally inherited.

The same variant had already been described in the literature (2, 33) and reported as causative of a BFNE phenotype in a female patient with maternal inheritance (2).

Our patient, with his overall good seizure-responsivity despite impaired neurodevelopment, does not show all the typical characteristics of BFNE or NEE. Even if no evidence of an inborn error of VitB6 was available for our patient (ruling out the diagnosis of a PDE), his seizures, scarcely controlled by AEDs, revealed a good and immediate electro-clinical response to the initiation of intramuscular PN. Interestingly, this effect did not cease after switching to PN oral administration, neither after the discontinuation of AEDs, strengthening the diagnostic hypothesis of PN-responsive epilepsy (PRE).

The second patient, after a sudden and severe onset of neonatal seizures, requiring plural hospitalizations, and failed attempts with AEDs, such as Pb and VPA, and with PN too, demonstrated an immediate clinical benefit from the initiation of PLP, and, over time, to folic acid as well.

In this case, a *de novo* disease-causing KCNQ2 variant was detected (c.740C>T; p.Ser247Leu), and the good clinical response to PLP and folic acid were supported, respectively, by elevated levels of pipecolic acid both in serum and urine and by reduced CSF folates level. Moreover, genetic testing resulted negative for ALDH7A1 and PNPO pathological variants. These data supported the possibility to classify this clinical phenotype into the PRE spectrum.

Moreover, even though the clear effect of PLP reduced over time, other AEDs (i.e., Pb and VPA) proved to be ineffective, and the neurocognitive outcome of the patient is quite poor, she still presents an overall good clinical control, with seizures being years apart.

Summarizing, regardless of the several divergences between these 2 cases, both of them may fit into the category of PRE, particularly within the subgroup of KCNQ2-related ones.

Data from the literature have demonstrated the usefulness of VitB6, either as PN or, even better, as PLP, in certain types of neonatal-onset epilepsies (13, 19). In addition, recent reports have been unraveling a potential correlation between KCNQ2-related epilepsies and VitB6 responsiveness (18). To date, several cases of patients carrying a pathogenic variant of KCNQ2 trialed with VitB6 (either in the form of PN or PLP) have been reported in the literature. Unfortunately, the effects of VitB6 have not been accurately described for all of them. Additionally, several cases have been extracted from studies focusing on other than the KCNQ2-PN correlation, making it arduous to infer the exact impact of VitB6 on the clinical picture (6, 22, 26). Five reports have openly disclosed various degrees of a successful response to PN/PLP in KCNQ2-related epilepsies (5, 16, 18, 23, 27). Interestingly, despite their small number, all patients share a neuro-cognitive impairment in the lack of genetic data confirming/denying the PN-dependency/responsiveness, in line with ours. All cases are reported in **Table 1** (and detailed in the complete version of the table—see **Supplementary Material**).

Currently, the etiopathogenic mechanism underlying the PN responsiveness of certain neonatal seizures, and particularly of those KCNQ2-related, remains unclear. However, some hypotheses have been proposed [(18); **Figure 2**].

First of all, VitB6, particularly as PLP, is notably implicated as a cofactor of hundreds of enzymatic reactions, having a role in several functions, such as in the metabolism of amino-acids and the synthesis of neurotransmitters (42). In this regard, PLP is notably a cofactor of glutamic acid decarboxylase (GAD), an enzyme involved in the synthesis of gamma-amino butyric acid (GABA) from glutamate (GLUT). These two are, respectively, the key inhibitory and excitatory neurotransmitters of the CNS, and an imbalance between them has long been considered among the molecular mechanisms underlying epilepsy (43). The reduction of GABA deriving from low PLP levels has been proposed as a potential mechanism in the genesis of PDE, but it is

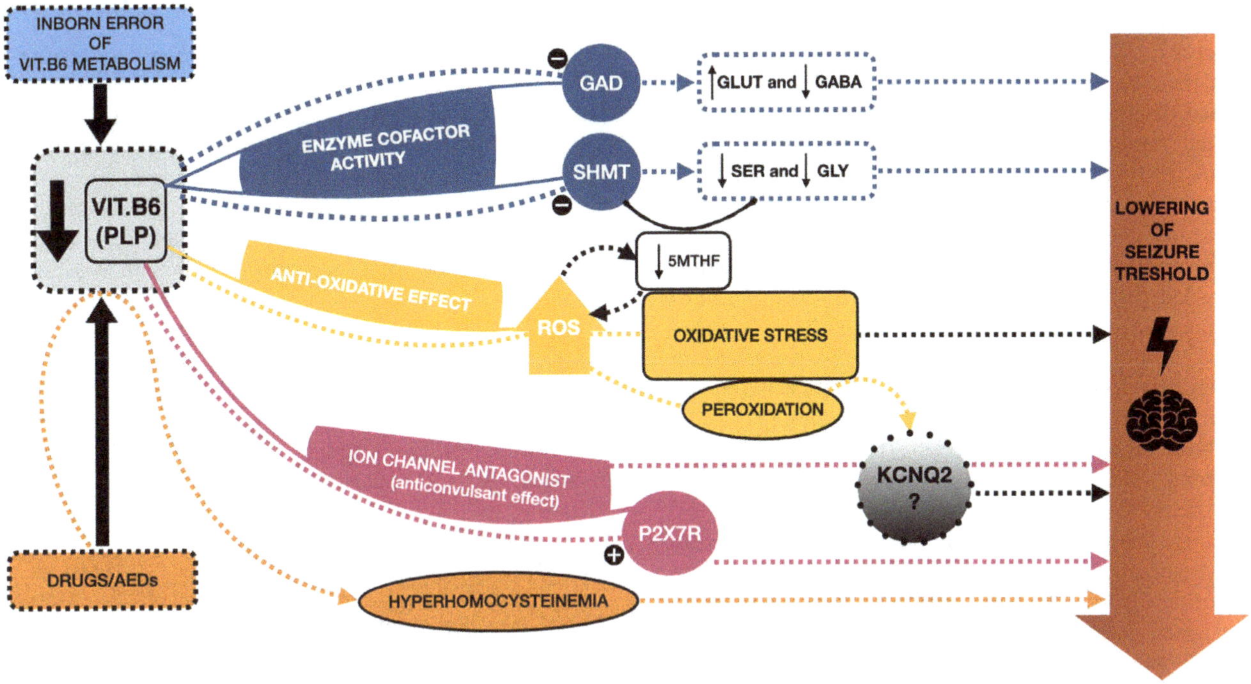

FIGURE 2 | Schematic representation of the mechanisms proposed to explain seizure responsiveness to vitamin B6 and the potential link with KCNQ2. Several etiopathogenic mechanisms have been proposed to explain the responsiveness of certain neonatal seizures to vitamin B6 (VitB6), and particularly to its active form, pyridoxal 5′ phosphate (PLP). PLP acts as a cofactor of several enzymes, such as Glutamic acid decarboxylase (GAD), regulating the synthesis of gamma-amino butyric acid (GABA) from Glutamate (GLUT). A reduction of PLP may determine an imbalance between these two (in favor of GLUT), hence decreasing the seizure threshold. PLP is also involved in the synthesis of serine (SER) and glycine (GLY), modulating the serine hydroxymethyltransferase (SHMT) activity; thus, a reduction of PLP may determine lower levels of these two amino-acids, whose reduction has been related to epileptic phenotypes. SHMT is involved in the metabolic pathway, eventually leading to the formation of the main circulating form of folates, the 5-methyltetrahydrofolate (5-mTHF), a reduction of which has been reported in some patients suffering from pyridoxine-dependent epilepsies (PDE). Furthermore, the reduction of 5-mTHF may fall into another proposed mechanism underlying epilepsy, namely oxidative stress, with excessive production of reactive oxygen species (ROS). This may be a consequence of low levels of VitB6 (anti-oxidative agent) and, at the same time, a cause of folates depletion. Additionally, ROS contribute to the peroxidation of several molecules, also affecting ion channels, hence potentially KCNQ2. PLP also acts as an antagonist of specific ion channels, as P2X7R, with a possible anticonvulsant effect, which could not occur when PLP levels are low. A similar antagonist action on KCNQ2, with possible analogous effects, has been proposed. Finally, some drugs, especially antiepileptic ones (AEDs), may be responsible for the depletion of VitB6 and, indirectly, hyperhomocysteinemia, which is known to lower the seizure threshold. Overall, these mechanisms may explain the responsiveness of some neonatal seizures to VitB6 treatment and help shed light on the potential link with KCNQ2-related epilepsies.

widespread among the authors the opinion that this cannot be the only one (43–45). Ramos et al. (45) have recently highlighted that conflicting data have been reported on GLUT and GABA levels in the CSF of patients suffering from VitB6 deficiency, supporting this hypothesis (45). In this regard, they carried out a study on a model system of VitB6-deficient Neuro-2a cells, revealing a significant reduction in the *de novo* synthesis of serine and, consequently, glycine, whose reduction has been related to epileptic phenotypes, suggesting a potential role of these two (45, 46).

Additionally, it is noteworthy to mention that glycine synthesis from serine depends on the enzyme serine hydroxymethyltransferase (SHMT), which requires PLP as a cofactor. SHMT is involved in the metabolic pathway which encompasses the enzyme methylenetetrahydrofolate reductase (MTHFR) as well, eventually leading to 5-methyltetrahydrofolate (5-mTHF) formation, the main circulating form of folate (45). This is particularly interesting since low levels of 5-mTHF in CSF have already been reported in our second patient and some PDE patients (18, 47).

In particular, the patient described by Reid et al. (18) and ours reported a positive response to VitB6 treatment, both in the presence of low folates and of different isolated lab findings suggestive for VitB6 disorders (respectively, a high plasma-to-CSF PLP ratio in the former, and an elevation of pipecolic acid both in serum and urine in the latter), though in the absence of a genetic confirmation of inborn errors of VitB6 metabolism. Although these findings cannot be fully explained, and no clear evidence on the topic is yet available, all this suggests not only a potential role of folates in PREs and PDEs, but also that there is much more to find out.

Besides, when it comes to folates, it is not possible to state whether their involvement in PDEs/PREs, and, in general, in epilepsy may be a causative factor, a consequence, or both. Their involvement in these conditions may be mutually related to another proposed mechanism underlying epilepsy, namely the excessive production of reactive oxygen species (ROS) (17, 18). Several studies have demonstrated an excessive ROS production in epilepsy, so they outgrow the capability of endogenous antioxidants to contrast their effect (43). Besides, the excess of ROS may determine a depletion of folates, which are known to exhibit antioxidant functions acting as ROS scavengers (18, 48).

Overall, high levels of ROS may have detrimental effects, including the peroxidation of structures and molecules (i.e., enzymes and components of cell membranes), potentially affecting ion channels indirectly as well (43). Moreover, given the demonstrated anti-oxidative effects of VitB6 (49) and the potential effect of ROS on ion channels, one could speculate that there may be a close, albeit yet unknown, relation between VitB6 and channelopathies, such as KCNQ2-related ones.

Anyhow, when ROS production is excessive, the result is a strong oxidative stress and an imbalance favoring the excitotoxicity (43).

Another possible mechanism may involve the recently demonstrated antagonist action of PLP toward P2X-receptors (and particularly the subtype P2X7R) (50). These receptors are a class of ligand-gated ion channels, activated by ATP, contributing to neuro- and glio-transmission and lately associated with epileptic conditions, such as status epilepticus (51). Since P2X7R antagonists have recently been reported as having anticonvulsant effects, this may apply as well to PLP, explaining at least partly its role in controlling seizures (52).

Given the above, Reid et al. (18) proposed that PLP may as well have a direct antagonist effect on ion channels, including the one encoded by KCNQ2. However, further evidence is needed to confirm this hypothesis.

Other potential mechanisms explaining PDE and PRE may relate to secondary defects of VitB6, for instance drug-induced ones. Several drugs, such as carbamazepine, phenytoin, and PB, may reduce VitB6 levels and indirectly lead to hyperhomocysteinemia (which is known to lower seizure threshold) (53, 54). It is likely that the same effect may apply to other AEDs and that it may partly explain the VitB6 responsiveness of certain patients, even when temporary. Unfortunately, it is not possible to confirm or deny this hypothesis for our patients.

Our study presents some limitations, such as its retrospective nature, with consequent possible information biases and lack of specific data (such as details about treatments and diagnostic assessment taking place in different centers from ours, or the correlation between AEDs modification and concomitant levels of VitB6 and homocysteine), as well as the small sample of patients, making it difficult to generalize our findings.

In the light of the above, further studies focusing on the correlation between types of AEDs used, treatment duration, concomitant plasma levels of VitB6, homocysteine and folates, and possibly considering the eventual disease-causing variants associated (and in particular KCNQ2 ones), may help unravel new evidence on the topic.

Prospective studies are needed to analyze and compare the effects of standardized treatment protocols with VItB6 in neonatal epilepsies in general and in those KCNQ2-related in particular.

All this is particularly important when considering the widespread resort to VitB6 trials in neonatal epilepsies in NICUs, where this treatment is quickly taken into account, though not devoid of risks. In fact, high doses of PN and PLP have been reported as causative of peripheral neuropathy and liver toxicity, respectively (14, 18). In our opinion, this sets some limits on the advisability of resorting to a blanket VitB6 treatment. Therefore, our suggestion would be to initiate it as soon as possible in all those cases in which clinical features and/or genetic testing and lab findings suggest, or, even better, clearly demonstrate a VitB6 disorder (preferably after excluding liver diseases and nerve conduction defects). Otherwise, we would instead reserve VitB6 treatment for peculiar situations, such as drug-resistant NEEs, including those with an already proven pathogenic KCNQ2 variant.

CONCLUSIONS

Despite the limits of our study, our data contribute to adding new evidence on the potential beneficial effect of VitB6 treatment in KCNQ2-neonatal epilepsies, in apparent lack of inborn errors of VitB6 metabolism. Further studies should be conducted to elucidate the mechanisms underlying the variability of VitB6 effects in these patients, to help discriminate whether to include or not KCNQ2 (besides ALDH7A1 and PNPO) in the genetic testing of neonatal-onset seizures responsive to PN/PLP, and, finally, to define appropriate clinical guidelines and treatment protocols.

ETHICS STATEMENT

Ethical review and approval was not required for the study on human participants in accordance with the local legislation and institutional requirements. Written informed consent to participate in this study was provided by the participants' legal guardian/next of kin. Written informed consent was obtained from the minor(s)' legal guardian/next of kin for the publication of any potentially identifiable images or data included in this article. Written informed consent was obtained from the participant for the publication of this case report.

AUTHOR CONTRIBUTIONS

AN and GD conceived planned and supervised the study. GA and AB wrote the first draft of the manuscript. GA, AB, and FC prepared the tables. GA and FC designed the figures. GS, GV, MS, and VS helped supervise the project. All authors contributed to manuscript revision, read, and approved the submitted version.

REFERENCES

1. Singh NA, Charlier C, Stauffer D, DuPont BR, Leach RJ, Melis R, et al. A novel potassium channel gene, KCNQ2, is mutated in an inherited epilepsy of newborns. *Nat Genet.* (1998) 18:25–9. doi: 10.1038/ng0198-25
2. Zara F, Specchio N, Striano P, Robbiano A, Gennaro E, Paravidino R, et al. Genetic testing in benign familial epilepsies of the first year of life: clinical and diagnostic significance. *Epilepsia.* (2013) 54:425–36. doi: 10.1111/epi.12089
3. Allen NM, Mannion M, Conroy J, Lynch SA, Shahwan A, Lynch B, et al. The variable phenotypes of KCNQ-related epilepsy. *Epilepsia.* (2014) 55:e99–105. doi: 10.1111/epi.12715
4. Spoto G, Saia MC, Amore G, Gitto E, Loddo G, Mainieri G, et al. Neonatal seizures: an overview of genetic causes and treatment options. *Brain Sci.* (2021) 11:1295. doi: 10.3390/brainsci11101295
5. Weckhuysen S, Mandelstam S, Suls A, Audenaert D, Deconinck T, Claes LRF, et al. KCNQ2 encephalopathy: Emerging phenotype of a neonatal epileptic encephalopathy. *Ann Neurol.* (2012) 71:15–25. doi: 10.1002/ana.22644
6. Milh M, Boutry-Kryza N, Sutera-Sardo J, Mignot C, Auvin S, Lacoste C, et al. Similar early characteristics but variable neurological outcome of patients with a *de novo* mutation of KCNQ2. *Orphanet J Rare Dis.* (2013) 8:80. doi: 10.1186/1750-1172-8-80
7. Kato M, Yamagata T, Kubota M, Arai H, Yamashita S, Nakagawa T, et al. Clinical spectrum of early onset epileptic encephalopathies caused by KCNQ2 mutation. *Epilepsia.* (2013) 54:1282–7. doi: 10.1111/epi.12200
8. Orhan G, Bock M, Schepers D, Ilina EI, Reichel SN, Löffler H, et al. Dominant-negative effects of KCNQ2 mutations are associated with epileptic encephalopathy. *Ann Neurol.* (2014) 75:382–94. doi: 10.1002/ana.24080
9. Miceli F, Soldovieri MV, Ambrosino P, De Maria M, Migliore M, Migliore R, Taglialatela M. Early-onset epileptic encephalopathy caused by gain-of-function mutations in the voltage sensor of Kv7.2 and Kv7.3 potassium channel subunits. *J Neurosci.* (2015) 35:3782–93. doi: 10.1523/JNEUROSCI.4423-14.2015
10. Hunt AD Jr, Stokes J Jr, Mccrory WW, Stroud HH. Pyridoxine dependency: report of a case of intractable convulsions in an infant controlled by pyridoxine. *Pediatrics.* (1954) 13:140–5.
11. Baxter P. Pyridoxine-dependent and pyridoxine-responsive seizures. *Dev Med Child Neurol.* (2001) 43:416–20. doi: 10.1017/s0012162201000779
12. Mills PB, Struys E, Jakobs C, Plecko B, Baxter P, Baumgartner M, et al. Mutations in antiquitin in individuals with pyridoxine-dependent seizures. *Nat Med.* (2006) 12:307–9. doi: 10.1038/nm1366
13. Wang HS, Kuo MF, Chou ML, Hung PC, Lin KL, Hsieh MY, et al. Pyridoxal phosphate is better than pyridoxine for controlling idiopathic intractable epilepsy. *Arch Dis Child.* (2005) 90:512–5. doi: 10.1136/adc.2003.045963
14. Mills PB, Camuzeaux SS, Footitt EJ, Mills KA, Gissen P, Fisher L, et al. Epilepsy due to PNPO mutations: genotype, environment and treatment affect presentation and outcome. *Brain.* (2014) 137(Pt 5):1350–60. doi: 10.1093/brain/awu051
15. Gospe SM Jr. Pyridoxine-dependent epilepsy - ALDH7A1. In: Adam MP, Ardinger HH, Pagon RA, Wallace SE, Bean LJH, Gripp KW, editors. *GeneReviews®*. Seattle, WA: University of Washington (1993–2022). Available online at: https://www.ncbi.nlm.nih.gov/books/NBK1486/
16. Mefford HC, Cook J, Gospe SM Jr. Epilepsy due to 20q13.33 subtelomere deletion masquerading as pyridoxine-dependent epilepsy. *Am J Med Genet Part A.* (2012) 158A:3190–5. doi: 10.1002/ajmg.a.35633
17. Footitt EJ, Heales SJ, Mills PB, Allen GF, Oppenheim M, Clayton PT. Pyridoxal 5'-phosphate in cerebrospinal fluid; factors affecting concentration. *J Inherit Metab Dis.* (2011) 34:529–38. doi: 10.1007/s10545-011-9279-7
18. Reid ES, Williams H, Stabej P, James C, Ocaka L, Bacchelli C, et al. Seizures due to a KCNQ2 mutation: treatment with vitamin B6. *JIMD Rep.* (2016) 27:79–84. doi: 10.1007/8904_2015_460
19. Ohtahara S, Yamatogi Y, Ohtsuka Y. Vitamin B(6) treatment of intractable seizures. *Brain Dev.* (2011) 33:783–9. doi: 10.1016/j.braindev.2011.01.010
20. Millichap JJ, Park KL, Tsuchida T, Ben-Zeev B, Carmant L, Flamini R, et al. KCNQ2 encephalopathy: features, mutational hot spots, and ezogabine treatment of 11 patients. *Neurol Genet.* (2016) 2:e96. doi: 10.1212/NXG.0000000000000096
21. Sands TT, Balestri M, Bellini G, Mulkey SB, Danhaive O, Bakken EH, et al. Rapid and safe response to low-dose carbamazepine in neonatal epilepsy. *Epilepsia.* (2016) 57:2019–30. doi: 10.1111/epi.13596
22. Mulkey SB, Ben-Zeev B, Nicolai J, Carroll JL, Grønborg S, Jiang YH, et al. Neonatal nonepileptic myoclonus is a prominent clinical feature of KCNQ2 gain-of-function variants R201C and R201H. *Epilepsia.* (2017) 58:436–45. doi: 10.1111/epi.13676
23. Sharawat IK, Kasinathan A, Sahu JK, Sankhyan N. Response to carbamazepine in KCNQ2 related early infantile epileptic encephalopathy. *Indian J Pediatr.* (2019) 86:301–2. doi: 10.1007/s12098-018-2796-8
24. Spagnoli C, Salerno GG, Iodice A, Frattini D, Pisani F, Fusco C. KCNQ2 encephalopathy: a case due to a *de novo* deletion. *Brain Dev.* (2018) 40:65–8. doi: 10.1016/j.braindev.2017.06.008
25. Vilan A, Mendes Ribeiro J, Striano P, Weckhuysen S, Weeke LC, Brilstra E, et al. A distinctive ictal amplitude-integrated electroencephalography pattern in newborns with neonatal epilepsy associated with KCNQ2 mutations. *Neonatology.* (2017) 112:387–93. doi: 10.1159/000478651
26. Pisano T, Numis AL, Heavin SB, Weckhuysen S, Angriman M, Suls A, et al. Early and effective treatment of KCNQ2 encephalopathy. *Epilepsia.* (2015) 56:685–91. doi: 10.1111/epi.12984
27. Klotz KA, Lemke JR, Korinthenberg R, Jacobs J. Vitamin B6-responsive epilepsy due to a novel KCNQ2 mutation. *Neuropediatrics.* (2017) 48:199–204. doi: 10.1055/s-0037-1601857
28. Borgatti R, Zucca C, Cavallini A, Ferrario M, Panzeri C, Castaldo P, et al. A novel mutation in KCNQ2 associated with BFNC, drug resistant epilepsy, and mental retardation. *Neurology.* (2004) 63:57–65. doi: 10.1212/01.wnl.0000132979.08394.6d
29. Dedek K, Fusco L, Teloy N, Steinlein OK. Neonatal convulsions and epileptic encephalopathy in an Italian family with a missense mutation in the fifth transmembrane region of KCNQ2. *Epilepsy Res.* (2003) 54:21–7. doi: 10.1016/S0920-1211(03)00037-8
30. Martin HC, Kim GE, Pagnamenta AT, Murakami Y, Carvill GL, Meyer E, et al. Clinical whole-genome sequencing in severe early-onset epilepsy reveals new genes and improves molecular diagnosis. *Hum Mol Genet.* (2014) 23:3200–11. doi: 10.1093/hmg/ddu030
31. Numis AL, Angriman M, Sullivan JE, Lewis AJ, Striano P, Nabbout R, et al. KCNQ2 encephalopathy: delineation of the electroclinical phenotype and treatment response. *Neurology.* (2014) 82:368–70. doi: 10.1212/WNL.0000000000000060
32. Saitsu H, Kato M, Koide A, Goto T, Fujita T, Nishiyama K, et al. Whole exome sequencing identifies KCNQ2 mutations in Ohtahara syndrome. *Ann Neurol.* (2012) 72:298–300. doi: 10.1002/ana.23620
33. Lindy AS, Stosser MB, Butler E, Downtain-Pickersgill C, Shanmugham A, Retterer K, et al. Diagnostic outcomes for genetic testing of 70 genes in 8565 patients with epilepsy and neurodevelopmental disorders. *Epilepsia.* (2018) 59:1062–71. doi: 10.1111/epi.14074
34. Kopanos C, Tsiolkas V, Kouris A, Chapple CE, Albarca Aguilera M, Meyer R, et al. VarSome: the human genomic variant search engine. *Bioinformatics.* (2019) 35:1978–80. doi: 10.1093/bioinformatics/bty897
35. Stenson PD, Mort M, Ball EV, Chapman M, Evans K, Azevedo L, et al. The Human Gene Mutation Database (HGMD®): optimizing its use in a clinical diagnostic or research setting. *Hum Genet.* (2020) 139:1197–207. doi: 10.1007/s00439-020-02199-3
36. Baldridge D, Heeley J, Vineyard M, Manwaring L, Toler TL, Fassi E, et al. The Exome clinic and the role of medical genetics expertise in the interpretation of exome sequencing results. *Genet Med.* (2017) 19:1040–8. doi: 10.1038/gim.2016.224
37. Freibauer A, Jones K. KCNQ2 mutation in an infant with encephalopathy of infancy with migrating focal seizures. *Epilept Disord.* (2018) 20:541–4. doi: 10.1684/epd.2018.1011
38. Palmer EE, Schofield D, Shrestha R, Kandula T, Macintosh R, Lawson JA, et al. Integrating exome sequencing into a diagnostic pathway for epileptic encephalopathy: evidence of clinical utility and cost effectiveness. *Mol Genet Genomic Med.* (2018) 6:186–99. doi: 10.1002/mgg3.355
39. Lee IC, Chang TM, Liang JS, Li SY. KCNQ2 mutations in childhood nonlesional epilepsy: variable phenotypes and a novel mutation in a case series. *Mol Genet Genomic Med.* (2019) 7:e00816. doi: 10.1002/mgg3.816
40. Papuc SM, Abela L, Steindl K, Begemann A, Simmons TL, Schmitt B, et al. The role of recessive inheritance in early-onset epileptic encephalopathies: a combined whole-exome sequencing and copy number study. *Eur J Hum Genet.* (2019) 27:408–21. doi: 10.1038/s41431-018-0299-8
41. Malerba F, Alberini G, Balagura G, Marchese F, Amadori E, Riva A, et al. Genotype-phenotype correlations in patients with

de novo KCNQ2 pathogenic variants. *Neurol Genet.* (2020) 6:e528. doi: 10.1212/NXG.0000000000000528
42. Parra M, Stahl S, Hellmann H. Vitamin B6 and its role in cell metabolism and physiology. *Cells.* (2018) 7:84. doi: 10.3390/cells7070084
43. Kim JE, Cho KO. Functional nutrients for epilepsy. *Nutrients.* (2019) 11:1309. doi: 10.3390/nu11061309
44. Gospe SM Jr, Olin KL, Keen CL. Reduced GABA synthesis in pyridoxine-dependent seizures. *Lancet.* (1994) 343:1133–4. doi: 10.1016/s0140-6736(94)90236-4
45. Ramos RJ, Pras-Raves ML, Gerrits J, van der Ham M, Willemsen M, Prinsen H, et al. Vitamin B6 is essential for serine *de novo* biosynthesis. *J Inherit Metab Dis.* (2017) 40:883–91. doi: 10.1007/s10545-017-0061-3
46. Almannai M, El-Hattab AW. Inborn errors of metabolism with seizures: defects of glycine and serine metabolism and cofactor-related disorders. *Pediatr Clin North Am.* (2018) 65:279–99. doi: 10.1016/j.pcl.2017.11.007
47. van Karnebeek CD, Tiebout SA, Niermeijer J, Poll-The BT, Ghani A, Coughlin CR II, et al. Pyridoxine-dependent epilepsy: an expanding clinical spectrum. *Pediatric Neurol.* (2016) 59:6–12. doi: 10.1016/j.pediatrneurol.2015.12.013
48. Joshi R, Adhikari S, Patro BS, Chattopadhyay S, Mukherjee T. Free radical scavenging behavior of folic acid: evidence for possible antioxidant activity. *Free Radic Biol Med.* (2001) 30:1390–9. doi: 10.1016/s0891-5849(01)00543-3
49. Chumnantana R, Yokochi N, Yagi T. Vitamin B6 compounds prevent the death of yeast cells due to menadione, a reactive oxygen generator. *Biochim Biophys Acta.* (2005) 1722:84–91. doi: 10.1016/j.bbagen.2004.11.013
50. Thériault O, Poulin H, Thomas GR, Friesen AD, Al-Shaqha WA, Chahine M. Pyridoxal-5'-phosphate (MC-1), a vitamin B6 derivative, inhibits expressed P2X receptors. *Can J Physiol Pharmacol.* (2014) 92:189–96. doi: 10.1139/cjpp-2013-0404
51. Henshall DC, Diaz-Hernandez M, Miras-Portugal MT, Engel T. P2X receptors as targets for the treatment of status epilepticus. *Front Cell Neurosci.* (2013) 7:237. doi: 10.3389/fncel.2013.00237
52. Jimenez-Pacheco A, Mesuret G, Sanz-Rodriguez A, Tanaka K, Mooney C, Conroy R, et al. Increased neocortical expression of the P2X7 receptor after status epilepticus and anticonvulsant effect of P2X7 receptor antagonist A-438079. *Epilepsia.* (2013) 54:1551–61. doi: 10.1111/epi.12257
53. Schwaninger M, Ringleb P, Winter R, Kohl B, Fiehn W, Rieser PA, et al. Elevated plasma concentrations of homocysteine in antiepileptic drug treatment. *Epilepsia.* (1999) 40:345–50. doi: 10.1111/j.1528-1157.1999.tb00716.x
54. Attilakos A, Papakonstantinou E, Schulpis K, Voudris K, Katsarou E, Mastroyianni S, et al. Early effect of sodium valproate and carbamazepine monotherapy on homocysteine metabolism in children with epilepsy. *Epilepsy Res.* (2006) 71:229–32. doi: 10.1016/j.eplepsyres.2006.06.015

Case Report: Effect of Targeted Therapy with Carbamazepine in KCNQ2 Neonatal Epilepsy

Robertino Dilena[1], Eleonora Mauri[1], Alessio Di Fonzo[2], Cristina Bana[1], Paola Francesca Ajmone[3], Claudia Rigamonti[3], Tamara Catenio[4], Silvana Gangi[5], Pasquale Striano[6,7] and Monica Fumagalli[5]*

[1] Neurophysiopathology Unit, Department of Neuroscience and Mental Health, Foundation IRCCS Ca' Granda Ospedale Maggiore Policlinico, Milan, Italy, [2] Neurology Unit, Department of Neuroscience and Mental Health, Foundation IRCCS Ca' Granda Ospedale Maggiore Policlinico, Dino Ferrari Centre, University of Milan, Milan, Italy, [3] Child and Adolescent Neuropsychiatic Unit (UONPIA), Foundation IRCCS Ca' Granda Ospedale Maggiore Policlinico, Milan, Italy, [4] Grioni Center, Danelli Onlus Foundation, Lodi, Italy, [5] Foundation IRCCS Cà Granda Ospedale Maggiore Policlinico, University of Milan, Neonatology and NICU, Milan, Italy, [6] Pediatric Neurology and Muscular Diseases Unit, IRCCS 'G. Gaslini' Institute, Genoa, Italy, [7] Department of Neurosciences, Rehabilitation, Ophthalmology, Genetics, Maternal and Child Health, University of Genoa, Genoa, Italy

***Correspondence:**
Robertino Dilena
robertino.dilena@policlinico.mi.it

We present a family case of neonatal-onset *KCNQ2*-related epilepsy due to a novel intronic mutation. Three members of an Italian family (father and offspring) presented with neonatal-onset asymmetric tonic and clonic seizures with peculiar video-electroencephalography and aEEG features referring to sequential seizures. The father and the first son underwent standard of care treatments in line with current neonatal intensive care unit protocols, with a prolonged hospitalization before reaching full seizure control with carbamazepine. After the experience acquired with her family and the latest advances in the literature, the younger daughter was directly treated with carbamazepine, obtaining rapid seizure control and short hospitalization. They all had normal development. Carbamazepine is rarely administered as a first-line option in neonatal seizures. Recent evidence suggests that neonatal intensive care unit protocols should implement a trial with sodium channel blockers such as carbamazepine as first-option anti-seizure medication and a fast access to genetic testing in neonates with sequential seizures without structural brain injury or acute causes. Moreover, we report and discuss the laboratory studies performed on a novel causative intronic mutation in *KCNQ2* (c.1525+5 G>A in IVS13), since pathogenicity may be difficult to prove for intronic variants.

Keywords: *KCNQ2, SCN2A*, self-limited neonatal epilepsy, carbamazepine (CBZ), developmental and epileptic encephalopathy (DEE), EEG, sodium channel blocker, intronic mutation

INTRODUCTION

Seizures are the most frequent neurological sign observed in the neonatal intensive care unit (NICU) (1), and according to etiology, seizures can be classified into structural, metabolic, toxic, infectious, and genetic (2). Early recognition of the specific etiology has a significant impact on therapeutic management of neonatal seizures and neonatal epilepsies.

Genetic neonatal-onset epilepsies (13% of all neonatal seizures) (3) can be further subclassified into structural, metabolic, and functional (4). Functional genetic neonatal-onset epilepsy (8% of all neonatal seizures) (5) may be due to defects in channels, cell signaling, or synaptic transmission (4) with a phenotypic spectrum ranging from self-limited neonatal epilepsy (SLNE, previously referred as benign familial/non-familial neonatal epilepsy) to developmental and epileptic encephalopathy (DEE) (4, 6). Over 80% of SLNE cases are due to mutations in *KCNQ2* (7), and less commonly in *SCN2A* and *KCNQ3* (7).

KCNQ2, *KCNQ3*, and *SCN2A* channelopathies typically present with sequential seizures (2, 4). According to the ILAE consensus sequential seizures are defined by a repetitive succession of asymmetric tonic posturing alternating side, clonic movements, and/or apnea/cyanosis (2, 4). In correspondence to this clinical semiology, video EEG shows a typical sequence (2): electrical decrement (tonic phase) often from one hemisphere (alternating side) is followed by spikes and rhythmic delta-theta activity (clonic phase) and subsequent EEG depression (8). A distinctive ictal pattern has also been observed on aEEG consisting of rapid upper and lower margin rise followed by amplitude depression (8, 9).

This characteristic electroclinical seizure pattern can be encountered both in benign presentations (SLNE) or not (DEE). Interictal EEG with normal background, sleep-wake cycles and physiological graphoelements address a favorable outcome (SLNE) (6), while EEG disorganization with absence of sleep-wake cycles, random attenuation and abundant epileptiform abnormalities, or burst-suppression pattern suggests an unfavorable outcome with disability (DEE) (4). Moreover, DEE is commonly associated with encephalopathy signs, while SLNE is associated with normal neurological examination and positive family history, although it may also have a sporadic presentation (4–6).

Sodium channel blockers and anti-seizure medications such as phenytoin, carbamazepine (CBZ), oxcarbazepine, and lacosamide have been proved effective in neonates with channel-related epilepsy that may be refractory to other therapy (7, 10–14), and around 80% of *KCNQ2*- and *SCN2A*-related epilepsies have a full response to sodium channel blockers. Recognition of sequential seizures addresses diagnosis and treatment early.

Here, we report a family with *KCNQ2*-related epilepsy with a novel intronic mutation and the results of different Neonatal Intensive Care Unit (NICU) therapeutic approaches performed in the different family members due to the evolving knowledge on neonatal-onset epilepsies in the last years and the experiences progressively acquired in the family.

Abbreviations: NICU, neonatal intensive care unit; VUS, variant of unknown significance; SLNE, self-limited neonatal epilepsy; DEE, developmental and epileptic encephalopathy; CBZ, carbamazepine; IVS, intervening sequence or intron.

CASE REPORT

Sibling I

The first son was born at term with an unremarkable perinatal history. From the 2nd day of life, he presented seizures characterized by asymmetric tonic posturing, clonic movements shifting laterality, and apnea up to 15 times a day (**Figure 1A**). aEEG (**Figure 2A**) traces showed high-amplitude peaks enclosed by short depressions in correspondence to clinical seizures. Ictal EEG showed electrical decrement for a few seconds, and then rhythmic theta-delta activity with the focus changing in laterality, lasting 60–120 s (**Figures 2B,C**), whereas background EEG activity was normal. Brain MRI was unremarkable. Phenobarbital was used with partial efficacy. Then, phenytoin was effective during intravenous administration although requiring frequent blood tests to adjust doses and keep therapeutic blood concentrations, but after switching to oral phenytoin administration, seizure relapse occurred and plasma drug levels could not be reached. Finally, oral carbamazepine (5 mg/kg twice a day) was introduced obtaining stable plasma drug levels and was fully effective in seizure control, thus he was finally discharged from neonatal intensive care unit (NICU) (**Figure 1A**). Carbamazepine was withdrawn after 1.5 years without further relapses.

KCNQ2 sequencing revealed the novel variant c.1525+5 G>A in the intron or intervening sequence (IVS) 13, which was inherited from the father and considered at that time a variant of unknown significance (VUS). At 2 years of age the general developmental quotient determined by the Griffiths Mental Development Scale was 95 (within normal values, average 100, standard deviation 15). At 6 years of age, psychomotor development was normal, and he was seizure-free.

Father

The father, in the neonatal age, had epileptic tonic and clonic seizures treated with phenobarbital without full control, and then ACTH was also used. Seizure remission occurred at 8 months of age. At 7 years of age he presented childhood epilepsy with centro-temporal spikes, responsive to carbamazepine, withdrawn at the age of 11 without relapse. Brain MRI was not performed. His neurodevelopment was normal.

Sibling II

The second sibling was a girl without a remarkable perinatal history. On the 2nd day of life, she manifested a couple of doubtful paroxysmal events suspicious of seizures. An EEG was performed, but it was normal, so she was discharged. At home, new more clear and frequent events suggestive of seizures occurred, so she was again admitted, and the video EEG monitoring demonstrated repetitive sequential seizures, so she was directly treated with oral CBZ 5 mg/kg twice a day with immediate seizure control, allowing discharge from hospital in only 5 days (**Figure 1B**). Brain MRI did not reveal structural abnormalities or acute brain injuries. She had an epilepsy panel,

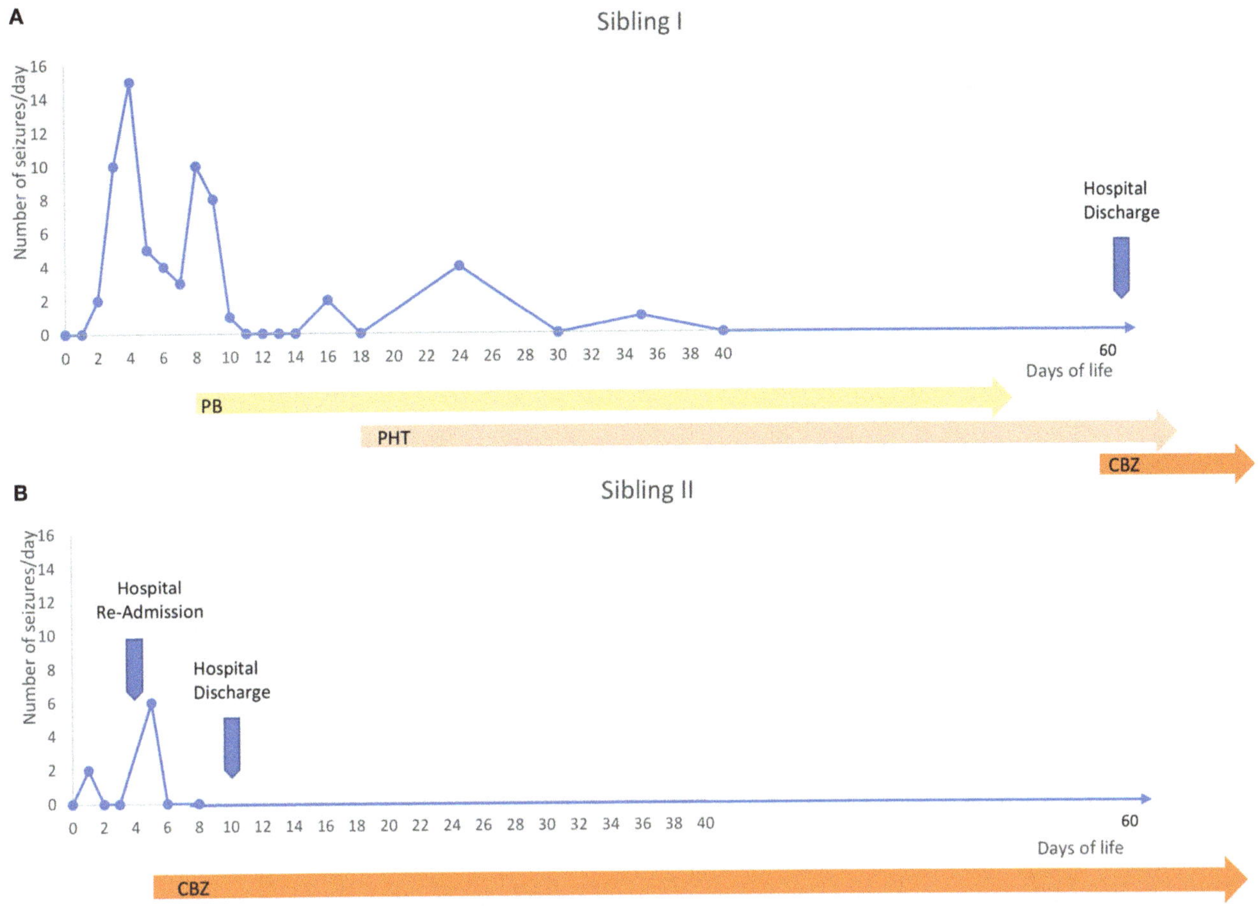

FIGURE 1 | Timeline. **(A)** The first sibling manifested sequential seizures from the second day of life and up to 15 seizures per day in the next days. He was firstly treated with phenobarbital with partial efficacy, so phenytoin was then trialed and it was effective, but seizures relapsed when blood levels were low due to difficulties in maintaining stable drug concentrations in the chronic stage, especially with oral use, so many blood tests were needed to check blood concentrations. Carbamazepine was finally introduced (5 mg/kg twice) at 2 months of age, obtaining stable seizure control. **(B)** One year later, a second sibling was born and had a couple of doubtful paroxysmal events on the second day of life suspicious to be a seizure, so an EEG was performed, but it was normal, so she was discharged. Then, at home, new more clear and frequent events suggestive of seizures occurred, so she was again admitted and the VideoEEG monitoring demonstrated repetitive sequential seizures, so, she was treated with carbamazepine as first choice (5 mg/kg twice) with immediate full seizure control and just five days after she was discharged.

but only the same intronic mutation was found, and other mutations in other genes involved in epilepsy were excluded. CBZ was withdrawn at 1 year without seizure relapses.

At 10 months of age, her general developmental quotient determined by the Griffiths Mental Development Scale was 100 (within normal values, average 100, standard deviation 15). At 4 years of age, the follow-up of her psychomotor development was normal, and she was seizure free.

Laboratory

The c.1525+5 G>A IVS13 variant was found in the family in 2015 by *KCNQ2* Sanger sequencing, but at that time, it was considered a VUS. After the second sibling was born, a 72-gene Next Generation Sequencing epilepsy-panel was performed to exclude other mutations, reporting only the same heterozygous variant, segregating within the affected relatives and confirmed by Sanger.

In order to study the effect of the intronic variant found in our family, a transcript expression study on RNA extracted from patient peripheral leukocytes was performed to replicate a study previously applied in another published intronic KCNQ2 mutation (15). A two-round PCR approach was used to overcome the very low expression in blood of *KCNQ2* transcripts, which are brain-specific. However, the transcript sequence analysis on blood-derived cDNA failed to detect splicing aberrations probably because of the limitation of the two-round PCR approach in being able to detect a null transcript or large intron retention as a pathogenetic consequence of the variant.

This variant was absent from clinical and population databases (ClinVar, gnomAD). An *in silico* analysis predicted a high pathogenic probability affecting the normal splicing.

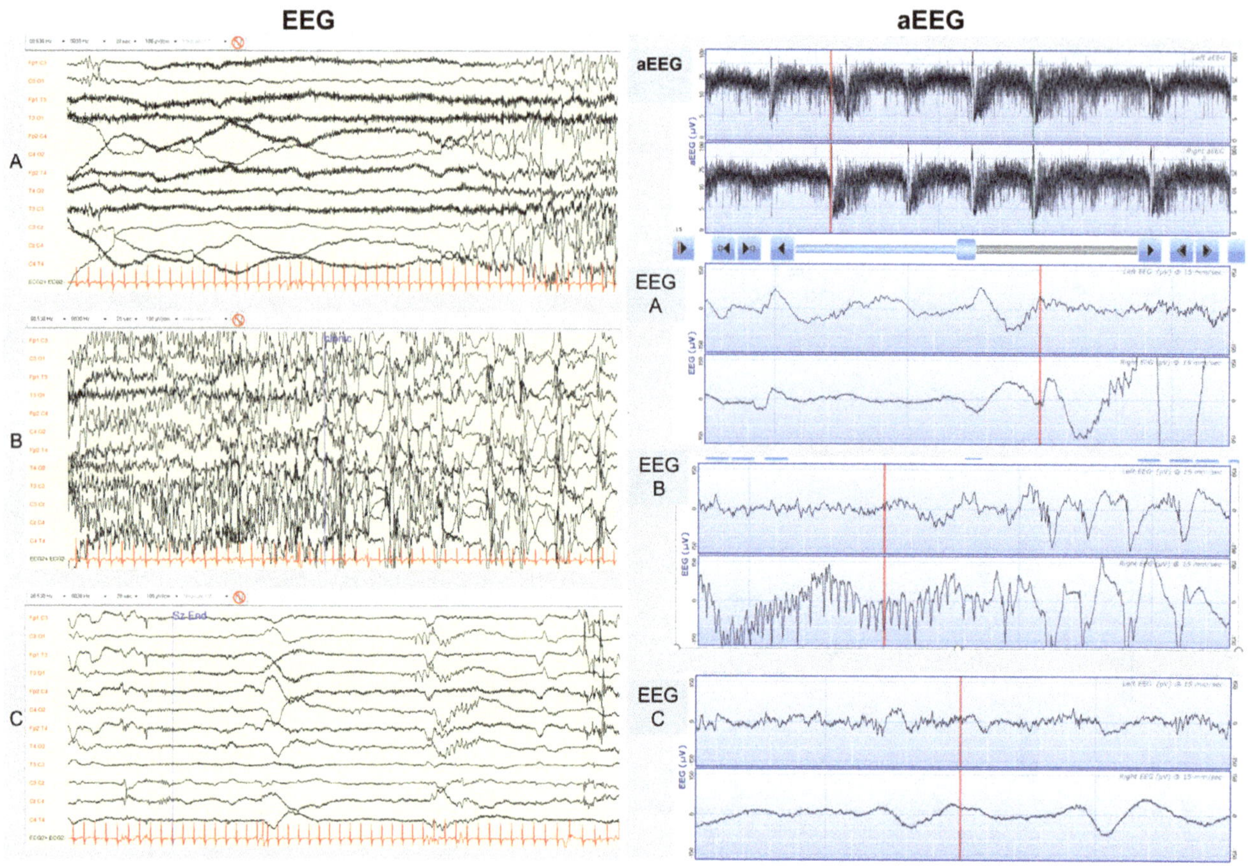

FIGURE 2 | EEG (on the left). Conventional EEG traces of a typical seizure of KCNQ2-related neonatal epilepsy. **(A)** The initial tonic phase is characterized by ictal low-amplitude EEG appearance mixed with muscle artifact. **(B)** The following clonic phase is characterized by rhythmic high-amplitude spike-wave activity. **(C)** Post-ictal low-amplitude depression phase. aEEG (on the right). 2-channel-aEEG (and corresponding EEG raw traces) in KCNQ2-related neonatal epilepsy. Cluster of KCNQ2-related seizures typically characterized by high amplitude peaks enclosed by short troughs. In addition to the first KCNQ2-seizure aEEG pattern description by Vilan et al. we underline the frequent typical appearance in KCNQ2 seizures of a trough preceding the aEEG peak during the initial tonic phase, corresponding in the raw EEG trace to a low-amplitude high-frequency EEG pattern **(EEG A)**, followed by the aEEG peak pattern during the clonic phase, corresponding in the raw EEG to a high-amplitude rhythmic low-frequency spike **(EEG B)**, and finally another trough following the peak during the post-ictal depression phase, corresponding to a low-amplitude EEG pattern **(EEG C)**.

On VarSome platform (a search engine, aggregator and impact analysis platform for human genetic variations, that aims at sharing global expertise on human variants) (16), the variant is predicted to be likely pathogenetic, as result of the combination of the strong criterium of pathogenicity PP3 (as the variant is predicting a novel splicing site in gene KCNQ2, for which loss-of-function is a known mechanism of disease) and the moderate criterium of pathogenicity PM2 (as the position is moderately conserved).

DISCUSSION

We report a family with a novel intronic mutation, c.1525+5 G>A, of the *KCNQ2* gene associated with a self-limited neonatal epilepsy phenotype and a specific response to sodium channel blocker and anti-seizure medications. Since pathogenicity may be difficult to prove for intronic variants, this report may hasten the diagnosis and better treatment in future patients. The report also illustrates how clinical management of functional genetic neonatal epilepsy has greatly changed in the last 8 years thanks to recent scientific advances in clinical, neurophysiological, genetic and pharmacological knowledge (2–14) with a profound impact on patient and family quality of life, although at the moment there is no proof of an improved neurodevelopmental outcome.

Nowadays, the distinction between genetic neonatal-onset epilepsy and provoked seizures could be performed very early (8). The role of neurophysiological evaluation and monitoring by conventional EEG and aEEG has become crucial in clinical practice (17). The recognition of a typical sequential seizure pattern with a prominent tonic onset on video-EEG in a neonate without structural brain damage or acute etiology is an accessible and reliable marker of genetic epilepsy due to *KCNQ2/KCNQ3/SCN2A* channelopathies, allowing for a tailored diagnostic workup and early targeted effective treatment (2–14). Indeed, independently from the neurodevelopmental evolution into SLNE or DEE, neonatal epilepsy associated with channelopathies, *KCNQ2*- or *SCN2A*-related, shows a better response to sodium-channel blockers (2–14) such as phenytoin, oxcarbazepine, and CBZ. In this family, the first son, after 2 months of hospitalization and different anti-seizure medications, obtained full control only after CBZ was started. The second neonate was immediately treated with CBZ with prompt efficacy, markedly shortening hospitalization and preventing complications related to the NICU setting (separation from the mother, infections, and discomfort). The 6-year follow-up of this family also proved normal neurodevelopment after early use of CBZ. Oral CBZ has traditionally been rarely prescribed in neonates (<1% of all neonatal seizures, never as a first-line treatment) (18). There are no specific data on the safety of CBZ use in neonates or infants in comparison with other anti-seizure medications, whereas there are studies on safety of anti-seizure medications during pregnancy (19). Apparently, there is no reason to hypothesize that there could be more side effects with CBZ in neonatal age in comparison with other ages, and studies reporting on the efficacy of CBZ in *KCNQ2* and *SCN2A* neonatal epilepsies did not raise any safety concerns regarding reactions or neurodevelopmental outcomes (2–14). Oral phenytoin is not suitable for chronic use in neonates as plasma drug levels cannot often be achieved by oral administration, as shown in our case and as described by pharmacokinetic studies on phenytoin in neonates (20). The only downside of CBZ is that a parenteral formulation is not available, so in case of status epilepticus with need to rapidly control seizures, initial use of intravenous phenytoin followed by a switch to CBZ oral syrup is suggested (12). An oral alternative to CBZ with a more favorable side effect profile may be represented by oxcarbazepine given its better profile of enzyme induction properties, but not all countries have the availability of oxcarbazepine syrup formulation suitable for infants. A new sodium channel blocker very promising for neonatal seizures is represented by lacosamide, a manageable drug with a good safety profile for which both intravenous and oral syrup formulations have been produced. Lacosamide has been very recently used as an alternative third-option anti-seizure medication for refractory neonatal seizures in some centers (21). Lacosamide has also been demonstrated effective in two neonates with *SCN2A*-related intractable seizures (14). A multicenter randomized controlled study to evaluate efficacy and safety of lacosamide in neonatal seizures described on clinicalTrials.gov (22) is currently recruiting patients. The results of lacosamide trials on neonatal seizures could potentially change the management of neonatal seizures, possibly allowing for its consideration as a first- or second-option targeted treatment for *KCNQ2* or *SCN2A* neonatal epilepsy.

CONCLUSIONS

Early identification of *KCNQ2* variants in patients with epilepsy raises prognostic issues toward optimal management (23). We report a novel intronic mutation of *KCNQ2* associated with familial self-limited neonatal epilepsy. *KCNQ2* and *SCN2A* neonatal epilepsies can be early suspected on the basis of typical clinical, EEG, and aEEG features (sequential seizures with prominent tonic onset semiology) in the absence of acute causes and structural abnormalities. In addition, in inherited cases, family history strongly points to the diagnosis. On the basis of the literature of the last 8 years and experience at our center, we suggest that in suspected *KCNQ2* and *SCN2A* neonatal epilepsies, NICUs should implement fast genetic testing for neonatal epileptic channelopathies and a trial with CBZ. In severe epileptic presentations with status epilepticus, phenytoin could be first started to rapidly obtain seizure control and then in case of positive response, switch to CBZ or oxcarbazepine, as they are more suitable for long-term maintenance. A further promising alternative could be lacosamide given the availability of intravenous and oral formulations and anecdotal evidence showing a good potential for neonatal seizures and channel-related neonatal epilepsies, but larger studies are warranted.

ETHICS STATEMENT

The research was conducted ethically following the World Medical Association Declaration of Helsinki and its amendments. Subjects involved and their parents (for minors) have given their written informed consent to publish their case. This study protocol was reviewed and approved by Comitato Etico Milano Area 2 protocol n.0050696.

AUTHOR CONTRIBUTIONS

RD conceptualized and wrote the manuscript, performed the neurologic evaluations, collected the clinical history, and performed the neurophysiological assessments. EM conceptualized and wrote the manuscript, collected the clinical, and neurophysiological data. AD performed the genetic analysis and reviewed the manuscript. CB performed the neurophysiological examinations and reviewed the manuscript. CR and TC performed the neuropsychological tests and reviewed the manuscript. SG performed the pediatric evaluation and follow-up and reviewed the manuscript. PS and MF contributed in intellectual content and supervision and reviewed the manuscript. All authors contributed to the article and approved the submitted version.

ACKNOWLEDGMENTS

The authors would like to thank the family members for their cooperation. This work was developed within the framework of the DINOGMI Department of Excellence of MIUR 2018–2022 (legge 232 del 2016).

REFERENCES

1. Volpe JJ. Neurology of the Newborn (5th edition): Elsevier Ltd, Oxford, Philadelphia (2008).
2. Pressler RM, Cilio MR, Mizrahi EM, Moshé SL, Nunes ML, Plouin P, et al. The ILAE classification of seizures and the epilepsies: Modification for seizures in the neonate. Position paper by the ILAE task force on neonatal seizures. *Epilepsia.* (2021) 62:615–28. doi: 10.1111/epi.16815
3. Glass HC, Shellhaas RA, Wusthoff CJ, Chang T, Abend NS, Chu CJ, et al. Neonatal seizure registry study group. Contemporary profile of seizures in neonates: a prospective cohort study. *J Pediatr.* (2016) 174:98–103. doi: 10.1016/j.jpeds.2016.03.035

4. Cornet MC, Cilio MR. Genetics of neonatal-onset epilepsies. *Handb Clin Neurol.* (2019) 162:415–33. doi: 10.1016/B978-0-444-64029-1.00020-5 PMID: 31324323.
5. Shellhaas RA, Wusthoff CJ, Tsuchida TN, Glass HC, Chu CJ, Massey SL, et al. Profile of neonatal epilepsies: characteristics of a prospective US cohort. *Neurology.* (2017) 89:893–9. doi: 10.1212/WNL.0000000000004284
6. Zuberi SM, Wirrell E, Yozawitz E, Wilmshurst JM, Specchio N, Riney K, et al. ILAE classification and definition of epilepsy syndromes with onset in neonates and infants: position statement by the ILAE task force on nosology and definitions. *Epilepsia.* (2022) 63:1349–397. doi: 10.1111/epi.17239
7. Sands TT, Balestri M, Bellini G, Mulkey SB, Danhaive O, Bakken EH, et al. Rapid and safe response to low-dose carbamazepine in neonatal epilepsy. *Epilepsia.* (2016) 57:2019–30. doi: 10.1111/epi.13596
8. Cornet MC, Morabito V, Lederer D, Glass HC, Ferrao Santos S, Numis AL, et al. Neonatal presentation of genetic epilepsies: early differentiation from acute provoked seizures. *Epilepsia.* (2021) 62:1907–20. doi: 10.1111/epi.16957
9. Vilan A, Mendes Ribeiro J, Striano P, Weckhuysen S, Weeke LC, Brilstra E, et al. A distinctive ictal amplitude-integrated electroencephalography pattern in newborns with neonatal epilepsy associated with KCNQ2 mutations. *Neonatology.* (2017) 112:387–93. doi: 10.1159/000478651
10. Numis AL, Angriman M, Sullivan JE, Lewis AJ, Striano P, Nabbout R, et al. KCNQ2 encephalopathy: delineation of the electroclinical phenotype and treatment response. *Neurology.* (2014) 82:368–70. doi: 10.1212/WNL.0000000000000060 Epub 2013 Dec 26. PMID: 24371303
11. Pisano T, Numis AL, Heavin SB, Weckhuysen S, Angriman M, Suls A, et al. Early and effective treatment of KCNQ2 encephalopathy. *Epilepsia.* (2015) 56:685–91. doi: 10.1111/epi.12984
12. Dilena R, Striano P, Gennaro E, Bassi L, Olivotto S, Tadini L, et al. Efficacy of sodium channel blockers in SCN2A early infantile epileptic encephalopathy. *Brain Dev.* (2017) 39:345–8. doi: 10.1016/j.braindev.2016.10.015
13. Wolff M, Johannesen KM, Hedrich UBS, Masnada S, Rubboli G, Gardella E, et al. Genetic and phenotypic heterogeneity suggest therapeutic implications in SCN2A-related disorders. *Brain.* I2017 140:1316–36. doi: 10.1093/brain/awx054
14. Flor-Hirsch H, Heyman E, Livneh A, Reish O, Watemberg N, Litmanovits I, et al. Lacosamide for SCN2A-related intractable neonatal and infantile seizures. *Epileptic Disord.* (2018) 20:440–6. doi: 10.1684/epd.2018.1001
15. de Haan G-J, Pinto D, Carton D, Bader A, Witte J, Peters E, et al. A novel splicing mutation in KCNQ2 in a multigenerational family with BFNC followed for 25 years. *Epilepsia.* (2006) 47:851–9. doi: 10.1111/j.1528-1167.2006.00552.x
16. Kopanos C, Tsiolkas V, Kouris A, Chapple CE, Albarca Aguilera M, Meyer R, et al. The human genomic variant search engine. *Bioinformatics.* (2019) 35:1978–80. doi: 10.1093/bioinformatics/bty897
17. Dilena R, Raviglione F, Cantalupo G, Cordelli DM, De Liso P, Di Capua M, et al. Consensus protocol for EEG and amplitude-integrated EEG assessment and monitoring in neonates. *Clin Neurophysiol.* (2021) 132:886–903. doi: 10.1016/j.clinph.2021.01.012
18. Ahmad KA, Desai SJ, Bennett MM, Ahmad SF, Ng YT, Clark RH, et al. Changing antiepileptic drug use for seizures in US neonatal intensive care units from 2005 to 2014. *J Perinatol.* (2017) 37:296–300. doi: 10.1038/jp.2016.206
19. Thangaratinam S, Marlin N, Newton S, Weckesser A, Bagary M, Greenhill L, et al. AntiEpileptic drug Monitoring in PREgnancy (EMPiRE): a double-blind randomised trial on effectiveness and acceptability of monitoring strategies. *Health Technol Assess.* (2018) 22:1–152. doi: 10.3310/hta22230
20. Painter MJ, Pippenger C, MacDonald H, Pitlick W. Phenobarbital and diphenylhydantoin levels in neonates with seizures. *J Pediatr.* (1978) 92:315–9. doi: 10.1016/s0022-3476(78)80034-1
21. Keene JC, Morgan LA, Abend NS, Bates SV, Bauer Huang SL, Chang T, et al. Treatment of neonatal seizures: comparison of treatment pathways from 11 neonatal intensive care units. *Pediatr Neurol.* (2022) 128:67–74. doi: 10.1016/j.pediatrneurol.2021.10.004
22. Available online at: https://clinicaltrials.gov/ct2/show/NCT04519645
23. Malerba F, Alberini G, Balagura G, Marchese F, Amadori E, Riva A, et al. Genotype-phenotype correlations in patients with de novo KCNQ2 pathogenic variants. *Neurol Genet.* (2020) 6:e528. doi: 10.1212/NXG.0000000000000528

30

Case Report: A Case of Epileptic Disorder Associated with a Novel *CNTN2* Frameshift Variant in Homozygosity due to Maternal Uniparental Disomy

Wenjie Chen[1,2†], *Fei Chen*[3], *Yiping Shen*[3,4,5,6*†], *Zhixian Yang*[7] *and Jiong Qin*[1*†]

[1]*Department of Paediatrics, Peking University People's Hospital, Beijing, China,* [2]*Department of Neurology, Guangzhou Women and Children's Medical Center, Guangzhou, China,* [3]*The Maternal and Child Health Care Hospital of Guangxi Zhuang Autonomous Region, Guangxi Birth Defects Prevention and Control Institute, Guangxi, China,* [4]*Department of Medical Genetics, Shanghai Children's Medical Center, Shanghai Jiao Tong University School of Medicine, Shanghai, China,* [5]*Division of Genetics and Genomics, Boston Children's Hospital, Boston, MA, United States,* [6]*Department of Neurology, Harvard Medical School, Boston, MA, United States,* [7]*Department of Pediatrics, Peking University First Hospital, Beijing, China*

***Correspondence:**
Jiong Qin
qinjiong@pkuph.edu.cn
Yiping Shen
yiping.shen@childrens.harvard.edu

[†]**ORCID**:
Wenjie Chen
orcid.org/0000-0001-9884-2270
Jiong Qin
orcid.org/0000-0002-9109-3286
Yiping Shen
orcid.org/0000-0001-5820-0839

Background: Contactin 2, encoded by *CNTN2* on chromosome 1q32.1, is a neural-specific glycoprotein and plays important roles in neurodevelopment. A deleterious homozygous variant in the *CNTN2* gene was previously reported to cause autosomal recessive cortical myoclonic tremor and epilepsy. Since then, there has been no further report confirming the association of *CNTN2* and epilepsy. Here, we reported one new case, who presented with epilepsy, carrying a novel homozygous frameshift variant in *CNTN2*. The clinical and genetic features of the patient were reviewed.

Case presentation: The male patient presented with preschool age-of-onset neurodevelopmental impairment and focal seizures of temporal origin, and responded to valproate. A trio-whole exome sequencing revealed a novel homozygous frameshift variant in *CNTN2* (c.2873_c.2874delCT, p.Thr958Thrfs). The patient's mother was a heterozygous carrier while his father was wild-type; they were both unaffected and non-consanguineous. Further study revealed that maternal uniparental disomy (1q32.1) unmasked the heterozygous variant of *CNTN2* in the proband.

Conclusions: This case enhanced the gene–disease relationship between *CNTN2* and epilepsy, which will help to further understand this emerging disorder.

Keywords: *CNTN2*, epilepsy, uniparental disomy (UPD), neurodevelopmental disorder (NDD), genotype-phenotype correlation

BACKGROUND

One deleterious homozygous mutation in the contactin two gene (*CNTN2*) was previously reported to be associated with epilepsy, familial adult myoclonic, 5 (FAME5, OMIM 615400) (Stogmann et al., 2013). The reported patients were from a consanguineous Egyptian family. He presented with early adolescence onset focal epilepsy which responded well to carbamazepine treatment. Myoclonus developed soon after seizure; he also presented with neuropsychiatric symptoms and borderline cognitive level. However, controversy exists about the diagnosis of "familial cortical myoclonic tremor with epilepsy" (FCMTE) that Stogmann et al. established in the report (Striano et al., 2013). Striano et al. have challenged about the nature of tremors that Stogmann et al. described as cortical origin. In addition, Striano et al. also inquired the difference of inheritance pattern presenting in the family compared with the previous patients with FCMTE (Striano et al., 2013).

Given the small number of mutations and lack of phenotypic information, the relationship between *CNTN2* and epileptic disorder is of limited support at this time. Reporting of additional case can further enhance the causal relationship and better understand the genotypic and phenotypic spectra. Herein, we presented a Chinese patient with cognitive and behavior deficit, neuropsychiatric disorders, and pediatric epilepsy of temporal origin, who carried a novel homozygous frameshift variant p.Thr958Thrfs in *CNTN2* gene. Moreover, we also reported an unusual inheritance of the *CNTN2* variant involving maternal uniparental disomy (UPD).

CASE PRESENTATION

The 7-year-old boy was born at full term by cesarean section; his parents were healthy and non-consanguineous Chinese Han. The parents denied any family history of neurologic disease. The boy had his first attack of generalized tonic-clonic seizure at the age of 5 years. Seizures lasted for 4–5 min and 2–3 times per month at initiation.

Levetiracetam (LEV) was given 4 months later after the first seizure and seizure was free. However, 3 months later, seizure was recurrent and was refractory to control even with the highest dose of LEV (50 mg/kg/day). Since then, seizure became frequent and focal seizure types evolved including 1) attacks with presentation of fear or panic followed by a scared scream, hand holding and scratching, foot pedaling, then loss of awareness, followed by swallow and eye blink that lasted for 30–90 s, which occurred up to 6–7 attacks per day; and 2) pause in activity, gazing, then loss of awareness, followed by swallow or jerking of left facial muscle that lasted for 10 s to 1 min, several times a day. Oxcarbazepine (OXC, 30 mg/kg/day) was added 6 months later, yet it was still ineffective.

He had a history of development delay before seizure onset, mainly presenting in learning ability, and seizures had been exacerbating his poor academic performance based on the description of his parents. On examination at the age of 7 years, his cognitive function was impaired at mild-moderate level, including learning difficulties, memory deficits, hyperactivity, and attention deficit, and could not handle well with schoolwork. In addition, he also behaved aggressively and impulsively. The previous VEEG showed left temporal-PG1-frontal interictal epileptiform discharges, ictal suggesting temporal and frontal lobe origin. Brain MRI revealed no abnormality. We prescript valproate (VPA) to the patient and ordered a trio-exome sequencing.

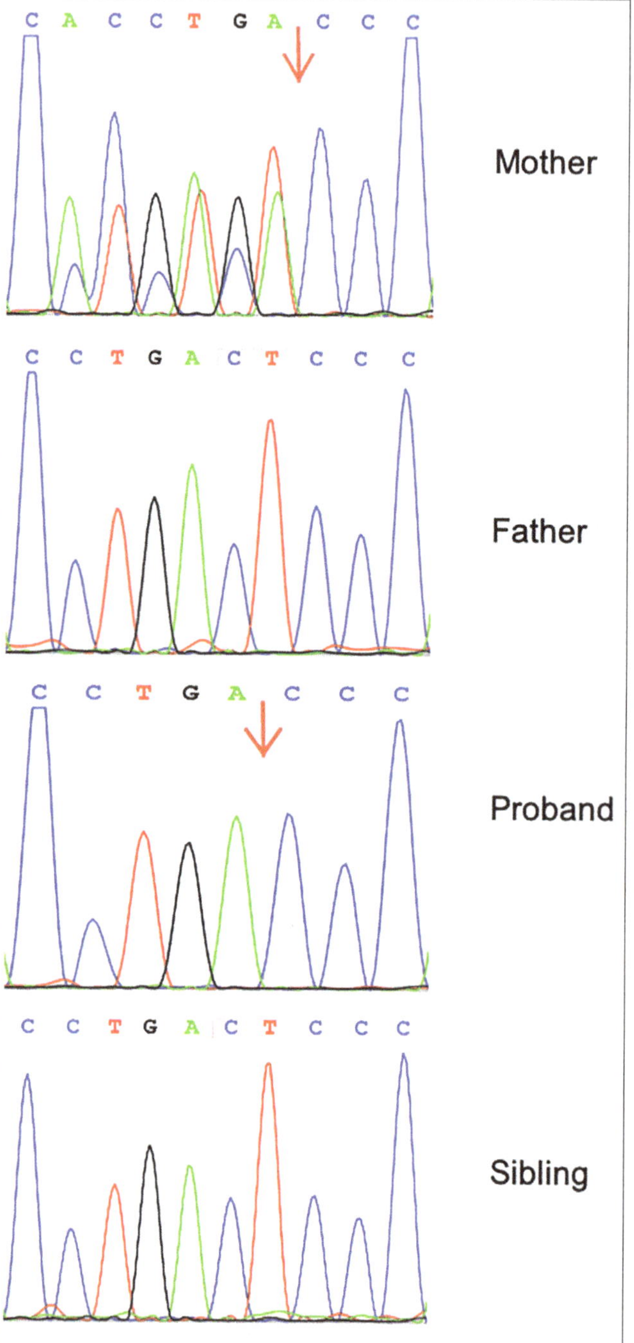

FIGURE 1 | Sequence analysis of *CNTN2* gene from the family. Chromatograms showing that the mother is heterozygous for c.2873_c.2874delCT (p.Thr958Thrfs*17). The proband shows a homozygosity of the mutation; his father and little brother have wild-type sequence.

SEQUENCING METHODS

Genomic DNA was extracted from peripheral blood samples of the proband and his parents. We planned a proband–parent trio approach. Exome data processing, variant calling, and variant annotation were performed by the Chigene Translational Medicine Research Center (Beijing, China) as a clinical service. For whole-exome sequencing (WES), sequencing library was created by Agilent SureSelect Human All Exon V6 Kit (Agilent Technologies, Santa Clara, CA) in accordance with

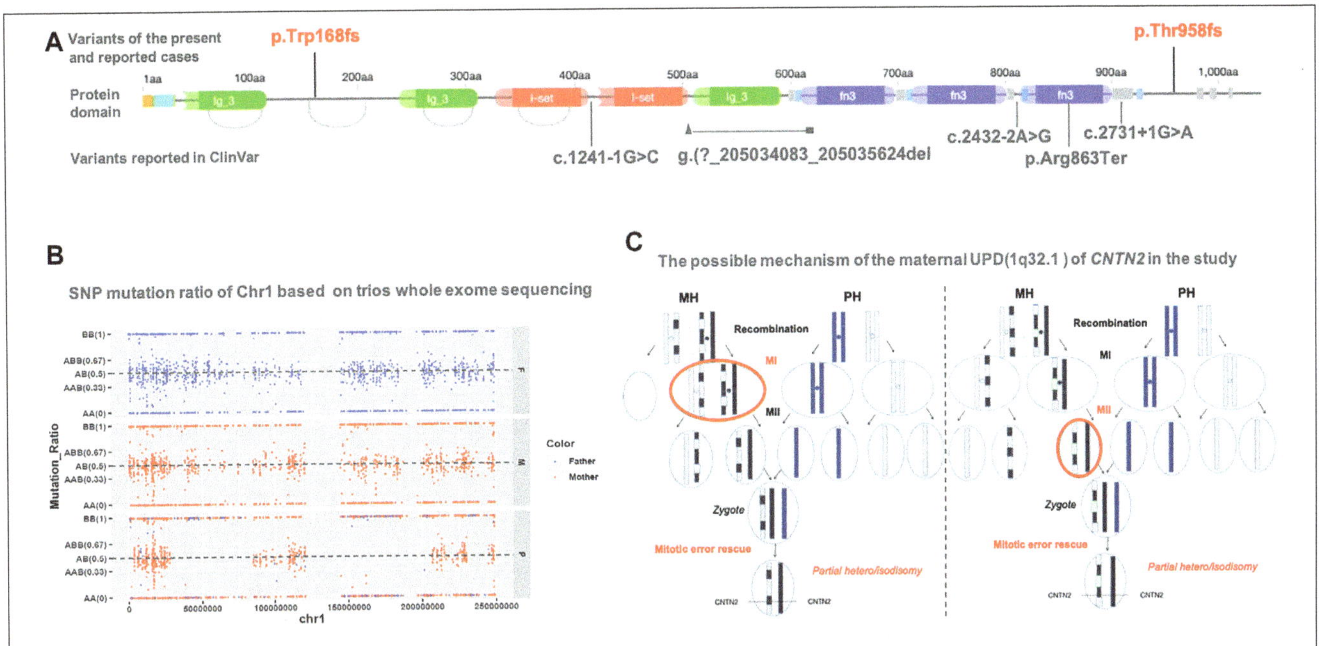

FIGURE 2 | (A) Protein structure of CNTN2 and localization of variants reported in the present study, previous literature (red), and ClinVar database (gray). This present variant (red: c.2873_c.2874delCT, p.T958Tfs*17) is in the second last exon but within the last 50aa. There is only one publication (NM_005076.5: c.504del, p.Trp168fs) reported with FAME5. Another five reported loss-of-function variants in ClinVar lack detailed clinical information. The origin graph of protein domain is cited from DECIPHER (https://www.deciphergenomics.org/). **(B)** SNP analysis reveals the altered regions on chromosome 1, including maternal heterodisomy at chr1: 1-26488019, chr1: 79411951-150123132, and chr1:206230986-249250621; and maternal isodisomy at chr1: 26488019-49511248, chr1: 50957509-79411951, and chr1: 150123132-206230986 **(C)** Based on the results of SNP analysis, the possible mechanism that results in the mixture pattern of uniparental disomy (UPD) is recombination of maternal homologs (MH) before Meiosis I, then LEFT: chromosome segregation error at Meiosis I (MI), or RIGHT: chromosome segregation error at Meiosis II (MII), and then a rescuing segregation error in the zygote. For simplicity, we only show the chromatid of chromosome pair for UPD with partial hetero/isodisomy. Paternal homologs (PH).

the manufacturer's protocol. The prepared libraries were sequenced with a HiSeq2500 (Illumina, San Diego, CA). The Genome Analysis Toolkit (GATK) was used for variant calling (GATK HaplotypeCaller) (McKenna et al., 2010). A total of >99% of reads were mapped to genomic targets, with 20× coverage for >95% of bases. In the proband, a total of 118,818 variants were identified in exonic and splice site regions. "Rare deleterious" mutations were defined as those that met the following criteria: 1) their alternative allele frequencies were ≤0.5% in gnomAD database and our local database; 2) the severity of the impact on the protein should be high, such as a stop-gain, stop-loss, nonsense, frameshift, or splice-site mutation. The standard of missense mutation is REVEL ≥0.75 or all the prediction tools score as Damaging; 3) the clinical manifestations of the patient should closely associate with the disease phenotype. All of the mutations were classified following the ACMG/AMP guidelines to define (Richards et al., 2015). We comprehensively evaluated the pathogenicity, frequency, and clinical manifestations of the mutation. Sanger sequencing was used to verify the authenticity of the mutations.

SEQUENCING RESULTS

We identified 11,287 variants existing in genes that matched with known phenotypes. Variants from 1,683 genes associated with epilepsy were subsequently extracted, leading to the identification of a novel homozygous frameshift variant (c.2873_c.2874delCT, p.Thr958Thrfs*17) in the *CNTN2* gene (RefSeq NM_005076) (**Supplementary Table 1**). Parental WES data and Sanger analysis of the mutation revealed that one copy of the variant was inherited from his unaffected mother; the other variant was not detected in the father's genome. He has a healthy little brother who carried no variant at this locus (**Figure 1**).

This variant is not in gnomAD. It is located in the second last exon but not within the last 50aa; this frameshift variant is expected to result in a null product due to nonsense-mediated decay. On investigation, only one loss-of-function variant of *CNTN2* has been reported in an individual with a similar presentation as our patient (Stogmann et al., 2013). Five loss-of-function variants (c.1241-1G>C; c.2432-2A>G; g. (?205034083_205035624del; c.2587C>T; c.2731 + 1G > A) are reported in ClinVar as pathogenic or likely pathogenic (**Figure 2A**). In the HGMD database, six heterozygous variants including four missense, one splice, and one nonsense variant are recorded. The nonsense variant (p.Tyr585Ter) was reported to be associated with autosomal recessive intellectual disability (Harripaul et al., 2018). All other variants were not reported to be associated with a specific phenotype.

The frameshift variant detected in our patient can be classified as pathogenic following the ACMG/AMG guideline (PVS1, PM2_P, PM3_P). Given the atypical inheritance pattern in this case, possibilities including maternal UPD or a paternal deletion including the *CNTN2* locus (at least exon 22) were examined. WES-based copy number analysis of the father's

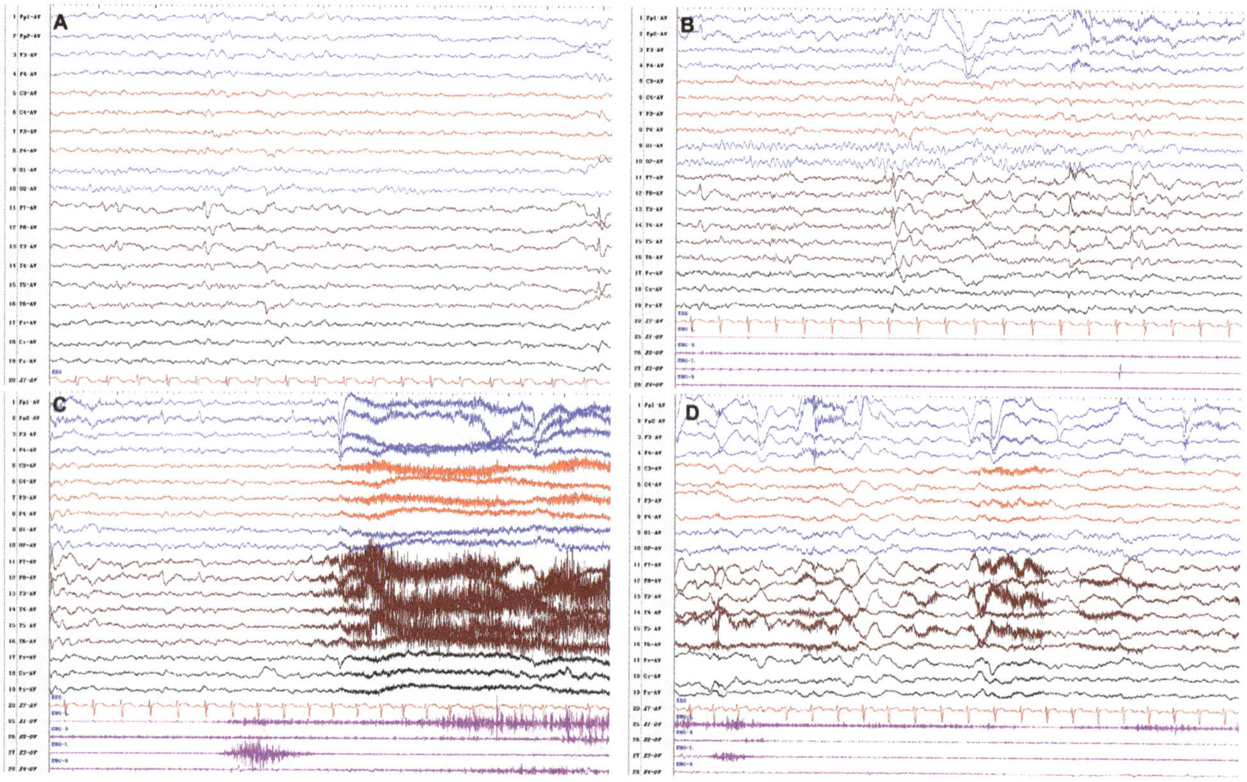

FIGURE 3 | VEEG after drug withdrawal at 10 years 8 months. Interictal **(A,B)**: bilateral frontal–temporal epileptiform discharges, **(B)** was the background a few seconds before the onset. Ictal **(C,D)** recorded a focal seizure (fear, closed eyes, vocalization, forward and backward movements of the hips, pedaling movements of lower limbs) in awake period.

genomic DNA yielded normal results and a further qPCR detecting genomic copy number abnormalities of exon 22 in *CNTN2* from his father.

As expected, SNP mutation ratio of Chr1 based on trios-WES showed the maternal UPD of chromosome 1 [UPD (1)mat] in the proband. It revealed the altered regions on chromosome one; maternal heterodisomy at chr1:1-26488019, chr1:79411951-150123132, and chr1:206230986-249250621; and maternal isodisomy at chr1: 26488019-49511248, chr1: 50957509-79411951, and chr1: 150123132-206230986 (**Figure 2B**). *CNTN2* is located on chromosome 1q32.1, from chr1: 205042937 to 205078289, exactly where the isodisomy of chr1: 150123132-206230986 occurred.

FOLLOW-UP

At the follow-up of 9 years old, he had been seizure free for 26 months since add-on therapy of VPA (9.3 mg/kg/day) with OXC remaining at 16.7 mg/kg/day, and LEV had been withdrawn 18 months earlier. The parents of the patient complained that the attack of behavior arrest occurred occasionally, which lasted for less than 10 s. However, EEG failed to monitor the ictal epileptiform discharges. By the last visit, the boy was 10 years 8 months; he had seizure relapse when his parents were trying to withdraw VPA and OXC. The seizure type and ictal EEG were similar as before (**Figure 3**), and a recurrent brain MRI did not show any abnormality. His seizure was under control with sufficient dose of VPA and OXC. He remained to have cognitive and behavioral deficits, as well as emotional regulation problem. He has normal growth.

DISCUSSION

We reported a non-consanguineous Han male with homozygous c.2873_c.2874delCT, p.T958Tfs*17 mutation in *CNTN2*, onset with generalized seizure and evolved into focal seizure (**Table 1**). At present, there was only one family reported worldwide with mutations in *CNTN2* and similar clinical presentation (Stogmann et al., 2013). According to the evidence accumulated from public databases such as HGMD, gnomAD, and ClinVar (**Figure 2A**), all the variants classified as pathogenic/likely pathogenic belong to loss-of-function.

This is a potentially important case for upgrading the gene–disorder relationship for this emerging seizure disorder. Similar to those patients reported by Stogmann et al. (2013), the patient showed focal seizures, which was indicative of a temporal origin in EEG, and cranial MRI revealing no abnormality. In addition, almost all patients demonstrated a non-progressive course on anti-epileptic therapy.

However, unlike previous patients with familial cortical myoclonic tremor with epilepsy (FCMTE) (Striano and Zara,

TABLE 1 | Summary of *CNTN2* mutations and main clinical features.

	Stogmann et al. (2013)					This report
Individual (sex)	1 (M)	2 (F)	3 (F)	4 (F)	5 (F)	6 (M)
Mutation (NM_005076.5)			p.Trp168fs			p.Thr958Thrfs*17
Age at seizure onset (years)	11	14	11	12	11	6
Age at follow-up (years)	39	37	29	24	21	10.7 (age at last follow-up)
Seizure type	GTCS, CPS	GTCS, CPS	GTCS, CPS	GTCS, CPS	GTCS, CPS	GTCS, CPS
Aura	–	–	–	–	–	-
Cortical tremor	+	+	+	+	+	-
Myoclonic jerks	–	+	+	+	–	-
Cognitive function	NA	IQ 85	IQ 86	IQ 79	IQ 78	Learning difficulties, memory deficits, ADHD traits
Mental disorder	–	–	–	Depressive symptoms	Depressive symptoms	Aggressive, impulsive
Cranial MRI/CT	Normal	Normal	Normal	Normal	MRI bilateral mS	Normal
EEG	–	Temporal IEDs	Normal	Tempoparietal IEDs	Temporal IEDs	T-F IEDs; ictal: T, F onset
AEDs	CBZ	CBZ	CBZ	CBZ, LTG	CBZ	VPA, OXC
Outcomes of AEDs	Good	Good	Good	Poor	Good	Good

M, male; F, female; GTCS, generalized tonic-clonic seizure; CPS, complex partial seizure; IQ, intelligence quotient; OXC, oxcarbazepine; VPA, valproate; LTG, lamotrigine; NA, not available; IED, interictal epileptic discharge; T, temporal; F, frontal; ADHD, attention-deficit hyperactivity disorder; mS, mesial sclerosis.

2016), the manifestation of myoclonus was not observed in our patient throughout the course of disease. It is unclear whether this symptom was an aspect of *CNTN2*-associated disorder or not.

Furthermore, by summarizing the clinical manifestation of the patients with homozygous mutation in *CNTN2*, we found that focal epilepsy is the main clinical feature, in conjunction with other neuropsychiatric symptoms, whereas our patient displayed more apparent cognitive impairment and emotional regulation problem than previous patients with FCMTE.

Evidence from Harripaul et al.'s study provide a suggestion that loss-of-function variants in *CNTN2* might be responsible for the neuropsychiatric symptoms. In that study, a nonsense variant (p.Tyr585Ter) of *CNTN2* was detected, although it was only supplemented as a candidate gene of autosomal recessive intellectual disability (Harripaul et al., 2018).

Rather than the only explanation of FCMTE, this spectrum of symptoms is more likely to be a consequence of clinical or genetic heterogeneity of *CNTN2*-associated disorder. Due to the limited number of such a rare disease, more cases will help to better understand the phenotype–genotype correlation.

The special autosomal recessive (AR) inheritance presenting in our case was finally confirmed to be a UPD (1)mat of *CNTN2* on 1q32.1. UPD is the presence of a chromosome pair derived only from one parent in a disomic cell line. So far, three types of UPD including isodisomy (UPiD, both copies of a single chromosome homolog are inherited from one parent), heterodisomy (UPhD, a pair of homologous chromosomes are inherited from one parent), and partial heterodisomy/partial isodisomy (segments of both isodisomy and heterodisomy are identified across the chromosome) have been reported (Benn, 2021).

UPD is rare in health populations. In fact, it could become a pathogenic event, when UPD involves imprinted chromosomal region or gene (chromosomes 6, 7, 11, 14, 15, or 20) (Eggermann, 2020), or results in the homozygosity of recessive mutation (Yamazawa et al., 2010). This occurs as a consequence of isodisomy, when one of the parents is a carrier for recessive disorder (Yamazawa et al., 2010).

Just in the case of our study, a mixture of partial heterodisomy and partial isodisomy was identified across the maternal chromosome one from the patient (**Figure 2B**). The homozygous state of *CNTN2* mutation was the result of maternal UPiD (1q32.1).

There are many possible mechanisms leading to UPD including meiotic non-disjunction with mitotic correction, gametic complementation, mitotic segregation error, or micronuclei (Conlin et al., 2010; Kearney et al., 2011; Benn P, 2020).

Mechanism for the formation of UPD in our case is supposed to be the initial chromosome segregation error during meiosis and a rescuing segregation error in the zygote (**Figure 2C**).

The occurrence of UPD in the inheritance of autosomal recessive disorder is not very rare (yet at least uncommon), and related studies have been reported since 1988 (Spence et al., 1988; Yamazawa et al., 2010; Soler-Palacín et al., 2018).

Based on the ChromosOmics Database (Liehr T., 2021), 32 records of maternal UPD (1) have been reported (clinical significance of seven cases are unavailable, one is irrelevant). Of the 24 cases with clinical findings, 20 have relevant phenotype with responsible genes located on the UPD, and almost of them are AR (19/20). The remaining four cases are neurodevelopmental disorders without associated pathogenic genes. Yet similar case of maternal UPD (1) of *CNTN2* has not been reported.

In brief, UPD (1) can cause disease not only through imprinting defects but also through homozygous exposure of recessive genes. For fetus with UPD (1) during pregnancy examinations, the recessive genes mapped on the chromosome should be analyzed with caution, and combined with other important clinical features, appropriate management for the genetic diagnosis and counseling should be made.

In recent years, SNP array is recommended in the detection of UPD; it was proven to play an important role in disclosing the mechanisms of UPD (Conlin et al., 2010; Kearney et al., 2011). With the advance of next-generation sequencing, a late work demonstrated that WES-based copy number analysis could also reveal UPD (Soler-Palacín et al., 2018).

Collectively, our study suggested that loss-of-function variants in *CNTN2* may be responsible for temporal epilepsy accompanied with neurodevelopmental impairment. Reporting of this new case will help to upgrade the gene–disease relationship for this emerging *CNTN2*-related disorder. We also provided clinical experience for additional choice of appropriate AEDs for *CNTN2*-related epilepsy. This case revealed a rare a mixture of maternal isodisomy and heterodisomy of chromosome one that unmasked a heterozygous variant.

ETHICS STATEMENT

The studies involving human participants were reviewed and approved by The Ethical Review Committee (ERC) of Peking University People's Hospital (PKUPH). Written informed consent to participate in this study was provided by the participants' legal guardian/next of kin.

AUTHOR CONTRIBUTIONS

WC: writing—original draft and study designing. FC: conducting bioinformatics analysis and study designing. ZY: providing the data of VEEG. JQ and YS: writing—review and editing. All authors contributed to the article and approved the submitted version.

ACKNOWLEDGMENTS

We thank the patient's family for participation in the study. We acknowledge Dr. Zhang G for graph edition and sequencing data verification.

REFERENCES

1. Benn, P. (2021). Uniparental Disomy: Origin, Frequency, and Clinical Significance. *Prenatal Diagn.* 41, 564–572. doi:10.1002/pd.5837
2. Conlin, L. K., Thiel, B. D., Bonnemann, C. G., Medne, L., Ernst, L. M., Zackai, E. H., et al. (2010). Mechanisms of Mosaicism, Chimerism and Uniparental Disomy Identified by Single Nucleotide Polymorphism Array Analysis. *Hum. Mol. Genet.* 19 (7), 1263–1275. doi:10.1093/hmg/ddq003
3. Eggermann, T. (2020). Prenatal Detection of Uniparental Disomies (UPD): Intended and Incidental Finding in the Era of Next Generation Genomics. *Genes* 11, 1454. doi:10.3390/genes11121454
4. Harripaul, R., Vasli, N., Mikhailov, A., Rafiq, M. A., Mittal, K., Windpassinger, C., et al. (2018). Mapping Autosomal Recessive Intellectual Disability: Combined Microarray and Exome Sequencing Identifies 26 Novel Candidate Genes in 192 Consanguineous Families. *Mol. Psychiatry* 23 (4), 973–984. doi:10.1038/ mp.2017.60
5. Kearney, H. M., Kearney, J. B., and Conlin, L. K. (2011). Diagnostic Implications of Excessive Homozygosity Detected by SNP-Based Microarrays: Consanguinity, Uniparental Disomy, and Recessive Single-Gene Mutations. *Clin. Lab. Med.* 31, 595–613. doi:10.1016/j.cll.2011.08.003
6. Liehr, T. (2021). Cases with Uniparental Disomy. Available at: http://cs-tl.de/DB/CA/UPD/0-Start.html. (Accessed 09, 2021).
7. McKenna, A., Hanna, M., Banks, E., Sivachenko, A., Cibulskis, K., Kernytsky, A., et al. (2010). The Genome Analysis Toolkit: a MapReduce Framework for Analyzing Next-Generation DNA Sequencing Data. *Genome Res.* 20 (9), 1297–1303. doi:10.1101/gr.107524.110
8. Richards, S., Aziz, N., Aziz, N., Bale, S., Bick, D., Das, S., et al. (2015). Standards and Guidelines for the Interpretation of Sequence Variants: a Joint Consensus Recommendation of the American College of Medical Genetics and Genomics and the Association for Molecular Pathology. *Genet. Med.* 17 (5), 405–423. doi:10.1038/gim.2015.30
9. Soler-Palacín, P., Garcia-Prat, M., Martín-Nalda, A., Franco-Jarava, C., Rivière, J. G., Plaja, A., et al. (2018). LRBA Deficiency in a Patient with a Novel Homozygous Mutation Due to Chromosome 4 Segmental Uniparental Isodisomy. *Front. Immunol.* 9, 2397. doi:10.3389/fimmu.2018.02397
10. Spence, J. E., Perciaccante, R. G., Greig, G. M., Willard, H. F., Ledbetter, D. H., Hejtmancik, J. F., et al. (1988). Uniparental Disomy as a Mechanism for Human Genetic Disease. *Am. J. Hum. Genet.* 42 (2), 217–226.
11. Stogmann, E., Reinthaler, E., Eltawil, S., El Etribi, M. A., Hemeda, M., El Nahhas, N., et al. (2013). Autosomal Recessive Cortical Myoclonic Tremor and Epilepsy: Association with a Mutation in the Potassium Channel Associated Gene CNTN2. *Brain* 136 (Pt 4), 1155–1160. doi:10.1093/brain/awt068
12. Striano, P., and Zara, F. (2016). Autosomal Dominant Cortical Tremor, Myoclonus and Epilepsy. *Epileptic Disord.* 18 (2), 139–144. doi:10.1684/epd.2016.0860
13. Striano, P., Zara, F., Striano, S., and Minetti, C. (2013). Autosomal Recessive Epilepsy Associated with Contactin 2 Mutation Is Different from Familial Cortical Tremor, Myoclonus and Epilepsy. *Brain* 136 (Pt 10), e253. doi:10.1093/brain/awt140
14. Yamazawa, K., Ogata, T., and Ferguson-Smith, A. C. (2010). Uniparental Disomy and Human Disease: An Overview. *Am. J. Med. Genet.* 154C, 329–334. doi:10.1002/ajmg.c.30270

31

Case Report: A Case of Eyelid Myoclonic Status with Tonic–Clonic Seizure and Literature Review

*Yujun Yuan, Fenghua Yang, Liang Huo, Yuying Fan, Xueyan Liu, Qiong Wu and Hua Wang**

Department of Pediatrics, Shengjing Hospital of China Medical University, Shenyang, China

***Correspondence:**
Hua Wang
wangh1@sj-hospital.org

Eyelid myoclonus with or without absence epilepsy is a rare and usually misdiagnosed disease in the neurology department. It is an idiopathic general epileptic syndrome, the onset period is 6–8 years, and is more common in girls. It is characterized by rapid abnormal eye blinking, accompanied by upward rolling of the eye and slight backward movement of the head, with eye closure sensitivity and photosensitivity. The seizure is frequent and short, dozens or even hundreds of times a day; a small number of patients may have eyelid myoclonus status. We report a patient who visits the hospital for the first time with eyelid myoclonic problem; the patient continued to wink the eyes, eye rolled up, and backward movement of the head, accompanied by impairment of consciousness. Video electroencephalography (VEEG) suggests continued spike slow-wave, polyspike slow-wave. After the patient had 2, 4, 6, 8, 10, 12, and 14 Hz of intermittent photic stimulation (IPS), her seizures and epileptic discharges reduced or stopped. Seven min after giving stimulation at 20 Hz, the child developed an occipital-initiated tonic–clonic seizure, which demonstrated that after sufficient IPS stimulation, the occiput cortex became excited and initiated a brain network, leading to diffuse brain discharge and tonic–clonic seizures. At 1 h after onset, the child developed a nonconvulsive state, with impairment of consciousness despite no eyelid myoclonic movements, and VEEG suggested a large number of epileptic discharges. After 10 min of administrating midazolam, the patient's EEG immediately became normal, and the patient regained consciousness. Therefore, this paper presents an eyelid myoclonus status patient with occipital origin seizure, we recorded the whole course of the disease and the treatment effect, and reviewed the literature accordingly.

Keywords: eyelid myoclonus, Jeavons syndrome, status epilepticus, photosensitiveness, eye closure sensitivity

INTRODUCTION

Eyelid myoclonus with absence (EMA) or Jeavons syndrome is a rare idiopathic generalized epilepsy (IGE) that occurs in childhood. The symptomatic features of eyelid myoclonus were first reported by Radovici et al. (1) more than 80 years ago. The study of epileptic discharges and seizures caused by closing the eyes was reported in 1955 (2). This epileptic syndrome was first fully described by Jeavons in 1977. It is characterized by eyelid myoclonus, with or without absence of seizures, eyelid closure induces epileptic discharge and/or seizures, and photosensitivity. Subsequently, EMA was again confirmed as an independent individual in IGE. Eyelid myoclonus is a hallmark of Jeavons syndrome. Usually, it is associated with repeated myoclonic jerks of the eyelids, eyeballs roll upward, and the head may move slightly backward. When accompanied by impairment of consciousness, it is named eyelid myoclonus with absence. Eyelid myoclonic status may be spontaneous or light stimulated. It consists of recurrent and discontinuous seizures of eyelid myoclonus, accompanied by mild absence (3). Many patients with IGE have visual precursors associated with photosensitive and focal epilepsy, EMA is common in IGE patients with photosensitivity. The occipital cortex can be activated by eye closure and IPS, and this excitability may spread to the brain stem, resulting in eyelid myoclonus. As the intensity of the photic stimulus increases, the excitability can be projected into the central frontal cortex via transcortical and thalamocortical pathways, and then generalized seizures and absence seizures may occur (4). However, focal epileptic discharge is also present in patients with IGE. Gungor-Tuncer et al. had demonstrated that epileptic discharges of focal origin can still occur in some IGE patients. The interictal focal discharge independent of localization in some patients suggests that there may be an overlap between focal epilepsy and generalized epilepsy (5). Eyelid myoclonus has some overlap with other seizures, especially photosensitive epilepsy, and reflex epilepsy; therefore, the differential diagnosis of EMA is very important. Patients with eyelid myoclonic status are even less common in clinical practice. Giuliano et al. (6) found that 17.6% of patients with eyelid myoclonus had epileptic status. Striano (1) also reported that one in five patients might experience eyelid myoclonus status. We input the keywords "eyelid myoclonic status" when searching in PubMed. There were only three reported cases (7–9). Valproate is widely recognized as the most effective treatment for photosensitive epilepsies (10). Therefore, we present a very rare case of eyelid myoclonus status followed by an occipital origin of tonic–clonic seizure with the clinical manifestations, electroencephalogram (EEG) characteristics, differential diagnosis, and therapeutic effect in detail, and reviewed the literature.

CASE REPORT

A 12-year-old girl was admitted to the hospital (*Department of Pediatrics, Shengjing Hospital of China Medical University, Shenyang, China*) with the main complaint of "frequent blinking for 4 h." Her main manifestations were continuous blinking, upward rolling of the eyeball, backward movement of the head, and accompanied by decreased consciousness. Physical examination showed poor condition, continuous eyelid blinking with unclear consciousness; neck strength (–), Babinski sign (–), limb muscle tone was normal, and muscle strength grade V. Physical examination of other nervous systems was normal. After hospitalization, video electroencephalography (VEEG) was performed immediately. It showed persistent spike–wave, polyspike–wave discharge (**Figure 1**), especially when the eyes were closed. At the same time, the patient had low response ability, slow speech, and slow action. However, she could answer the questions accurately. It suggested that the patient had an eyelid myoclonus status accompanied by absence. The patient had an IPS test; when at 2, 4, 6, 8, 10, 12, and 14 Hz frequency, the seizures and epileptic discharges reduced or stopped (**Figure 2**). However, after the patient had 16, 18, and 20 Hz, the epileptic discharges increased and blinking started again. Seven min after 20 Hz, the VEEG found a tonic–clonic seizure starting from the occipital region (**Figure 3**). That indicated that the patient had photosensitivity. After a seizure, her eyelid myoclonus symptoms disappeared, and simultaneously, EEG discharge decreased significantly. However, the girl was heavily drowsy, and slow-wave increased. 30 minutes after onset, the VEEG showed that epileptic discharges increased again and after 1 hour of onset, the epileptic discharge increased to the initial state-continuous discharge. We hypothesized the girl was experiencing a non-convulsive status; therefore, we gave her midazolam 5 mg via intravenous injection immediately and then 2 ml/h (0.05 mg/kg/h) of intravenous fluid. After 10 min, the EEG showed that the epileptic discharge disappeared and started recovering to normal state (**Figure 4**). Besides, the consciousness of children returned to normal, speaking speed and action were as usual. She had a history of convulsions. Each convulsion is manifested as loss of consciousness, backward movement of the head, teeth closed, limbs stiff and shaking, no second incontinence, lasting for about 1 min, and can be relieved by itself. She was tired and went to sleep after convulsion. During the month prior to admission, the child developed frequent eyelid blinking and decreased consciousness following frequent eye closure. Combined with the patient's clinical manifestations, EEG, closed eye sensitivity, photosensitivity, and history, we diagnosed the patient as with eyelid myoclonic status. She has no positive family history.

After admission, the biochemical examination was completed. There was no significant abnormality on her biochemical examination, and no abnormality on her head MRI. When we arranged the IQ test for the patient, the family members thought that the daughter did not show cognitive impairment with normal life, and no mental decline was found. So the IQ test was refused. After being diagnosed, the girl was given sodium valproate 1.5 ml bid orally, and the patient responded well to valproic acid, without obvious side effects. On the 8th day of admission, the child had no convulsions and was discharged. In addition, we recommended to the patient to check the liver and kidney function, blood routine, and blood drug concentration detection regularly, drug increase or decrease according to clinical manifestations, and EEG examination. Moreover, mental tests should be performed to determine whether the cognitive aspects of the patient are affected. She was also told to watch for if other types of epilepsies occur and avoid light stimulation. The patient was followed-up by a call for 2 years. She had no recurrence. The girl is now in junior high school and has no obvious adverse reactions or cognitive changes.

DISCUSSION

Eyelid myoclonus with or without absences (EMA, Jeavons syndrome) has episodic EEG that is typically characterized by extensive high-amplitude polyspike slow-wave discharges of 3–6 Hz lasting for 1.5–6 s. Epileptic discharges occur during or before eyelid myoclonus. Most studies have shown that Jeavons syndrome has eye closure sensitivity (ECS) and photosensitivity.

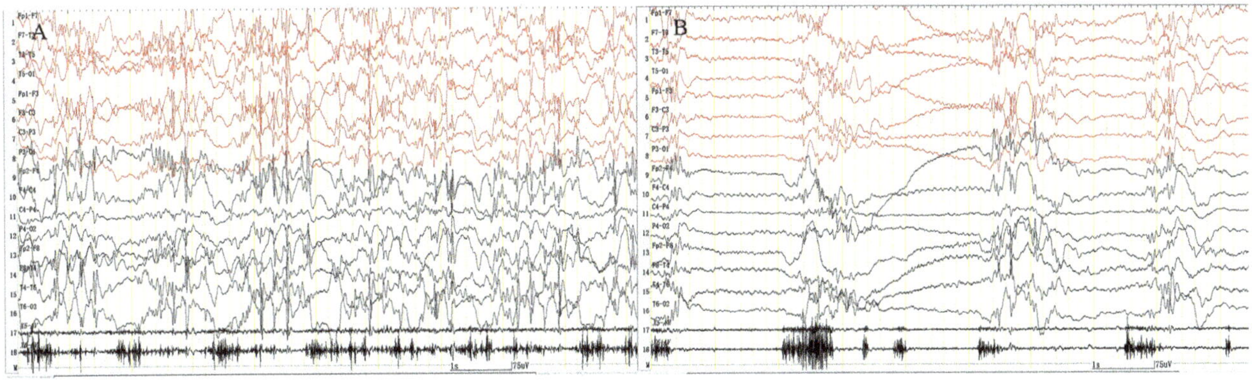

FIGURE 1 | Eyelid myoclonic status. The patient was continuously blinking with upward rolling of the eyeball and backward movement of the head; VEEG: sustained and extensive 3- to 6-Hz high-amplitude spike–slow wave, polyspike–slow wave discharge. **(A)** Fast blinking movement. **(B)** Slow blinking movement. X5, outer eyelid; X6, upper eyelid. SEN: 15 μV; HF: 70; TC: 0.3.

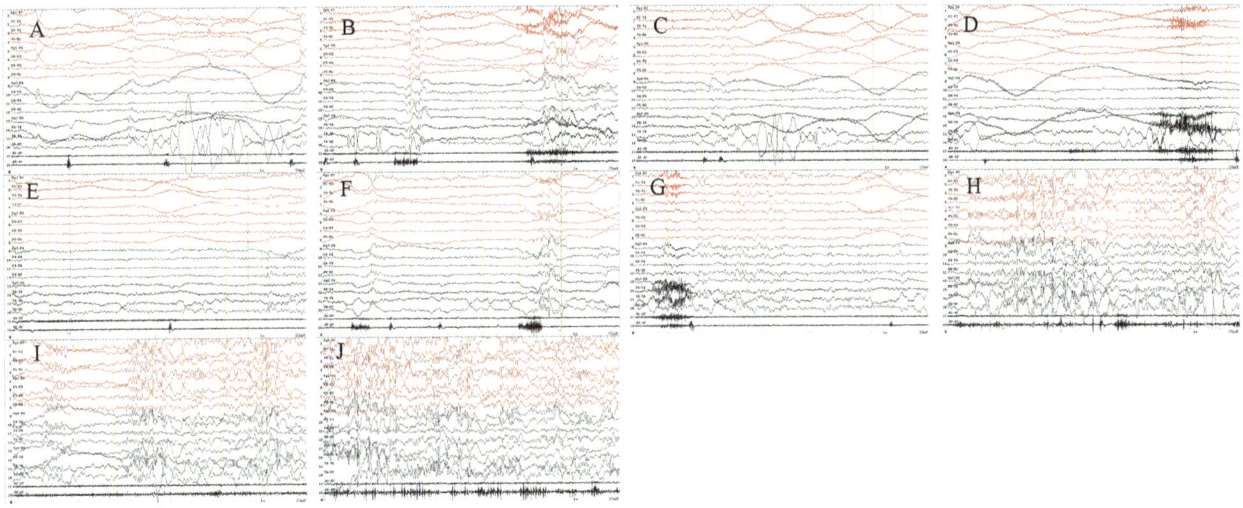

FIGURE 2 | Intermittent photic stimulation (IPS). After the patient had 2 Hz **(A)**, 4 Hz **(B)**, 6 Hz **(C)**, 8 Hz **(D)**, 10 Hz **(E)**, 12 Hz **(F)**, and 14 Hz **(G)**, the epileptic discharges reduced or stopped. But after 16 Hz **(H)**, 18 Hz **(I)**, and 20 Hz **(J)**, the epileptic discharges increased and blinking started again. X5, outer eyelid; X6, upper eyelid. SEN: 15 μV; HF: 70; TC: 0.3.

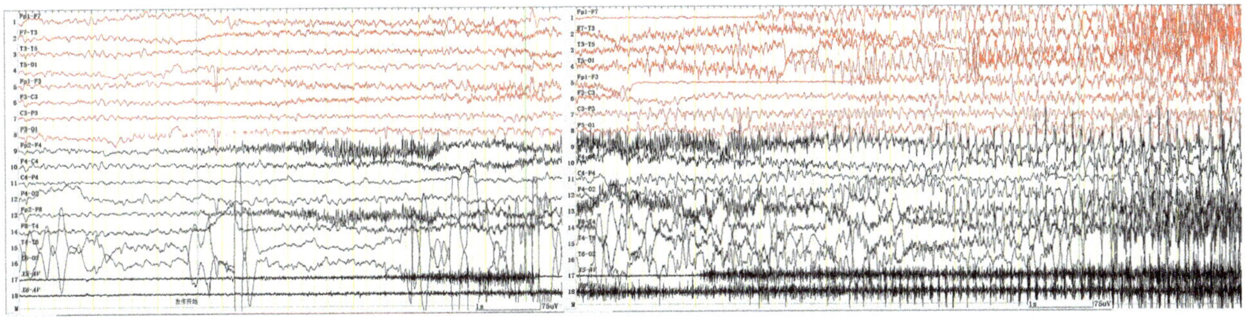

FIGURE 3 | Tonic clonic seizures beginning in the occipital region 7 min after IPS. X5, outer eyelid; X6, upper eyelid. SEN: 15 μV; HF: 70; TC: 0.03.

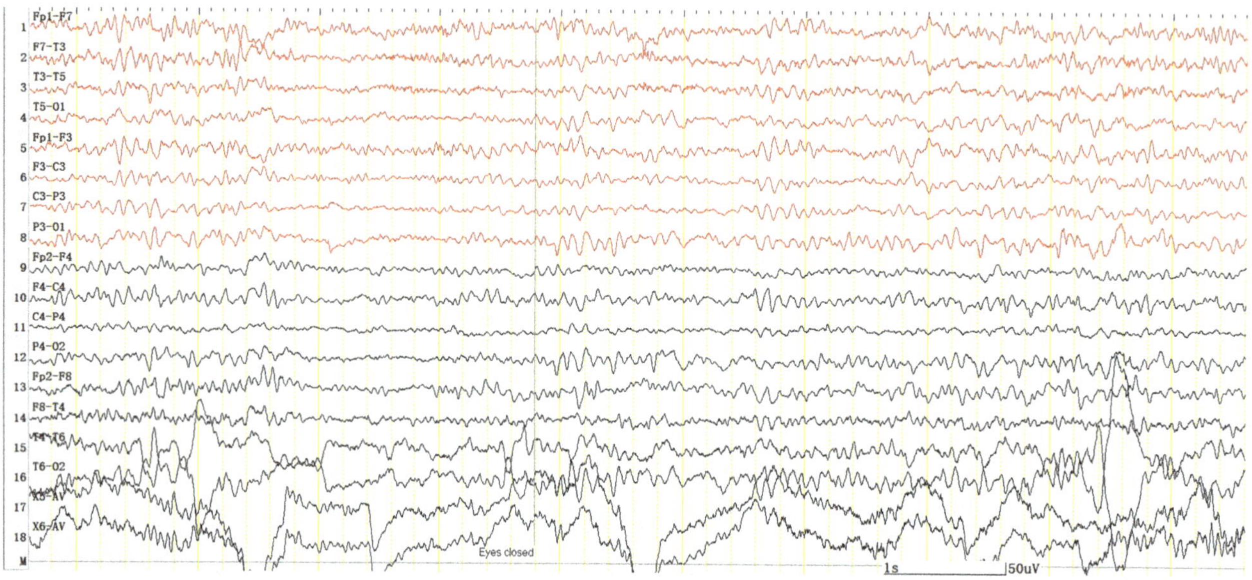

FIGURE 4 | There was no epileptic discharge in VEEG 10 min after the administration of midazolam, and the background rhythm was about 8 Hz. X5, outer eyelid; X6, upper eyelid. SEN: 10 μV; HF: 70; TC: 0.1.

The characteristic epileptic discharge appears within 1–3 s after eye closure and lasts 1–4 s. However, the discharge does not last for the whole time after eye closure. This is a called ECS, and it is different from fixation-off sensitivity (FOS). In FOS, the epileptic discharges persist for the whole duration of eye closure and disappear till eye opening (11). In this case, the abnormal discharges persisted and became more pronounced after eye closure. Vaudano et al. (12) conducted a detailed study of the eyelid myoclonus visual system and found that patients with EMA had abnormal changes at the anatomical and functional level. In patients with EMA, the gray matter content in bilateral peripheral calcarine cortex increased, demonstrating hyperexcitability of the primary visual cortex and impaired intracortical inhibition in photosensitive patients (13). The increased activity of the posterior thalamus and dysfunction of the occipital cortex are involved in the pathogenesis of ECS (14). In patients with EMA, hemodynamic demands of the parietal cortex increase during eye movement, especially around the intraparietal sulcus, which is a network structure that participates in the photoparoxysmal response (PPR) (15). Combined with this case, the patient had eyelid myoclonus status accompanied by continuous blinking or eye closing, so the ECS phenomenon exists in continuous discharge and was covered by a mass of abnormal discharges. We speculated that the frequent blinking action was both manifestation and triggering factors in myoclonic eyelid status.

The eyelid myoclonus patients are photosensitive. That is a characteristic, an abnormal EEG change called photoparoxysmal response, and occurs in about 75% of patients. It can cause episodic symptoms (10). Prolonged IPS stimulation may induce generalized seizures, so patients with a lower IPS onset threshold should be closely monitored. Patients may have one or more IPS-related seizures, such as juvenile myoclonic epilepsy (JME), absence seizures, childhood epilepsy with occipital paroxysms, generalized tonic–clonic seizures, etc. However, routine IPS may not be sufficient to provoke photosensitive seizures. Therefore, the positive rate can be increased by sleep deprivation or prolonged IPS (16). Siniatchkin et al. (17) demonstrated that PPR is associated with increased excitability in the occipital cortex. The increased excitability in the occipital cortex may explain the abnormal response of the occipital cortex to visual input, including super excitation of the occipital cortex during IPS. Surprisingly, after the patient had 2, 4, 6, 8, 10, 12, 14, and 16-Hz IPS, her seizures and epileptic discharges reduced or stopped. We had three extrapolations: First, the frequent blinking action was both a manifestation of eyelid myoclonic seizures and a triggering factor, continuous blinking action led to repeated eye closing movements, resulting in continuous epileptic discharge. When performing IPS, the patients kept their eyes open (we ask patients to keep their eyes open as much as possible), so the blinking movement, epileptic discharges, and seizures reduced. This was consistent with the report of Dede et al. (18). Moreover, a previous study suggested that the eye closure mechanism may be a more potent precipitating factor than photosensitivity in the pathophysiology of EMA (8). Second, because of the neuronal exhaustion during SE, the patient could not respond to IPS. Third, it is just a coincidence because there are natural fluctuations during SE. Therefore, further investigation of the eyelid myoclonic status is urgently needed.

As the intensity of the IPS increases, the cortical excitability of the patient increases, leading to increased epileptic discharges. Just like this case, the patient had eye blinking movement again after 16 Hz and besides, 7 min. After given the stimulation at 20 Hz, the children developed an occipital initiated tonic–clonic seizures called photo-convulsive responses. It demonstrated that after sufficient IPS stimulation, the occiput cortex became excited and initiated a brain network, including the thalamic–cortex and brainstem, leading to diffuse brain discharge and tonic–clonic seizures (5, 19). So the discovery of focal discharges interictal and ictal posterior in eyelid myoclonus patients had led to the hypothesis that EMA was a generalized epilepsy induced by the occipital cortex (4). This hypothesis was validated by Dr. Lee's report of a patient with eyelid myoclonus who developed occipital tonic–clonic seizures following photic stimulation (19). Many epilepsies or epileptic syndromes have a visual aura. Gungor-Tuncer et al. had observed 11 cases of IGE patients with visual aura, including absence of seizures, eyelid myoclonia, eyelid myoclonia with absences, juvenile absence epilepsy, juvenile myoclonic epilepsy, and visual reflex seizures. One of the patients showed up with occipital-originating ictal after IPS (5). Viravan et al. had found two electroencephalographic features in EMA patients in their study; in males, there were predominant epileptic discharges in the frontal, and the clinical manifestations were eyelid myoclonia, and the eyes were rolling up. In the female group, there were predominant epileptic discharges in the occipital with eyelid myoclonia alone, but their eyelid myoclonia is associated with eyes rolling up or absences when their epileptic discharges spread to involve the frontal lobe. However, both the frontal and occipital lobes could trigger generalized discharges and generalized epileptic seizures through either transcortical or thalamocortical pathways (20). Taylor et al. had reported the coexistence of patients with idiopathic generalized epilepsies and photosensitive occipital lobe epilepsy in the same family, and also reported electroclinical features that suggest overlap between idiopathic generalized epilepsies and photosensitive occipital lobe epilepsy. these diseases share common genetic determinants and complex genetic characteristics. the coexistence of generalized and focal seizures within families suggests that rigid clinical distinctions between these groups may not hold true (21, 22).

After patients had a seizure onset, the eyelid myoclonus status symptoms disappeared, the epileptic discharge on EEG also decreased significantly, and even disappeared completely. However, 30 min after onset, the patient's EEG showed epileptic discharge again and gradually increased to the initial state-continuous discharge (1 hour after onset) but the patient's clinical symptom is not obvious with eyelid jerk, but patient drowsiness and consciousness impairment, indicating that the patient was experiencing a non-convulsive status. So we gave the patient midazolam intravenous. The discharge showed in EEG improved significantly after 3 min and completely disappeared after 10 min. The patient had a complete recovery of symptoms, normal communication, normal behavior, and activities. Epileptic status (SE) is a condition resulting from the failure of the mechanisms responsible for seizure termination or the initiation of mechanisms, leading to abnormally prolonged seizures defined by the International Anti-Epilepsy Alliance (23). In other words, it is caused by excessive excitement or the loss of endogenous inhibition mechanisms during seizures. These changes led to the transformation of a single epileptic seizure into the epileptic status and drug resistance (24). Two operational time points, T1 and T2, for epileptic status are proposed. T1 represents the time to start treatment, and T2 represents the time when adverse outcomes (including neuronal death, neuronal damage, and changes in neuronal networks) are likely to occur. Based on preclinical and clinical studies, these two time points are 5 min for T1 and 30 min for T2 (23). SE is a neurological emergency requiring urgent antiepileptic therapy and rapid treatment. Benzodiazepines are the first choice for SE, then antiepileptic drugs and even anesthetics. The prognosis depends on the etiology, age, and course of the disease. Therefore, the patient should be carefully evaluated, and an appropriate treatment plan should selected (25). Apparently, this patient had a significant response to midazolam. She had obvious relief within 3 min after medication. The etiology of ES includes symptoms such as stroke, intoxication, malaria, encephalitis, etc., in the acute phase; posttraumatic, postencephalitic, poststroke, etc., in the remote phase; and brain tumor, Lafora's disease, dementias, neurodegenerative, metabolic, neurogenetic, malignant and neurocutaneous disease in the progressive phase. Idiopathic/cryptogenic SE is referred to as status epilepticus in a patient without a clear cause (23, 26).

Clinically, eyelid myoclonus with absence has some similarities with typical absence epilepsy. Absence epilepsy may also be accompanied by rhythmic eyelid twitching, but the blinking is not the first or most crucial movement, and the EEG in the seizure phase presents as a 3-Hz spike–slow wave, which flares up and stops with normal background activity (27). In typical absence epilepsy patients, absence seizures last longer than eyelid myoclonus and have a more severe impairment of consciousness. Eyelid myoclonus seizures with or without absence are often produced by eye closing or photo stimulation. In addition, the triggering neural network of the two seizures are different. Studies had shown that in absence patients, the epileptic discharges start in the thalamus before the cortex, and the triggering area was in a specific region of the thalamic–cortical system (28, 29). In EMA, PPR is produced from the occipital cortex or frontal cortex (12). Eye closure and IPS can activate the occipital cortex and spread the excitabilities to the brainstem to produce EM (4). However, recent studies have shown that absence epilepsy in children may be transformed into eyelid myoclonic epilepsy, and it is speculated that the sensitivity changes of brain networks in epilepsy patients have a specific time cycle, such as childhood and adolescence, and epilepsy syndrome can evolve dynamically with changes in age and different sensitivities. For example, absence epilepsy can evolve into juvenile myoclonic epilepsy, and eyelid myoclonic epilepsy can also evolve into juvenile myoclonic epilepsy (30).

Eyelid myoclonus with or without absence should be differentiated from other idiopathic, cryptogenic, or symptomatic epilepsy (12). Sunflower syndrome is a reflex seizure. The main clinical manifestations are typically eyelid myoclonia with or without absence seizures triggered when patients wave their hands in front of the sun. Eyelid myoclonus is a genetic disorder. Mutations or deletions of related genes have been reported in eyelid myoclonus, such as RORB gene (31),

KIAA2022 gene (32), GLUT1 gene (33), and NAA10 gene (34). Therefore, the pathogenic genes can be confirmed by genetic testing. Some photosensitive IGE needs to be differentiated from EMA, such as juvenile myoclonic epilepsy (JME). JME is a heterogenetic generalized epilepsy (GGE) syndrome that begins at puberty and characterized by myoclonic convulsions, mainly in the upper extremities. It can be accompanied by tonic-clonic seizures (TCS), absence, PPR, ECS, and EM. Myoclonus occurs after frequent awakening from sleep (35). The EEG is more likely to detect abnormalities in the morning, and sleep EEG always shows epileptic discharges (11). Idiopathic photosensitive occipital lobe epilepsy is a rare but well-defined syndrome in the group of idiopathic focal epilepsies. It is characterized by changes in vision, including hallucinations, complex hallucinations, blindness, or both. Simple vision is common (two thirds of cases); eyelid closure and blinking, secondary generalized tonic–clonic seizures (GTCs), and complex focal seizures have also been reported in patients with idiopathic photosensitive occipital lobe epilepsy. Intermittent luminous stimulation can also trigger epileptic seizures. Unlike EMA, interictal EEG showed that occipital paroxysms occur when the eyes are closed, and disappear or attenuated when eyes are opened. Therefore, electroencephalogram is a good test to distinguish between EMA and idiopathic photosensitive occipital lobe epilepsy (36).

Valproic acid monotherapy is the most effective treatment for eyelid myoclonus with or without absence, which should be considered early. Patients who cannot tolerate valproic acid, lamotrigine, or a combination should be considered. Previous studies had shown that levetiracetam monotherapy, even at high doses, was unlikely to be effective (37). Verrotti et al. first proved that VPA monotherapy was very effective for both seizure outcome and photosensitive (PS) reduction or abolition in adolescents with photosensitive epilepsy with generalized tonic–clonic seizures (EGTCS). In their study, seizures disappeared in 69.1% of patients, and PS disappeared in 52.7% of patients after 6 months of treatment. During valproic acid treatment, seizures were more easily controlled than PS, but the potential of epileptic discharge could be revealed by IPS. Consequently, they argued that control of PPR in EGTCS patients might be a prognostic factor for better seizure control. VPA therapy may be more effective in generalized seizures than PPR, since PPR is the initial point of occipital discharge (38). A recent retrospective analysis of GGE patients also showed that valproic acid effectively reduced spike–slow waves induced by spontaneous and hyperventilation, but not in inhibiting spike–slow wave induced by IPS (9). It has also been mentioned that EM was an age-related electrical clinical manifestation that tends to disappear between 15 and 18 years old, even if the patient previously had only a partial response to different treatments (35). Studies have shown that photosensitivity, ECS, and family history can be used as prognostic indicators of eyelid myoclonus. The persistence of photosensitivity and ECS indicates the possibility of an epileptic seizure, and positive family history is a benign indicator (6). Therefore, it demonstrates the importance of EEG in the diagnosis and prognosis evaluation of EMS.

Patients with eyelid myoclonic seizures are often getting the attention of the patient or family for generalized tonic–clonic seizures, which usually occur at age 12. It also proves that the early diagnosis of Jeavons can be easily missed or even misdiagnosed, leading to the wrong antiepileptic, such as carbamazepine, which could actually exacerbate the disease (24). Like the girl in this case, she had a history of four convulsions in the 1.5 years before this visit. However, the patient's family did not follow the doctor's advice for a systematic examination, and thus, no diagnosis was given, which eventually led to the patient's epileptic status. Therefore, the enlightenment to us is that doctors should actively educate, encourage, and guide patients and their families to actively face the disease because early recognition of the disease has a significant impact on the prognosis and treatment.

CONCLUSION

Eyelid myoclonus with or without absence epilepsy is a relatively rare type of epilepsy in clinical practice. It is necessary to enhance doctors' awareness about this disease and improve the detection rate. The occurrence of eyelid myoclonus status is rarer, and it is rarely reported.

AUTHOR CONTRIBUTIONS

YY and HW designed and guided the work. YY collected the case and drafted the article. FY and YF collected and analyzed the case. LH and QW analyzed and followed-up the case. XL guided interpretation and revision of manuscript. All authors contributed to the article and approved the submitted version.

REFERENCES

1. Striano S, Capovilla G, Sofia V, Romeo A, Rubboli G, Striano P, et al. Eyelid myoclonia with absences (Jeavons syndrome): a well-defined idiopathic generalized epilepsy syndrome or a spectrum of photosensitive conditions? *Epilepsia.* (2009) 50(Suppl. 5):15–9. doi: 10.1111/j.1528-1167.2009.02114.x
2. Green JB. Seizures on closing the eyes. Electroencephalographic studies. *Neurology.* (1968) 18:391–6. doi: 10.1212/WNL.18.4.391
3. Panayiotopoulos CP. Syndromes of idiopathic generalized epilepsies not recognized by the international league against epilepsy. *Epilepsia.* (2005) 46(Suppl. 9):57–66. doi: 10.1111/j.1528-1167.2005.00314.x
4. Viravan S, Go C, Ochi A, Akiyama T, Carter Snead 3rd O, Otsubo H. Jeavons syndrome existing as occipital cortex initiating generalized epilepsy. *Epilepsia.* (2011) 52:1273–9. doi: 10.1111/j.1528-1167.2011.03068.x
5. Gungor-Tuncer O, Baykan B, Altindag E, Bebek N, Gurses C, Gokyigit A. Prevalence and characteristics of visual aura in idiopathic generalized epilepsy. *Epilepsy Behav.* (2012) 25:573–6. doi: 10.1016/j.yebeh.2012.09.004
6. Giuliano L, Fatuzzo D, Mainieri G, Maira G, Elia M, Ferlazzo E, et al. Eyelid myoclonia with absences: electroclinical features and prognostic factors. *Epilepsia.* (2019) 60:1104–13. doi: 10.1111/epi.15157
7. Veggiotti P, Viri M, Lanzi G. Electrical status epilepticus on eye closure: acase report. *Neurophysiol Clin.* (1992) 22:281–6. doi: 10.1016/S0987-7053(05)80260-6
8. Wakamoto H, Nagao H, Manabe K, Kobayashi H, Hayashi M. Nonconvulsive status epilepticus in eyelid myoclonia with absences–evidence of provocation unrelated to photosensitivity. *Neuropediatrics.* (1999) 30:149–50. doi: 10.1055/s-2007-973481
9. Oguz Akarsu E, Tekturk P, Yapici Z, Tepgec F, Uyguner ZO, Baykan B. Eyelid myoclonic status epilepticus: a rare phenotype in spinal muscular atrophy

with progressive myoclonic epilepsy associated with ASAH1 gene mutation. *Seizure.* (2016) 42:49–51. doi: 10.1016/j.seizure.2016.09.007
10. Padmanaban V, Inati S, Ksendzovsky A, Zaghloul K. Clinical advances in photosensitive epilepsy. *Brain Res.* (2019) 1703:18–25. doi: 10.1016/j.brainres.2018.07.025
11. Seneviratne U, Cook MJ, D'Souza WJ. Electroencephalography in the diagnosis of genetic generalized epilepsy syndromes. *Front Neurol.* (2017) 8:499. doi: 10.3389/fneur.2017.00499
12. Vaudano AE, Ruggieri A, Tondelli M, Avanzini P, Benuzzi F, Gessaroli G, et al. The visual system in eyelid myoclonia with absences. *Ann Neurol.* (2014) 76:412–27. doi: 10.1002/ana.24236
13. Strigaro G, Prandi P, Varrasi C, Monaco F, Cantello R. Defective visual inhibition in photosensitive idiopathic generalized epilepsy. *Epilepsia.* (2012) 53:695–704. doi: 10.1111/j.1528-1167.2012.03411.x
14. Sevgi EB, Saygi S, Ciger A. Eye closure sensitivity and epileptic syndromes: a retrospective study of 26 adult cases. *Seizure.* (2007) 16:17–21. doi: 10.1016/j.seizure.2006.09.004
15. Wilkins AJ, Bonanni P, Porciatti V, Guerrini R. Physiology of human photosensitivity. *Epilepsia.* (2004) 45(Suppl. 1):7–13. doi: 10.1111/j.0013-9580.2004.451009.x
16. Okudan ZV, Ozkara C. Reflex epilepsy: triggers and management strategies. *Neuropsychiatr Dis Treat.* (2018) 14:327–37. doi: 10.2147/NDT.S107669
17. Siniatchkin M, Groppa S, Jerosch B, Muhle H, Kurth C, Shepherd AJ, et al. Spreading photoparoxysmal EEG response is associated with an abnormal cortical excitability pattern. *Brain.* (2007) 130(Pt 1):78–87. doi: 10.1093/brain/awl306
18. Dede HO, Bebek N, Emekli S, Baykan B, Yapici Z, Gokyigit A. The clinical significance and electrophysiologic findings of fixation-off and closure of the eyes sensitivity: Data from a prospective unselected population. *Epilepsy Res.* (2021) 170:106541. doi: 10.1016/j.eplepsyres.2020.106541
19. Giraldez BG, Serratosa JM. Jeavons syndrome as an occipital cortex initiated generalized epilepsy: further evidence from a patient with a photic-induced occipital seizure. *Seizure.* (2015) 32:72–4. doi: 10.1016/j.seizure.2015.09.003
20. Wang XL, Bao JX, Liang-Shi, Tie-Ma, Deng YC, Zhao G, et al. Jeavons syndrome in China. *Epilepsy Behav.* (2014) 32:64–71. doi: 10.1016/j.yebeh.2013.12.016
21. Koepp MJ, Caciagli L, Pressler RM, Lehnertz K, Beniczky S. Reflex seizures, traits, and epilepsies: from physiology to pathology. *Lancet Neurol.* (2016) 15:92–105. doi: 10.1016/S1474-4422(15)00219-7
22. Taylor I, Berkovic SF, Scheffer IE. Genetics of epilepsy syndromes in families with photosensitivity. *Neurology.* (2013) 80:1322–9. doi: 10.1212/WNL.0b013e31828ab349
23. Trinka E, Cock H, Hesdorffer D, Rossetti AO, Scheffer IE, Shinnar S, et al. Definition and classification of status epilepticus–Report of the ILAE task force on classification of status epilepticus. *Epilepsia.* (2015) 56:1515–23. doi: 10.1111/epi.13121
24. Betjemann JP, Lowenstein DH. Status epilepticus in adults. *Lancet Neurol.* (2015) 14:615–24. doi: 10.1016/S1474-4422(15)00042-3
25. Santamarina E, Abraira L, Toledo M. Update in status epilepticus. *Med Clin.* (2019) 153:70–7. doi: 10.1016/j.medcle.2019.05.002
26. Chiarello D, Duranti F, Lividini A, Maltoni L, Spadoni C, Taormina S, et al. Clinical characterization of status epilepticus in childhood: a retrospective study in 124 patients. *Seizure.* (2020) 78:127–33. doi: 10.1016/j.seizure.2020.03.019
27. Wolf P, Goosses R. Relation of photosensitivity to epileptic syndromes. *J Neurol Neurosurg Psychiatry.* (1986) 49:1386–91. doi: 10.1136/jnnp.49.12.1386
28. Duncan JS. Idiopathic generalized epilepsies with typical absences. *J Neurol.* (1997) 244:403–11. doi: 10.1007/s004150050113
29. Mazzocchetti C, Striano P, Verrotti A. How to select the appropriate pharmacotherapy for absence seizures in children. *Expert Opin Pharmacother.* (2018) 19:1045–7. doi: 10.1080/14656566.2018.1484902
30. Galli J, Micheletti S, Malerba L, Fazzi E, Giordano L. Childhood absence epilepsy evolving to eyelid myoclonia with absence epilepsy. *Seizure.* (2018) 61:1–3. doi: 10.1016/j.seizure.2018.07.009
31. Morea A, Boero G, Demaio V, Francavilla T, La Neve A. Eyelid myoclonia with absences, intellectual disability and attention deficit hyperactivity disorder: a clinical phenotype of the RORB gene mutation. *Neurol Sci.* (2021). doi: 10.1007/s10072-020-05031-y
32. Samanta D, Willis E. KIAA2022-related disorders can cause jeavons (eyelid myoclonia with absence) syndrome. *Acta Neurol Belg.* (2020) 120:205–7. doi: 10.1007/s13760-018-0887-y
33. Madaan P, Jauhari P, Chakrabarty B, Gulati S. Jeavons syndrome in a family with GLUT1-deficiency syndrome. *Seizure.* (2019) 71:158–60. doi: 10.1016/j.seizure.2019.07.011
34. Valentine V, Sogawa Y, Rajan D, Ortiz D. A case of de novo NAA10 mutation presenting with eyelid myoclonias (AKA Jeavons syndrome). *Seizure.* (2018) 60:120–2. doi: 10.1016/j.seizure.2018.06.008
35. Uchida C, de Carvalho KC, Guaranha M, Guilhoto L, de Araujo FG, Yacubian E. Prognosis of juvenile myoclonic epilepsy with eye-closure sensitivity. *Seizure.* (2018) 62:17–25. doi: 10.1016/j.seizure.2018.09.006
36. Khiari HM, Chehaider HB, Mrabet A. Childhood occipital epilepsy of gastaut: a case report. *Tunis Med.* (2010) 88:516–8. doi: 10.1016/j.jaac.2018.02.017
37. Baumer FM, Porter BE. Clinical and electrographic features of sunflower syndrome. *Epilepsy Res.* (2018) 142:58–63. doi: 10.1016/j.eplepsyres.2018.03.002
38. Verrotti A, Grosso S, D'Egidio C, Parisi P, Spalice A, Pavone P, et al. Valproate in adolescents with photosensitive epilepsy with generalized tonic-clonic seizures only. *Eur J Paediatr Neurol.* (2014) 18:13–8. doi: 10.1016/j.ejpn.2013.06.006

32

Case Report: Responsive Neurostimulation of the Centromedian Thalamic Nucleus for the Detection and Treatment of Seizures in Pediatric Primary Generalized Epilepsy

William P. Welch[1], *Jasmine L. Hect*[2] *and Taylor J. Abel*[2,3*]

[1] Division of Pediatric Neurology, Department of Pediatrics, University of Pittsburgh School of Medicine, Pittsburgh, PA, United States, [2] Department of Neurological Surgery, University of Pittsburgh School of Medicine, Pittsburgh, PA, United States, [3] Department of Bioengineering, University of Pittsburgh Swanson School of Engineering, Pittsburgh, PA, United States

***Correspondence:**
Taylor J. Abel
abeltj@upmc.edu

Up to 20% of pediatric patients with primary generalized epilepsy (PGE) will not respond effectively to medication for seizure control. Responsive neurostimulation (RNS) is a promising therapy for pediatric patients with drug-resistant epilepsy and has been shown to be an effective therapy for reducing seizure frequency and severity in adult patients. RNS of the centromedian nucleus of the thalamus may help to prevent loss of awareness during seizure activity in PGE patients with absence seizures. Here we present a 16-year-old male, with drug-resistant PGE with absence seizures, characterized by 3 Hz spike-and-slow-wave discharges on EEG, who achieved a 75% reduction in seizure frequency following bilateral RNS of the centromedian nuclei. At 6-months post-implant, this patient reported complete resolution of the baseline daily absence seizure activity, and decrease from 3–4 generalized convulsive seizures per month to 1 per month. RNS recordings showed well-formed 3 Hz spike-wave discharges in bilateral CM nuclei, further supporting the notion that clinically relevant ictal discharges in PGE can be detected in CM. This report demonstrates that CM RNS can detect PGE-related seizures in the CM nucleus and deliver therapeutic stimulation.

Keywords: case report, responsive neurostimulation, drug-resistant epilepsy, centromedian nucleus, pediatric generalized epilepsy, absence seizures

INTRODUCTION

Primary generalized epilepsy (PGE) accounts for ∼15–20% of all children diagnosed with epilepsy (1, 2). Of patients with PGE, 10–20% will meet criteria for drug-resistant epilepsy (3). Unfortunately, there are no FDA-approved neuromodulation treatment options for PGE. Absence seizures are commonly seen in patients with PGE in the form of behavioral arrest with impaired awareness, with concomitant variable motor or behavioral manifestations. Uncontrolled seizures are a significant source of morbidity in PGE, impacting development, academic performance, activities of daily living, and quality of life measures (4–7). Investigation and validation of neuromodulation treatment options for pediatric PGE are necessary to improve patient outcomes and quality of life.

Stimulation of the thalamic centromedian nucleus (CM) is associated with improved frequency and severity of generalized seizures in adult patients, including both deep brain (DBS) stimulation and responsive neurostimulation (RNS) system approaches (8, 9). There is supportive evidence for the use of deep brain stimulation (DBS) in pediatric epilepsy, although data is limited (10, 11). A limitation of DBS devices is that while they are able to deliver programmed stimulation in an open-loop system, they lack the functionality to record or respond to changes in brain activity and, therefore, cannot be programmed to deliver personalized therapy in response to patient-specific seizure patterns (12). The closed-loop RNS system has the functionality of recording and storing patient-specific neuronal activity and can be programmed to deliver stimulation in response to detected changes during seizure activity. RNS has been shown to be safe and effective in the treatment of drug-resistant epilepsy (13, 14). Here, we report the diagnostic utility and outcome of bilateral CMN thalamic RNS implantation in a single pediatric patient for the treatment of PGE.

PATIENT INFORMATION

A 16-year-old male diagnosed with childhood absence epilepsy (CAE) at 4 years of age presented for evaluation for uncontrolled seizures. At the time of diagnosis, he was an otherwise healthy and developmentally appropriate child with no family history of significant neurological disease or parental consanguinity. Genetic testing was not performed at our institution during his evaluation. Initial seizure semiology consisted of behavioral arrest, eye rolling, and variable impaired awareness, with rare progression to bilateral tonic-clonic seizure. Initial EEG captured typical absence seizures with correlating 3 Hz spike-and-slow-wave discharges, as well as interictal high-amplitude spike- and polyspike-and-slow-wave discharges. Repeat EEG over several years remained consistent with this diagnosis. Seizures proved resistant to treatment with ethosuximide, lamotrigine, topiramate, clobazam, valproate, and the modified Atkin's diet. At 12 years of age, repeat brain MRI detected a lesion in the right amygdala suggestive of dysembryoplastic neuroepithelial tumor (DNET). Repeat routine EEG while on medications again demonstrated generalized spike- and polyspike-and-slow-wave discharges and typical absence seizures, with new findings of independent bilateral centroparietal and centrotemporal epileptiform discharges. Additionally, a focal impaired awareness seizure with temporal semiology was captured on prolonged EEG which was electroclinically distinct from his typical absence seizures, with onset characterized by rhythmic theta activity over the left temporal head region and clinical accompaniment speech difficulty, confusion, and oral automatisms lasting over 9 min.

Due to new neuroradiologic and EEG findings, phase 2 pre-surgical evaluation was pursued. Fourteen sEEG electrodes were implanted targeting the right temporal lobe (including the right amygdala lesion) and cingulate, and left hippocampus. Prior to and during weaning of anti-seizure medications, numerous typical absence seizures were captured. Electrographic onset was not localizable, with diffuse onset of 2.5–3.0 Hz spike-wave morphology throughout the intracranial array, including the bilateral hippocampal electrodes. Interestingly, independent rare bursts of 2.5–3.0 Hz spike-wave discharges were detected in peri-lesional contacts in the right amygdala, but never evolving to electrographic seizures.

Robot-assisted stereotactic biopsy of the amygdala lesion was performed at the time of sEEG electrode removal, which was negative due to small sample size. However, given the progression of the lesion and presence of peri-lesional epileptiform activity, stereotactic laser ablation (SLA) of the lesion was performed with simultaneous redo stereotactic biopsy. The redo biopsy was consistent with a low grade glioneuronal neoplasm, however given the small volume of the biopsy, a more specified diagnosis (e.g., DNET was not achieved). A complete ablation of the lesion was achieved. After surgical recovery, the patient continued to have daily typical absence seizures, with occasional progression to bilateral tonic-clonic seizure, despite continuation of prior anti-seizure medications. Given continuance of seizures despite best medical management, vagus nerve stimulation (VNS) was discussed with the family, who were not interested in VNS. CM RNS was thus offered to the family and after discussion of the risks and potential benefits the patient and family elected to proceed.

THERAPEUTIC INTERVENTION

The patient was taken to the operating room for implantation of bilateral CM RNS electrodes. CM targeting was performed using indirect and direct targeting as previously described (10, 15–17). Briefly, MP2RAGE inversion images were merged to a preoperative thin-cut (1 mm) CT angiogram using the ROSA platform. Standard entry points near the coronal suture that would allow an avascular trajectory to the target were selected. Four-contact depth electrodes, with 3.5-mm spacing, were implanted with these trajectories using the ROSA robot (registered via bone fiducials), following previously published methods (18). Intraoperative O-Arm CT scan was used for both registration to bone fiducials and confirmation of final electrode lead position in the CM. RNS-electrodes were automatically pre-localized in native & template space using Lead-DBS software (19) (https://www.lead-dbs.org) and visualized in reference to thalamic nuclei defined by The Thalamus Atlas (20), see **Figure 1**. The patient recovered and was discharged home on postoperative day 1.

After implantation, the device was programmed to record scheduled electrocorticography (ECoG), and a broad detector was programmed (75% power change). Multiple ECoG recordings were saved for patient/caregiver event identification (via magnet swipe) over a period of 4 weeks postop. Review of saved ECoG in the Patient Data Management System (PDMS) revealed well-formed 3 Hz spike-wave discharges in the bilateral thalamic contacts, with highest amplitudes in the distal contacts bilaterally (**Figure 2**). Four weeks after implantation, the detection pattern was adjusted to reliably detect ictal discharges (channel 1: bandpass 2.0–41.7 Hz, amplitude threshold 4%, minimum duration 0.38 s; channel 3: bandpass

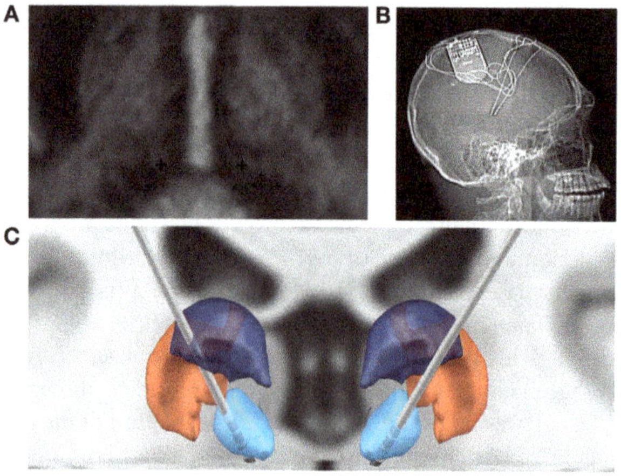

FIGURE 1 | Bilateral RNS CMN implantation. **(A)** Direct targeting of the bilateral CMN (crosses) in AC-PC orientation. **(B)** Post-implant x-ray of RNS system. **(C)** Coronal 3D reconstruction of bilateral RNS implantation targeting the CMN (blue), in relation to the posterior part of the ventral posterolateral nucleus (VPLp; red) and posterior dorsal part of the ventral lateral nucleus (VLpd; purple).

2.0–25 Hz, amplitude threshold 5%, minimum duration 0.38 s). Bipolar stimulation of most distal contacts (contact 1 and 2 bilaterally) was enabled at 0.2 $\mu C/Cm^2$ (0.2 mA, 125 Hz, 160 µS for 5,000 ms), in response to detected 3 Hz spike-wave discharges in these channels. Low charge density was used initially due to patient reporting non-painful left arm paresthesia during stimulation. Additionally, ECOG recordings captured prolonged absence seizure and generalized tonic-clonic seizure activity, see **Figure 3**.

FOLLOW-UP AND OUTCOMES

One month after turning on stimulation, the patient reported improved seizure frequency, although continued to experience multiple weekly absence seizures. At that time, our patient elected to increase stimulation and was willing to tolerate mild left arm paresthesia along with this this increase to 0.4 $\mu C/Cm^2$ (0.4 mA, 125 Hz, 160 µS for 5,000 ms). These paresthesias resolved within a few days of stimulation. Changes to other stimulation parameters were not considered due to the fact that this patient's symptoms were mild and temporary, but may be considered in other cases (21).

At most recent follow-up 6-months post-implant, the patient and family reported no noticeable absence seizures and reported 1 generalized convulsive seizure per month, improved from previous baseline of 3 to 4 per month. Our patient is tolerating increased stimulation parameters with a charge density of 1.5 $\mu C/Cm^2$ (1.5 mA, 125 Hz, 160 µS for 5,000 ms) without side effects, including resolution of left arm paresthesia. Long Episodes were detected at a rate of 4.4/month, with an average of 441 therapies delivered per day. Repeat scalp EEG has not yet been performed.

DISCUSSION

Here we describe the first pediatric PGE patient with absence seizures successfully recorded from bilateral CM RNS, and report on successful RNS targeting absence seizures in drug-resistant CAE. This patient experienced decreased seizure frequency at 1-month follow-up, and patient and family reports resolution of detectable absence seizures as well as 75% reduction in generalized convulsive seizures at 6-month follow up. Our findings suggest that CM RNS can prevent loss of consciousness through disruption of low-frequency thalamocortical ictal recruitment.

RNS is a promising technology which offers personalized therapy based on a patient's own seizure electrophysiology by recording and responding to neural activity through delivery of programmable stimulation directly to seizure foci. Several multi-center outcomes studies have demonstrated the efficacy of the RNS system for the treatment of drug-resistant mesial temporal or neocortical seizures, in which 70% of patients saw a 78% reduction in seizure frequency at 6 years (13, 22–24). While the data captured by the RNS system remains computationally intensive to interpret, there are considerable, promising advances being made in the field to improve RNS as a patient-specific therapy (12, 25). In line with this, bilateral centromedian/ventrolateral thalamic RNS in an adult patient was successful in the treatment of generalized epilepsy (eyelid myoclonia with absence) (26). We provide further evidence to support RNS therapy as a safe and effective treatment option for drug-resistant PGE for pediatric patients and the CM as a targetable foci.

The CM receives converging input from the cortex, basal ganglia, and brainstem and participates in cognition (attention and arousal) and sensorimotor coordination (27). Thalamocortical feedback loops regulate cortical input during wakefulness to maintain attention and awareness and its suppression is implicated in the pathogenesis of CAE (27–31). The loss of awareness associated with absence seizures is theorized to occur during electrical perturbations in this feedback loop, such as seen in the aberrant low frequency thalamocortical signaling that is characteristic of absence seizures (29, 30, 32, 33). Neurostimulation of the CM disrupts the low-frequency ictal thalamocortical recruitment and may therefore help to prevent loss of awareness during seizure activity (31, 34). Leveraging the diffuse connectivity profile of this region, the CM has been successfully targeted by DBS for the treatment of drug-resistant PGE (8, 9, 15, 35, 36). RNS stimulation of the CM has been applied in adult patients for the treatment of drug-resistant regional neocortical epilepsy (37), generalized epilepsy (26), Lennox-Gastaut Syndrome (10, 38), and drug-resistant focal onset-seizures (39). Seizure frequency of patients with implanted RNS systems often continues to improve over months to years, which implicates the role of neural plasticity induced by programmable closed-loop stimulation (16, 23). Further research is needed to better understand the mechanisms underlying the clinical benefits of RNS CM stimulation for the treatment of CAE. We show here that the RNS targeting of the CM in this pediatric patient was able to reliably identify ictal discharges and

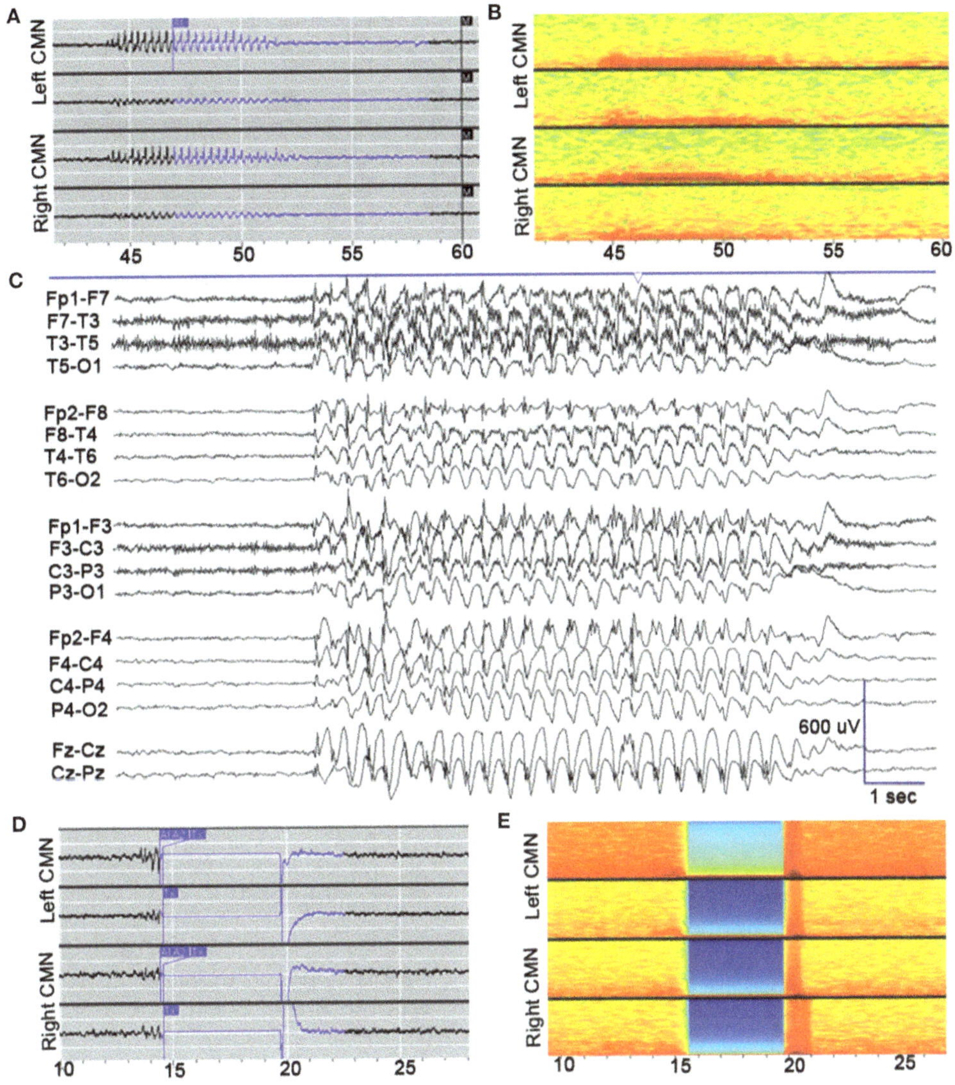

FIGURE 2 | Electrophysiological seizure characteristics. **(A)** Example of an electroclinical seizure stored the NeuroPace Patient Data Management System, detected by device (*A1*) and noted by patient's family with magnet swipe (*M*). Well-formed 3 Hz spike-and-wave discharges are detected maximally in channels 1 (LCM1–LCM2; top row) and 3 (RCM1–RCM2; third row). **(B)** Spectrogram of identical epoch. **(C)** Pre-implantation scalp EEG, capturing electroclinical typical absence seizure (TAS) with behavioral arrest. EEG demonstrates generalized 3 Hz spike- and polyspike-and-wave discharges (longitudinal bipolar montage; sensitivity: 30 μV/mm; timebase 30 mm/s). **(D)** Example of an electroclinical seizure stored the NeuroPace Patient Data Management System, detected by device (*A1, A2*) again detected maximally in channels 1 and 3, with responsive therapy delivered (*Tx*), subsequent amplifier artifact lasting 5 s, and return to electrographic baseline. Therapy delivered to channels 1 and 3: bipolar, current 0.4 mA, frequency 125 Hz, pulse width 160 μs, burst duration 5,000 ms, charge density 0.4 μC/cm^2. **(E)** Spectrogram of identical epoch.

improve seizure frequency through neurostimulation. Other groups have performed RNS of other targets (i.e., anterior thalamic nucleus) for the treatment of generalized epilepsy and the relative efficacy of subcortical RNS targets remains a topic for further investigation (40).

Electrophysiologic studies reveal that clinically relevant ictal discharges can be detected in the CM nucleus (16, 26). Kokkinos et al. (26), performed direct recording of the CM nucleus via RNS showing 3–5 Hz spike and wave activity consistent with their patient's preoperative EEG pattern. Warren et al. (16), performed simultaneous EEG and CM recordings during DBS implantation to examine the relationship between generalized paroxysmal fast activity (GPFA) and slow spike wave (SSW) on EEG and from direct CM recordings. In this study, 86% of GPFA events were seen in both on both scalp EEG and CM, whereas 25% of SSW was observed from both recordings. Interestingly, these recordings suggested that epileptiform activity occurred in cortex prior to CM. Further work will elucidate the interactions of cortex and CM in generalized epilepsy, but these findings suggest that clinically relevant ictal discharges are present in the CM nucleus.

The CM was targeted in this report using indirect and direct technique as previously described (10, 15–17). The CM remains difficult to demarcate on standard neuroimaging (36), however

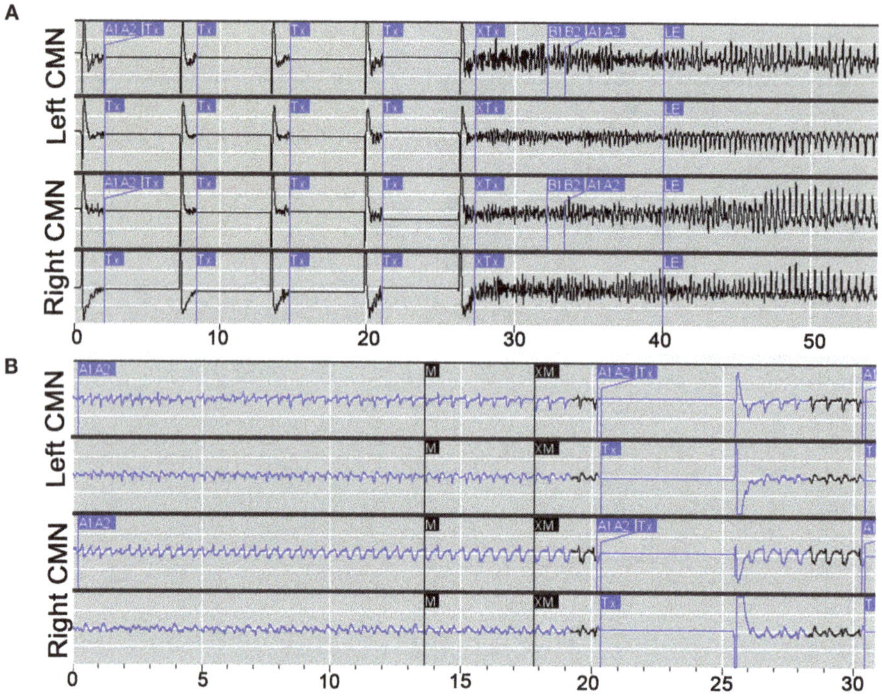

FIGURE 3 | Electrophysiological characteristics of prolonged absence and GTC seizures. **(A)** Example of an electroclinical generalized tonic clonic (GTC) seizure stored the NeuroPace Patient Data Management System, detected by device (A1, A2) and noted by patient's family with magnet swipe (M), with responsive therapy delivered (Tx). **(B)** Example of a prolonged electroclinical absence seizure stored the NeuroPace Patient Data Management System, detected by device (A1, A2) and noted by patient's family with magnet swipe (M), with responsive therapy delivered (Tx).

studies have shown that inverse MP2RAGE and quantitative susceptibility mapping (QSM) can be used to identify the nucleus with good reliability (16, 41). Confirmation of electrode placement using intraoperative microelectrode recording (MER) evaluation of the CMN neurophysiological signature has shown mixed results, given the presence of low frequency firing rate while sedated, considerable interpatient variability, and subtle differences in neural signatures between adjacent thalamic nuclei (16). Further research is needed to improve techniques for identifying thalamic subnuclei.

While this case highlights the promising utility of RNS for the treatment of complex, pediatric, drug-resistant PGE with absence seizures, the conclusions drawn are limited by the single patient sample size, short follow-up duration, and the potential under-reporting of absence seizure frequency. Repeat scalp EEG has not been performed in our patient since placement of RNS device, resulting in reliance on patient and family report for clinical absence seizure frequency. Our patient did have other seizure types emerge throughout his course, which precludes classifying his case as pure PGE, and presented unique challenges to his treatment plan. However, he originally presented with and continued to suffer from clearly well-defined typical absence seizures, which are the primary target of his RNS therapy. Successful treatment in our patient's case may highlight the possible role for thalamic RNS therapy in patients with primary generalized epilepsy as well as other cases of complex epilepsy in which cortico-thalamic networks are thought to play a large role.

The development of novel therapies for the treatment of pediatric drug-resistant PGE remain an important area of investigation. Children with PGE experience considerable burden on their quality of life and often experience cognitive, behavioral, and developmental deficits as a result of uncontrolled epilepsy during this critical period of brain development (4–7). Neocortical RNS implantation has been used successfully for the treatment of pediatric drug-resistant seizures in a few cases (42–45). Together, these provide preliminary evidence that RNS is a viable therapeutic option for patients with drug-resistant epilepsy who are not candidates for resective epilepsy surgery.

AUTHOR CONTRIBUTIONS

All authors listed have made a substantial, direct and intellectual contribution to the work, and approved it for publication.

ACKNOWLEDGMENTS

The authors acknowledge the patient and their family.

REFERENCES

1. Kwan P, Arzimanoglou A, Berg AT, Brodie MJ, Allen Hauser W, Mathern G, et al. Definition of drug resistant epilepsy: consensus proposal by the *ad hoc* task force of the ILAE commission on therapeutic strategies. *Epilepsia.* (2010) 51:1069–77. doi: 10.1111/j.1528-1167.2009.02397.x
2. Kwan P, Brodie MJ. Early identification of refractory epilepsy. *N Engl J Med.* (2000) 342:314–9. doi: 10.1056/NEJM200002033420503
3. Schuele SU, Lüders HO. Intractable epilepsy: management and therapeutic alternatives. *Lancet Neurol.* (2008) 7:514–24. doi: 10.1016/S1474-4422(08)70108-X
4. Cowan J, Baker GA. A review of subjective impact measures for use with children and adolescents with epilepsy. *Q Life Res.* (2004) 13:1435–43. doi: 10.1023/B:QURE.0000040796.54498.69
5. Caplan R, Siddarth P, Stahl L, Lanphier E, Vona P, Gurbani S, et al. Childhood absence epilepsy: behavioral, cognitive, linguistic comorbidities. *Epilepsia.* (2008) 49:1838–46. doi: 10.1111/j.1528-1167.2008.01680.x
6. Conway L, Smith ML, Ferro MA, Speechley KN, Connoly MB, Snead OC, et al. Correlates of health-related quality of life in children with drug resistant epilepsy. *Epilepsia.* (2016) 57:1256–64. doi: 10.1111/epi.13441
7. Schraegle WA, Titus JB. Executive function and health-related quality of life in pediatric epilepsy. *Epilepsy Behav.* (2016) 62:20–6. doi: 10.1016/j.yebeh.2016.06.006
8. Klinger N, Mittal S. Deep brain stimulation for seizure control in drug-resistant epilepsy. *Neurosurg Focus.* (2018) 45:E4. doi: 10.3171/2018.4.FOCUS1872
9. Zangiabadi N, Ladino LD, Sina F, Orozco-Hernández JP, Carter A, Téllez-Zenteno JF. Deep brain stimulation and drug-resistant epilepsy: a review of the literature. *Front Neurol.* (2019) 10:601. doi: 10.3389/fneur.2019.00601
10. Velasco AL, Velasco F, Jiménez F, Velasco M, Castro G, Carrillo-Ruiz JD, et al. Neuromodulation of the centromedian thalamic nuclei in the treatment of generalized seizures and the improvement of the quality of life in patients with lennox-gastaut syndrome. *Epilepsia.* (2006) 47:1203–12. doi: 10.1111/j.1528-1167.2006.00593.x
11. Yan H, Toyota E, Anderson M, Abel TJ, Donner E, Kalia SK, et al. A systematic review of deep brain stimulation for the treatment of drug-resistant epilepsy in childhood. *J Neurosurg Pediatr.* (2018) 23:274–84. doi: 10.3171/2018.9.PEDS18417
12. Sisterson ND, Wozny TA, Kokkinos V, Constantino A, Richardson RM. Closed-loop brain stimulation for drug-resistant epilepsy: towards an evidence-based approach to personalized medicine. *Neurotherapeutics.* (2019) 16:119–27. doi: 10.1007/s13311-018-00682-4
13. Jobst BC, Kapur R, Barkley GL, Bazil CW, Berg MJ, Bergey GK, et al. Brain-responsive neurostimulation in patients with medically intractable seizures arising from eloquent and other neocortical areas. *Epilepsia.* (2017) 58:1005–14. doi: 10.1111/epi.13739
14. Morrell MJ, On behalf of the RNS System in Epilepsy Study Group. Responsive cortical stimulation for the treatment of medically intractable partial epilepsy. *Neurology.* (2011) 77:1295–304. doi: 10.1212/WNL.0b013e3182302056
15. Valentín A, García Navarrete E, Chelvarajah R, Torres C, Navas M, Vico L, et al. Deep brain stimulation of the centromedian thalamic nucleus for the treatment of generalized and frontal epilepsies. *Epilepsia.* (2013) 54:1823–33. doi: 10.1111/epi.12352
16. Warren AEL, Dalic LJ, Thevathasan W, Roten A, Bulluss KJ, Archer J. Targeting the centromedian thalamic nucleus for deep brain stimulation. *J Neurol Neurosurg Psychiatry.* (2020) 91:339–49. doi: 10.1136/jnnp-2019-322030
17. Son BC, Shon YM, Choi JG, Kim JW, Kim SH, Lee SH. Clinical outcome of patients with deep brain stimulation of the centromedian thalamic nucleus for refractory epilepsy and location of the active contacts. *Stereotactic Funct Neurosurg.* (2016) 94:187–97. doi: 10.1159/000446611
18. Abel TJ, Osorio RV, Amorim-Leite R, Mathieu F, Kahane P, Minotti L, et al. Frameless robot-assisted stereoelectroencephalography in children: technical aspects and comparison with Talairach frame technique. *J Neurosurg Pediatr.* (2018) 22:37–46. doi: 10.3171/2018.1.PEDS17435
19. Horn A, Kühn AA. Lead-DBS: a toolbox for deep brain stimulation electrode localizations and visualizations. *NeuroImage.* (2015) 107:127–35. doi: 10.1016/j.neuroimage.2014.12.002
20. Krauth A, Blanc R, Poveda A, Jeanmonod D, Morel A, Székely G. A mean three-dimensional atlas of the human thalamus: generation from multiple histological data. *NeuroImage.* (2010) 49:2053–62. doi: 10.1016/j.neuroimage.2009.10.042
21. Hixon AM, Brown MG, McDermott D, Destefano S, Abosch A, Ojemann S, et al. RNS modifications to eliminate stimulation-triggered signs or symptoms (STS): Case series and practical guide. *Epilepsy Behav.* (2020) 112:107327. doi: 10.1016/j.yebeh.2020.107327
22. Heck CN, King-Stephens D, Massey AD, Nair DR, Jobst BC, Barkley GL, et al. Two-year seizure reduction in adults with medically intractable partial onset epilepsy treated with responsive neurostimulation: final results of the RNS System Pivotal trial. *Epilepsia.* (2014) 55:432–41. doi: 10.1111/epi.12534
23. Bergey GK, Morrell MJ, Mizrahi EM, Goldman A, King-Stephens D, Nair D, et al. Long-term treatment with responsive brain stimulation in adults with refractory partial seizures. *Neurology.* (2015) 84:810–7. doi: 10.1212/WNL.0000000000001280
24. Geller EB, Skarpaas TL, Gross RE, Goodman RR, Barkley GL, Bazil CW, et al. Brain-responsive neurostimulation in patients with medically intractable mesial temporal lobe epilepsy. *Epilepsia.* (2017) 58:994–1004. doi: 10.1111/epi.13740
25. Gummadavelli A, Zaveri HP, Spencer DD, Gerrard JL. Expanding brain–computer interfaces for controlling epilepsy networks: novel thalamic responsive neurostimulation in refractory epilepsy. *Front Neurosci.* (2018) 12:474. doi: 10.3389/fnins.2018.00474
26. Kokkinos V, Urban A, Sisterson ND, Li N, Corson D, Richardson RM. Responsive neurostimulation of the thalamus improves seizure control in idiopathic generalized epilepsy: a case report. *Neurosurgery.* (2020) 87:E578–83. doi: 10.1093/neuros/nyaa001
27. Ilyas A, Pizarro D, Romeo AK, Riley KO, Pati S. The centromedian nucleus: anatomy, physiology, clinical implications. *J Clin Neurosci.* (2019) 63:1–7. doi: 10.1016/j.jocn.2019.01.050
28. Kim SH, Lim SC, Yang DW, Cho JH, Son BC, Kim J, et al. Thalamo-cortical network underlying deep brain stimulation of centromedian thalamic nuclei in intractable epilepsy: a multimodal imaging analysis. *Neuropsychiatr Dis Treatment.* (2017) 13:2607–19. doi: 10.2147/NDT.S148617
29. Carney PW, Jackson GD. Insights into the mechanisms of absence seizure generation provided by EEG with functional MRI. *Front Neurol.* (2014) 5:162. doi: 10.3389/fneur.2014.00162
30. Kostopoulos GK. Involvement of the thalamocortical system in epileptic loss of consciousness. *Epilepsia.* (2001) 42:13–9. doi: 10.1046/j.1528-1157.2001.042suppl.3013.x
31. Blumenfeld H. The thalamus and seizures. *Arch Neurol.* (2002) 59:135–7. doi: 10.1001/archneur.59.1.135
32. Gloor, P. Generalized cortico-reticular epilepsies some considerations on the pathophysiology of generalized bilaterally synchronous spike and wave discharge. *Epilepsia.* (1968) 9:249–63. doi: 10.1111/j.1528-1157.1968.tb04624.x
33. Makinson CD, Tanaka BS, Sorokin JM, Wong JC, Christian CA, Goldin AL, et al. Regulation of thalamic and cortical network synchrony by Scn8a. *Neuron.* (2017) 93:1165–79.e6. doi: 10.1016/j.neuron.2017.01.031
34. Gummadavelli A, Motelow JE, Smith N, Zhan Q, Schiff ND, Blumenfeld H. Thalamic stimulation to improve level of consciousness after seizures: evaluation of electrophysiology and behavior. *Epilepsia.* (2015) 56:114–24. doi: 10.1111/epi.12872
35. Cukiert A, Cukiert CM, Burattini JA, Mariani PP. Seizure outcome during bilateral, continuous, thalamic centromedian nuclei deep brain stimulation in patients with generalized epilepsy: a prospective, open-label study. *Seizure Eur J Epilepsy.* (2020) 81:304–9. doi: 10.1016/j.seizure.2020.08.028
36. Cukiert A, Lehtimäki K. Deep brain stimulation targeting in refractory epilepsy. *Epilepsia.* (2017) 58:80–4. doi: 10.1111/epi.13686
37. Burdette DE, Haykal MA, Jarosiewicz B, Fabris RR, Heredia G, Elisevich K, et al. Brain-responsive corticothalamic stimulation in the centromedian nucleus for the treatment of regional neocortical epilepsy. *Epilepsy Behav.* (2020) 112:107354. doi: 10.1016/j.yebeh.2020.107354
38. Kwon C, Schupper AJ, Fields MC, Marcuse LV, La Vega-Talbott M, Panov F, et al. Centromedian thalamic responsive neurostimulation for lennox-gastaut epilepsy and autism. *Ann Clin Transl Neurol.* (2020) 7:2035–40. doi: 10.1002/acn3.51173
39. Nair DR, Laxer KD, Weber PB, Murro AM, Park YD, Barkley GL, et al. Nine-year prospective efficacy and safety of brain-responsive neurostimulation for focal epilepsy. *Neurology.* (2020) 95:e1244–56. doi: 10.1212/WNL.0000000000010154

40. Herlopian A, Cash SS, Eskandar EM, Jennings T, Cole AJ. Responsive neurostimulation targeting anterior thalamic nucleus in generalized epilepsy. *Ann Clin Translat Neurol.* (2019) 6:2104–9. doi: 10.1002/acn3.50858
41. Li J, Li Y, Gutierrez L, Xu W, Wu Y, Liu C, et al. Imaging the centromedian thalamic nucleus using quantitative susceptibility mapping. *Front Human Neurosci.* (2019) 13:447. doi: 10.3389/fnhum.2019.00447
42. Panov F, Ganaha S, Haskell J, Fields M, Vega-Talbott ML, Wolf S, et al. Safety of responsive neurostimulation in pediatric patients with medically refractory epilepsy. *J Neurosurg Pediatr.* (2020) 26:525–32. doi: 10.3171/2020.5.PEDS20118
43. Kokoszka MA, Panov F, Vega-Talbott ML, McGoldrick PE, Wolf SM, Ghatan S. Treatment of medically refractory seizures with responsive neurostimulation: 2 pediatric cases. *J Neurosurg Pediatr.* (2018) 21:421–7. doi: 10.3171/2017.10.PEDS17353
44. Bercu MM, Friedman D, Silverberg A, Drees C, Geller EB, Dugan PC, et al. Responsive neurostimulation for refractory epilepsy in the pediatric population: a single-center experience. *Epilepsy Behav.* (2020) 112:107389. doi: 10.1016/j.yebeh.2020.107389
45. Singhal NS, Numis AL, Lee MB, Chang EF, Sullivan JE, Auguste KI, et al. Responsive neurostimulation for treatment of pediatric drug-resistant epilepsy. *Epilepsy Behav Case Rep.* (2018) 10:21–4. doi: 10.1016/j.ebcr.2018.02.002

33

Case Report: Distinctive EEG Patterns in SCARB-2 Related Progressive Myoclonus Epilepsy

Mostafa Hotait†*, Maya Dirani*†*, Tarek El Halabi and Ahmad Beydoun**

Department of Neurology, American University of Beirut Medical Center, Beirut, Lebanon

***Correspondence:**
Ahmad Beydoun
ab29@aub.edu.lb

†These authors have contributed equally to this work

Action myoclonus-renal failure syndrome (AMRF) is a rare, recessively inherited form of progressive myoclonus epilepsy (PME) caused by mutations in the SCARB2 gene and associated with end-stage renal failure. In addition to severe progressive myoclonus, the neurological manifestations of this syndrome are characterized by progressive ataxia and dysarthria with preserved intellectual capacity. Since its original description, an increasing number of "AMRF-like" cases without renal failure have been reported. We describe the case of a 29-year-old woman with progressive disabling myoclonus associated with dysarthria and ataxia who was found to have a novel homozygous frameshift mutation in the SCARB2 gene. In addition, this report emphasizes the presence of two EEG patterns, fixation-off phenomenon, and bursts of parasagittal spikes exclusively seen during REM sleep that appear to be characteristic of this condition.

Keywords: SCARB2, progressive myoclonus epilepsy, action myoclonus with renal failure (AMRF), fixation-off phenomenon, EEG

INTRODUCTION

The progressive myoclonus epilepsies (PME) consist of a group of genetic neurodegenerative disorders that accounts for <1% of all epilepsies (Bhat and Ganesh, 2018). They are characterized by a distinctive triad of progressive myoclonus, epileptic seizures, and neurologic deterioration. Most PME are inherited in an autosomal recessive manner and can be distinguished according to age at symptom onset and the predominant neurological abnormalities, particularly dementia, dysarthria, or ataxia (Scala et al., 2020).

Action myoclonus-renal failure syndrome (AMRF, OMIM 254900) is a rare, autosomal recessive form of PME associated with end-stage renal failure requiring dialysis or transplantation. This condition, first described by Andermann et al. in four French-Canadian patients (Andermann et al., 1986) was found in 2008 to be caused by mutations in the SCARB2 gene (Berkovic et al., 2008). SCARB2 encodes for a lysosomal membrane protein essential for maintaining endosomal transport and lysosomal biogenesis (Eskelinen et al., 2003). This syndrome is characterized by a progressive disabling myoclonus frequently associated with ataxia and dysarthria and preserved intellectual capacity (Hopfner et al., 2011). Its clinical features overlap with those of Unverricht-Lundborg disease (ULD), another PME resulting from mutations in the gene encoding cystatin B (CSTB). In fact, in a genetic study of 41 patients with clinical features suggestive of ULD but with no mutations in the CSTB gene, five patients were found to have a SCARB2 mutation (Dibbens et al., 2009).

We report a novel SCARB2 frameshift mutation in a patient with progressive disabling action myoclonus without renal failure and suggest that this condition is associated with characteristic EEG patterns.

CASE

A 29-year-old, left-handed Iraqi woman with normal neurodevelopment, born to first-degree cousins and a member of a dizygotic twin pregnancy, presented for refractory epilepsy. At the age of 19 years, she started experiencing spontaneous and action-induced myoclonus, which were often precipitated by external stimuli, predominantly light sources. One year later, she experienced a nocturnal bilateral tonic-clonic (BTC) seizure for which she was started on levetiracetam. Over the next 2 years, the BTC seizures abated along with improvement in the frequency and severity of the myoclonic jerks. Subsequently, the BTC seizures recurred and were refractory to different combinations of levetiracetam, valproate, and clonazepam. Her myoclonic jerks progressively worsened and were exacerbated by light sources, which resulted in her spending most of her time in darkened rooms. At the age of 27, the patient developed progressively worsening dysarthria and disabling ataxia.

Her neurologic examination was relevant for severe dysarthria with barely comprehensible speech, a prominent tremor and frequent spontaneous and action myoclonus. In addition, she was severely ataxic and could not ambulate without assistance. Her cognitive function, motor strength, and muscle tone were otherwise normal. An epilepsy protocol brain MRI revealed a mild generalized cerebral atrophy with no abnormalities detected on a post-acquisition voxel-based morphometric analysis.

The patient was admitted for long-term video/EEG monitoring. Her EEG revealed a normal posterior background as well as frequent bursts and fragments of generalized spike and polyspike and wave discharges (GPSWD) with an occipital amplitude predominance, commonly associated with myoclonic jerks (**Figure 1A**). Intermittent photic stimulation at a frequency of 14 Hz triggered bursts of posteriorly predominant repetitive spikes that were associated with multifocal myoclonus, following which the photic stimulation was aborted (**Figure 1B**). Although the patient felt scared and uncomfortable following stimulation at flash frequencies of 2, 4, 6, 8, 10, and 12 Hz, those were not associated with a photoparoxysmal response or with worsening of her myoclonic jerks. In addition, a fixation-off phenomenon was consistently noted following eye closure and was characterized by bilateral posteriorly predominant repetitive spikes associated with violent multifocal myoclonus. The epileptiform discharges and associated myoclonic jerks persisted as long as her eyes remained closed and were immediately aborted upon eye opening (**Figure 2A**). In addition, the patient experienced frequent prolonged myoclonic seizures as well as a myoclonic-tonic-clonic seizure characterized by crescendo multifocal myoclonus that evolved to a BTC seizure. During REM sleep, a peculiar pattern consisting of bursts of repetitive parasagittal spikes associated with fragmentary minimyoclonus of the hands was seen (**Figure 2B**).

On whole exome sequencing (WES), a novel mutation of the SCARB2 gene was detected, c.40dup p. (Leu14Profs*35), creating a shift in the reading frame starting at codon 14 and ending in a stop codon 34 positions downstream. The WES and Sanger sequencing were validated by Centogene. Biochemical investigations showed a normal serum creatinine, and a 24-h urine collection revealed a normal creatinine clearance with elevated proteinuria at 51.1 mg/dL (normal range: 0–20 mg/dL). Perampanel was added to her treatment regimen and was titrated to 4 mg daily without any significant improvement in the frequency of her myoclonic jerks. Because this drug was not available in Iraq, the dose was not increased, and the medication was stopped due to lack of efficacy.

DISCUSSION

In this report, we present a patient diagnosed with AMRF based on a homozygous frameshift mutation in the SCARB2 gene resulting in SCARB2 deficiency. This variant is novel and was not identified in the NHLBI Exome Sequencing Project (ESP) Exome Variant server (http://evs.gs.washington.edu/EVS).

Since its original description in 1986 (Andermann et al., 1986), a total of 27 cases of AMRF from 20 families have been reported (Tian et al., 2018). Although its name implies the development of renal failure, typically within 0–5.5 years following symptom onset, 13 of the 27 reported cases did not have evidence of renal dysfunction despite being followed for up to 15 years until death (Dibbens et al., 2009; Tian et al., 2018). Our patient did not have evidence of renal insufficiency 10 years into her illness although we did document the presence of proteinuria on a 24-h urine collection following the results of the genetic testing. In light of the increased number of "ULD-like" cases without renal involvement, it is becoming clear that renal failure is not an invariable accompaniment of PME due to SCARB2 mutations. Because the phenotypes of the classical AMRF and those without renal failure are otherwise indistinguishable (Tian et al., 2018), it is best to refer to this condition as a SCARB2-related PME.

The EEG findings in SCARB2-related PME have been overall poorly documented with the exception of one previous study (Rubboli et al., 2011). The abnormalities included a progressively slowed background with irregular theta and delta activity intermixed with alpha activity and associated with intermittent bursts of GSWD (Tian et al., 2018). However, we noticed two distinctive EEG patterns that appear to be characteristic of this condition and which were not previously emphasized (Rubboli et al., 2011; Tian et al., 2018). The first pattern consisted of eyes-closed/fixation-off sensitivity (FOS), a phenomenon induced by elimination of central vision and characterized by the appearance of focal occipital or generalized epileptiform discharges following eye closure and persisting as long as the eyes are closed (Koutroumanidis et al., 2009; Brigo et al., 2013). Our patient consistently experienced intense multifocal myoclonic jerks with her eyes closed. These were associated with biposterior bursts of repetitive spikes that immediately aborted following eye opening. FOS is a rare phenomenon, most commonly encountered in children with the occipital epilepsy

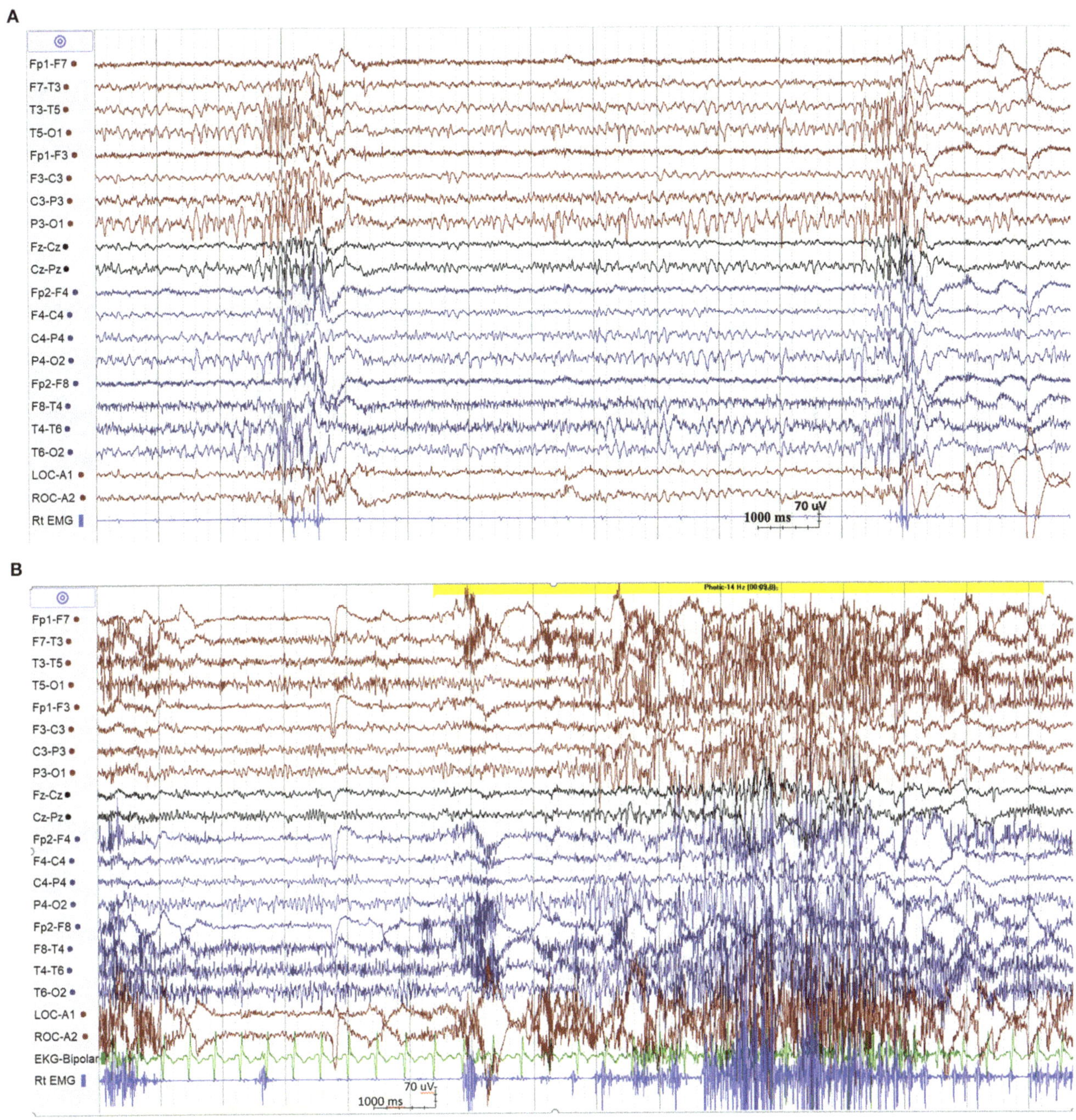

FIGURE 1 | (A) Spontaneous bursts of repetitive spikes with an occipital predominance associated with myoclonic jerks. **(B)** EEG showing normal posterior background and a non-sustained photoparoxysmal response associated with multifocal myoclonic jerks following stimulation at 14 Hz.

of Gastaut and the Panayiotopoulos syndrome, and anecdotally described in other focal or generalized epilepsy (Koutroumanidis et al., 2009; Brigo et al., 2013). It was, however, previously reported in two patients with SCARB2-related PME (Rubboli et al., 2011), but not in other types of PME with the exception of a single case of myoclonic epilepsy with red ragged fibers (Garcia Silva et al., 1987). More importantly, it has never been described in ULD, the condition resembling SCARB2-related PME at onset. In one patient with Lafora disease, the intractable myoclonic seizures were actually suppressed by fixation-off. In fact, neurophysiologic studies documented that fixation was the most important enhancer of myoclonus in this condition (Kumada et al., 2006). This is the opposite of what occurs in fixation-off sensitive epilepsies, a phenomenon described as inverted fixation-off sensitivity (Kumada et al., 2006).

The second EEG finding consisted of the exclusive appearance during REM sleep of bursts of bilateral repetitive polyspikes over the parasagittal derivations associated with subtle fragmentary

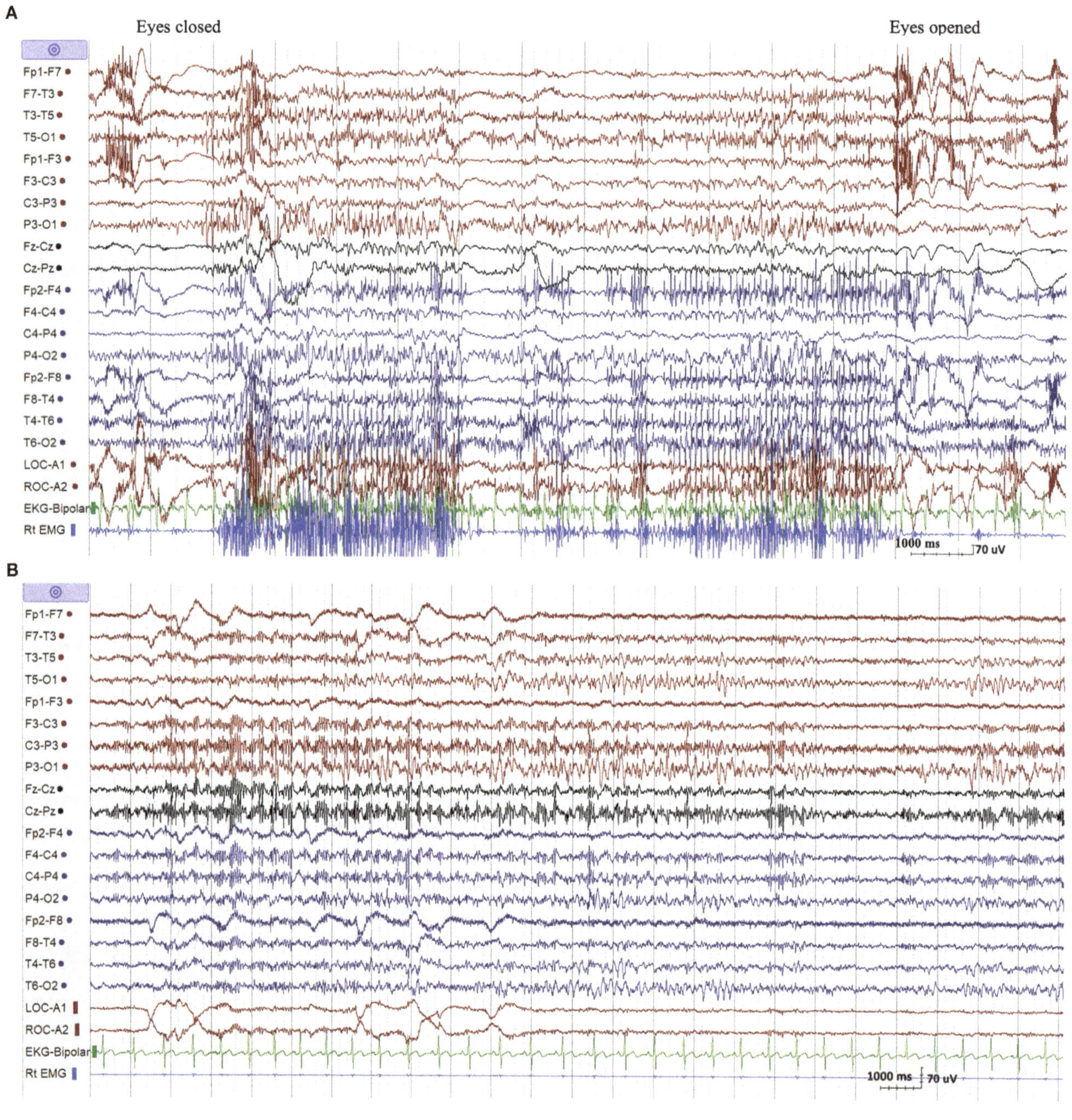

FIGURE 2 | (A) Fixation off sensitivity. **(B)** REM sleep. A peculiar pattern consisting of repetitive spikes over the parasagittal derivations associated with fragmentary minimyoclonus of the right hand.

myoclonus of the extremities. This pattern, initially described by Tassinari in 10 of 14 patients with ULD (Tassinari et al., 1974), was confirmed by other investigators and was believed to be one of the diagnostic clues of this disease (Ferlazzo et al., 2007; Avanzini et al., 2016). Our finding, which was also previously recorded on two patients with SCARB2-related PME (Rubboli et al., 2011), indicates that it is not specific for ULD but can also be seen in SCARB-2-related PME. Although those two EEG patterns are quite rare, their specificities in allowing distinguishing between the various forms of PMEs are yet undetermined. However, in the correct clinical setting, those EEG findings, especially the substantial worsening of myoclonus with eyes closed, should raise the suspicion of a SCARB-2-related PME.

We elected to add perampanel to the treatment regimen of our patient based on a previous positive experience with this drug in the treatment of Lafora disease and ULD (Dirani et al., 2014; Goldsmith and Minassian, 2016; Crespel et al., 2017). Although our patient did not titrate the perampanel dose beyond 4 mg daily, she did not notice any improvement while on this drug. The efficacy of perampanel needs to be tested in a cohort of patients before any conclusive determination of its value in SCARB-2-related PME.

We describe the third case of a patient of Arab descent to be diagnosed with a novel homozygous frameshift mutation of the SCARB-2 gene. This report emphasizes the presence of two EEG patterns, FOS and bursts of parasagittal spikes, exclusively seen during REM sleep that appear to be characteristic of this condition. Further studies are needed to confirm those findings.

ETHICS STATEMENT

Ethical approval was not provided for this study on human participants because this is a case report that does not require an ethical approval at our institution. The patients/participants provided their written informed consent to participate in this study. Written informed consent was obtained from the individual(s) for the publication of any potentially identifiable images or data included in this article.

AUTHOR CONTRIBUTIONS

MH and MD followed the patient clinically and were responsible for initial manuscript writing. TE reviewed the literature. AB was responsible for the final version of manuscript. All authors contributed to the article and approved the submitted version.

REFERENCES

1. Andermann, E., Andermann, F., Carpenter, S., Wolfe, L. S., Nelson, R., Patry, G., et al. (1986). Action myoclonus-renal failure syndrome: a previously unrecognized neurological disorder unmasked by advances in nephrology. *Adv. Neurol.* 43, 87–103. Available online at: https://www.ncbi.nlm.nih.gov/pubmed/3946122 (accessed July 02, 2020).
2. Avanzini, G., Shibasaki, H., Rubboli, G., Canafoglia, L., Panzica, F., Franceschetti, S., et al. (2016). Neurophysiology of myoclonus and progressive myoclonus epilepsies. *Epileptic Disord.* 18, 11–27. doi: 10.1684/epd.2016.0835
3. Berkovic, S. F., Dibbens, L. M., Oshlack, A., Silver, J. D., Katerelos, M., Vears, D. F., et al. (2008). Array-based gene discovery with three unrelated subjects shows SCARB2/LIMP-2 deficiency causes myoclonus epilepsy and glomerulosclerosis. *Am. J. Hum. Genet.* 82, 673–684. doi: 10.1016/j.ajhg.2007.12.019
4. Bhat, S., and Ganesh, S. (2018). New discoveries in progressive myoclonus epilepsies: a clinical outlook. *Expert Rev. Neurother.* 18, 649–667. doi: 10.1080/14737175.2018.1503949
5. Brigo, F., Rossini, F., Stefani, A., Nardone, R., Tezzon, F., Fiaschi, A., et al. (2013). Fixation-off sensitivity. *Clin. Neurophysiol.* 124, 221–227. doi: 10.1016/j.clinph.2012.07.017
6. Crespel, A., Gelisse, P., Tang, N. P., and Genton, P. (2017). Perampanel in 12 patients with Unverricht-Lundborg disease. *Epilepsia* 58, 543–547. doi: 10.1111/epi.13662
7. Dibbens, L. M., Michelucci, R., Gambardella, A., Andermann, F., Rubboli, G., Bayly, M. A., et al. (2009). SCARB2 mutations in progressive myoclonus epilepsy (PME) without renal failure. *Ann. Neurol.* 66, 532–536. doi: 10.1002/ana.21765
8. Dirani, M., Nasreddine, W., Abdulla, F., and Beydoun, A. (2014). Seizure control and improvement of neurological dysfunction in Lafora disease with perampanel. *Epilepsy Behav Case Rep.* 2, 164–166. doi: 10.1016/j.ebcr.2014.09.003
9. Eskelinen, E. L., Tanaka, Y., and Saftig, P. (2003). At the acidic edge: emerging functions for lysosomal membrane proteins. *Trends Cell Biol.* 13, 137–145. doi: 10.1016/S0962 8924(03)00005-9
10. Ferlazzo, E., Magaudda, A., Striano, P., Vi-Hong, N., Serra, S., and Genton, P. (2007). Long-term evolution of EEG in Unverricht-Lundborg disease. *Epilepsy Res.* 73, 219–227. doi: 10.1016/j.eplepsyres.2006. 10.006
11. Garcia Silva, M. T., Aicardi, J., Goutieres, F., and Chevrie, J. J. (1987). The syndrome of myoclonic epilepsy with ragged-red fibers. Report of a case and review of the literature. *Neuropediatrics* 18, 200–204. doi: 10.1055/s-2008-1052480
12. Goldsmith, D., and Minassian, B. A. (2016). Efficacy and tolerability of perampanel in ten patients with Lafora disease. *Epilepsy Behav.* 62, 132–135. doi: 10.1016/j.yebeh.2016.06.041
13. Hopfner, F., Schormair, B., Knauf, F., Berthele, A., Tolle, T. R., Baron, R., et al. (2011). Novel SCARB2 mutation in action myoclonus-renal failure syndrome and evaluation of SCARB2 mutations in isolated AMRF features. *BMC Neurol.* 11:134. doi: 10.1186/1471-2377-11-134
14. Koutroumanidis, M., Tsatsou, K., Sanders, S., Michael, M., Tan, S. V., Agathonikou, A., et al. (2009). Fixation-off sensitivity in epilepsies other than the idiopathic epilepsies of childhood with occipital paroxysms: a 12-year clinical-video EEG study. *Epileptic Disord.* 11, 20–36. doi: 10.1684/epd.2009.0235
15. Kumada, S., Kubota, M., Hayashi, M., Uchiyama, A., Kurata, K., and Kagamihara, Y. (2006). Fixation-sensitive myoclonus in Lafora disease. *Neurology* 66, 1574–1576. doi: 10.1212/01.wnl.0000216147.12172.39
16. Rubboli, G., Franceschetti, S., Berkovic, S. F., Canafoglia, L., Gambardella, A., Dibbens, L. M., et al. (2011). Clinical and neurophysiologic features of progressive myoclonus epilepsy without renal failure caused by SCARB2 mutations. *Epilepsia* 52, 2356–2363. doi: 10.1111/j.1528-1167.2011.03307.x
17. Scala, M., Bianchi, A., Bisulli, F., Coppola, A., Elia, M., Trivisano, M., et al. (2020). Advances in genetic testing and optimization of clinical management in children and adults with epilepsy. *Expert Rev. Neurother.* 20, 251–269. doi: 10.1080/14737175.2020.1713101
18. Tassinari, C. A., Bureau-Paillas, M., Grasso, E., and Roger, J. (1974). Electroencephalographic study of myoclonic cerebellar dyssynergia with epilepsy (Ramsay-Hunt syndrome). *Rev. Electroencephalogr. Neurophysiol. Clin.* 4, 407–428. doi: 10.1016/S0370-4475(74)80052-3
19. Tian, W. T., Liu, X. L., Xu, Y. Q., Huang, X. J., Zhou, H. Y., Wang, Y., et al. (2018). Progressive myoclonus epilepsy without renal failure in a Chinese family with a novel mutation in SCARB2 gene and literature review. *Seizure* 57, 80–86. doi: 10.1016/j.seizure.2018.03.015

Permissions

All chapters in this book were first published by Frontiers; hereby published with permission under the Creative Commons Attribution License or equivalent. Every chapter published in this book has been scrutinized by our experts. Their significance has been extensively debated. The topics covered herein carry significant findings which will fuel the growth of the discipline. They may even be implemented as practical applications or may be referred to as a beginning point for another development.

The contributors of this book come from diverse backgrounds, making this book a truly international effort. This book will bring forth new frontiers with its revolutionizing research information and detailed analysis of the nascent developments around the world.

We would like to thank all the contributing authors for lending their expertise to make the book truly unique. They have played a crucial role in the development of this book. Without their invaluable contributions this book wouldn't have been possible. They have made vital efforts to compile up to date information on the varied aspects of this subject to make this book a valuable addition to the collection of many professionals and students.

This book was conceptualized with the vision of imparting up-to-date information and advanced data in this field. To ensure the same, a matchless editorial board was set up. Every individual on the board went through rigorous rounds of assessment to prove their worth. After which they invested a large part of their time researching and compiling the most relevant data for our readers.

The editorial board has been involved in producing this book since its inception. They have spent rigorous hours researching and exploring the diverse topics which have resulted in the successful publishing of this book. They have passed on their knowledge of decades through this book. To expedite this challenging task, the publisher supported the team at every step. A small team of assistant editors was also appointed to further simplify the editing procedure and attain best results for the readers.

Apart from the editorial board, the designing team has also invested a significant amount of their time in understanding the subject and creating the most relevant covers. They scrutinized every image to scout for the most suitable representation of the subject and create an appropriate cover for the book.

The publishing team has been an ardent support to the editorial, designing and production team. Their endless efforts to recruit the best for this project, has resulted in the accomplishment of this book. They are a veteran in the field of academics and their pool of knowledge is as vast as their experience in printing. Their expertise and guidance has proved useful at every step. Their uncompromising quality standards have made this book an exceptional effort. Their encouragement from time to time has been an inspiration for everyone.

The publisher and the editorial board hope that this book will prove to be a valuable piece of knowledge for researchers, students, practitioners and scholars across the globe.

List of Contributors

Yulin Sun, Lin Wan, Huimin Yan and Zhichao Li
Department of Pediatrics, Chinese PLA General Hospital, Beijing, China
Department of Pediatrics, The First Medical Center, Chinese PLA General Hospital, Beijing, China

Guang Yang
Department of Pediatrics, Chinese PLA General Hospital, Beijing, China
Department of Pediatrics, The First Medical Center, Chinese PLA General Hospital, Beijing, China
The Second School of Clinical Medicine, Southern Medical University, Guangzhou, China

Konstantin L. Makridis and Angela M. Kaindl
Department of Pediatric Neurology, Charité – Universitätsmedizin Berlin, Berlin, Germany
Center for Chronically Sick Children, Charité – Universitätsmedizin Berlin, Berlin, Germany
Institute of Cell- and Neurobiology, Charité – Universitätsmedizin Berlin, Berlin, Germany

Christine Prager, Deniz A. Atalay and Sebastian Triller
Department of Pediatric Neurology, Charité – Universitätsmedizin Berlin, Berlin, Germany
Center for Chronically Sick Children, Charité – Universitätsmedizin Berlin, Berlin, Germany

Anna Tietze
Neuroradiology, Charité – Universitätsmedizin Berlin, Berlin, Germany

Christian E. Elger
Department of Pediatric Neurology, Charité – Universitätsmedizin Berlin, Berlin, Germany
Center for Chronically Sick Children, Charité – Universitätsmedizin Berlin, Berlin, Germany
Beta Neurologie – Kompetenzzentrum für Epilepsie, Beta Klinik GmbH, Bonn, Germany

Ulrich-Wilhelm Thomale
Pediatric Neurosurgery, Charité – Universitätsmedizin Berlin, Berlin, Germany

Jun-Hong Geng, Yang Zheng, Quan-Fu Li, Qun Hou, Xiao-Hang Wang and Yan Jiang
Department of Neurology, The First Affiliated Hospital of Zhejiang Chinese Medical University, Hangzhou, China

Ziqi Wei, Puming Zhang and Jun Zhao
School of Biomedical Engineering, Shanghai Jiao Tong University, Shanghai, China

Xiaolai Ye, Jiwen Xu and Qiangqiang Liu
Department of Neurosurgery, Clinical Neuroscience Center Comprehensive Epilepsy Unit, Ruijin Hospital, Shanghai Jiao Tong University School of Medicine, Shanghai, China
Clinical Neuroscience Center, Ruijin Hospital Luwan Branch, Shanghai Jiao Tong University School of Medicine, Shanghai, China

Changquan Wang
Clinical Neuroscience Center, Ruijin Hospital Luwan Branch, Shanghai Jiao Tong University School of Medicine, Shanghai, China

Jeff F. Zhang and Kevin Nickerson
Jacobs School of Medicine and Biomedical Sciences, University at Buffalo, Buffalo, NY, United States

Ravi Piryani and Anil K. Swayampakula
Division of Critical Care Medicine, Department of Pediatrics, John R. Oishei Children's Hospital, Buffalo, NY, United States

Osman Farooq
Division of Pediatric Neurology, John R. Oishei Children's Hospital, Buffalo, NY, United States

Coline Bouyer
Service de neurologie Centre Hospitalier de Cayenne, Cayenne, France

Bertrand de Toffol
Service de neurologie Centre Hospitalier de Cayenne, Cayenne, France
CIC Inserm 1424 CH Cayenne, Cayenne, France

Yuqing Lv
Department of Gastroenterology, Zhongnan Hospital of Wuhan University, Wuhan, China

Hui Xiang
Department of Critical Care Medicine, Zhongnan Hospital of Wuhan University, Wuhan, China

Marco Olivero and Gianluca Costamagna
Neuroscience Section, Dino Ferrari Centre, Department of Pathophysiology and Transplantation (DEPT), University of Milan, Milan, Italy

Delia Gagliardi, Stefania Corti and Megi Meneri
Neuroscience Section, Dino Ferrari Centre, Department of Pathophysiology and Transplantation (DEPT), University of Milan, Milan, Italy
Neurology Unit, Foundation IRCCS Ca' Granda Ospedale Maggiore Policlinico, Milan, Italy

Daniele Velardo
Neurology Unit, Foundation IRCCS Ca' Granda Ospedale Maggiore Policlinico, Milan, Italy

Francesca Magri
Neuromuscular and Rare Diseases Unit, Department of Neuroscience, Fondazione IRCCS Ca' Granda Ospedale Maggiore Policlinico, Milan, Italy

Fabio Triulzi and Giorgio Conte
Neuroradiology Unit, Fondazione IRCCS Ca' Granda Ospedale Maggiore Policlinico, Department of Pathophysiology and Transplantation, Università degli Studi Milano, Milan, Italy

Giacomo P. Comi
Neuroscience Section, Dino Ferrari Centre, Department of Pathophysiology and Transplantation (DEPT), University of Milan, Milan, Italy
Neuromuscular and Rare Diseases Unit, Department of Neuroscience, Fondazione IRCCS Ca' Granda Ospedale Maggiore Policlinico, Milan, Italy

Xiaoli Wang, Wenjuan Zhang and Yonghong Liu
Department of Neurology, Xijing Hospital, Fourth Military Medical University, Xi'an, China

Pengying Mu
Department of Neurology, Xijing Hospital, Fourth Military Medical University, Xi'an, China
Department of Neurology, Xing Yuan hospital of Yulin, Shaanxi, China

Ke Zhang, Shuang Xu, Yalan Zhou and Tangfeng Su
Department of Pediatrics, Tongji Hospital, Tongji Medical College, Huazhong University of Science and Technology, Wuhan, China

Elisa Micalizzi
Department of Brain and Behavioral Sciences, University of Pavia, Pavia, Italy

Anna Elisabetta Vaudano, Giulia Turchi and Leandra Giunta
Neurology Unit, Ospedale Civile di Baggiovara (OCB) Hospital, Azienda Ospedaliera-Universitaria, Modena, Italy

Giada Giovannini
Neurology Unit, Ospedale Civile di Baggiovara (OCB) Hospital, Azienda Ospedaliera-Universitaria, Modena, Italy
Department of Biomedical, Metabolic and Neural Science, University of Modena and Reggio Emilia, Modena, Italy
PhD Program in Clinical and Experimental Medicine, University of Modena and Reggio Emilia, Modena, Italy

Stefano Meletti
Neurology Unit, Ospedale Civile di Baggiovara (OCB) Hospital, Azienda Ospedaliera-Universitaria, Modena, Italy
Department of Biomedical, Metabolic and Neural Science, University of Modena and Reggio Emilia, Modena, Italy

Emmanuelle Hologne
Département de Neurologie, Centre Hospitalier Universitaire de Reims, Reims, France

Gabriela Hossu
IADI, U1254, Institut National de la Santé et de la Recherche Médicale et Université de Lorraine, Nancy, France
Centre d'Investigation Clinique-Innovation Technologique, Centre Hospitalier Régional Universitaire de Nancy, Nancy, France

Luca Fantin
IADI, U1254, Institut National de la Santé et de la Recherche Médicale et Université de Lorraine, Nancy, France
Laboratoire Développement Adaptation Handicap (DevAH) EA 3450, Nancy, France

Marc Braun
IADI, U1254, Institut National de la Santé et de la Recherche Médicale et Université de Lorraine, Nancy, France
Département de Neuroradiologie Diagnostique et Thérapeutique, Centre Hospitalier Universitaire de Nancy, Nancy, France

Cyril Husson
Pôle Hospitalo-Universitaire de Psychiatrie d'Adultes et d'Addictologie du Grand Nancy, Centre Psychothérapique de Nancy, Laxou, France

Louise Tyvaert
Département de Neurologie, Centre Hospitalier Universitaire de Nancy, Nancy, France
Centre de Recherche en Automatique de Nancy, U7039, Centre National de la Recherche Scientifique et Université de Lorraine, Nancy, France

Coraline Hingray
Pôle Hospitalo-Universitaire de Psychiatrie d'Adultes et d'Addictologie du Grand Nancy, Centre Psychothérapique de Nancy, Laxou, France
Département de Neurologie, Centre Hospitalier Universitaire de Nancy, Nancy, France

Ana Victoria Marco Hernández
Neuropediatrics Section, Hospital Universitari i Politècnic La Fe, Valencia, Spain
Genetics Unit, Hospital Universitari i Politècnic La Fe, Valencia, Spain

Miguel Tomás Vila
Neuropediatrics Section, Hospital Universitari i Politècnic La Fe, Valencia, Spain

Alfonso Caro Llopis and Francisco Martinez
Genetics Unit, Hospital Universitari i Politècnic La Fe, Valencia, Spain
Genomics Unit, La Fe Health Research Institute, Valencia, Spain

Sandra Monfort
Genomics Unit, La Fe Health Research Institute, Valencia, Spain

Sixian Li, Xiaodong Cai, Chen Yao, Yuanqing Wang, Xiaohua Xiao and Huafeng Yang
Department of Neurosurgery, Shenzhen Second People's Hospital, The First Affiliated Hospital of Shenzhen University, Shenzhen, China

Yi Yao
Department of Functional Neurosurgery, Xiamen Humanity Hospital, Xiamen, China

Lei Chen
Department of Neurology, West China Hospital in Sichuan University. Chengdu, China

Rui Ma, Jiaqi Han, Lehong Gao and Yuping Wang
Department of Neurology, Xuanwu Hosptial, Captial Medical University, Beijing, China
Beijing Key Laboratory of Neuromodulation, Beijing, China

Jing Ye
Department of Neurology, Xuanwu Hosptial, Captial Medical University, Beijing, China

Chaodong Wang
Department of Neurology, Xuanwu Hosptial, Captial Medical University, Beijing, China
National Clinical Research Center for Geriatric Diseases, Beijing, China

Sebastian Triller and Christine Prager
Charité - Universitätsmedizin Berlin, Department of Pediatric Neurology, Berlin, Germany
Charité - Universitätsmedizin Berlin, Center for Chronically Sick Children, Berlin, Germany

Marcin Siwek
Department of Affective Disorders, Jagiellonian University Medical College, Kraków, Poland

Aleksandra Gorostowicz and Dominika Dudek
Department of Psychiatry, Jagiellonian University Medical College, Kraków, Poland

Magdalena Bosak
Department of Neurology, Jagiellonian University Medical College, Krakow, Poland

Giorgia Sforza, Fabiana Ursitti, Michela Ada Noris Ferilli, Samuela Tarantino and Laura Papetti
Pediatric Headache Center, Department of Neuroscience, Bambino Gesù Children Hospital, Istituto di Ricovero e Cura a Carattere Scientifico, Rome, Italy

Claudia Ruscitto and Romina Moavero
Child Neurology and Psychiatry Unit, Tor Vergata University of Rome, Rome, Italy

Martina Balestri and Federico Vigevano
Child Neurology Unit, Bambino Gesù Children's Hospital, Istituto di Ricovero e Cura a Carattere Scientifico, Rome, Italy

Massimiliano Valeriani
Pediatric Headache Center, Department of Neuroscience, Bambino Gesù Children Hospital, Istituto di Ricovero e Cura a Carattere Scientifico, Rome, Italy
Center for Sensory-Motor Interaction, Aalborg University, Aalborg, Denmark

Huimin Li, Lina Xu, Fengbing Yang, Longbin Jia, Hongjiang Cheng and Wei Liu
Jincheng People's Hospital Affiliated to Shanxi Medical University, Jincheng, China

Giorgio Costagliola and Rita Consolini
Pediatric Immunology, Pediatric University Department, Azienda Ospedaliero Universitaria Pisana, University of Pisa, Pisa, Italy

Greta Depietri, Alice Bonuccelli and Alessandro Orsini
Pediatric Neurology, Pediatric University Department, Azienda Ospedaliero Universitaria Pisana, University of Pisa, Pisa, Italy

Alexandre Michev, Thomas Foiadelli, Salvatore Savasta and Gian Luigi Marseglia
Pediatric Clinic, Istituto di Ricovero e Cura a Carattere Scientifico (IRCCS) Policlinico San Matteo Foundation, University of Pavia, Pavia, Italy

Antonella Riva
Pediatric Neurology and Muscular Diseases Unit, IRCCS Istituto "Giannina Gaslini", Genova, Italy

Diego Peroni
Pediatric Immunology, Pediatric University Department, Azienda Ospedaliero Universitaria Pisana, University of Pisa, Pisa, Italy
Pediatric Neurology, Pediatric University Department, Azienda Ospedaliero Universitaria Pisana, University of Pisa, Pisa, Italy

M. C. Kravetz and M. S. Viola
Department of Pharmacology, Faculty of Farmacy and Biochemistry, University of Buenos Aires, Buenos Aires City, Argentina

J. Prenz and M. Curi
Department of Cardiology, Garrahan Hospital, Buenos Aires City, Argentina

G. F. Bramuglia
Department of Pharmacology, Faculty of Farmacy and Biochemistry, University of Buenos Aires, Buenos Aires City, Argentina
Fundacion Investigar, Buenos Aires City, Argentina

S. Tenembaum
Department of Neurology, Garrahan Hospital, Buenos Aires City, Argentina

Hideo Enoki, Shinji Itamura and Tohru Okanishi
Comprehensive Epilepsy Center, Seirei Hamamatsu General Hospital, Hamamatsu, Japan
Department of Child Neurology, Seirei-Hamamatsu General Hospital, Shizuoka, Japan

Petia Dimova
Epileptology Unit at Epilepsy Surgery Center, Department of Neurosurgery, St. Ivan Rilski University Hospital, Sofia, Bulgaria

Krassimir Minkin
Functional and Epilepsy Surgery Center, Department of Neurosurgery, St. Ivan Rilski University Hospital, Sofia, Bulgaria

Marcos García-Howard, María Urretavizcaya-Martínez and Josune Alegría-Echauri
Department of Pediatrics, CHN, Navarra Health Service Hospital, Pamplona, Spain

Mercedes Herranz-Aguirre
Pediatric Infectious Disease Unit, Department of Pediatrics, CHN, Navarra Health Service Hospital, Pamplona, Spain

Laura Moreno-Galarraga
NavarraBioMed and IdiSNA, Health Research Institute, Pamplona, Spain
Pediatric Respiratory Medicine, Department of Pediatrics, CHN, Navarra Health Service Hospital, Pamplona, Spain

Nerea Gorría-Redondo
Pediatric Neurology Unit, Department of Pediatrics, CHN, Navarra Health Service Hospital, Pamplona, Spain

Laura Planas-Serra and Agatha Schlüter
Neurometabolic Diseases Laboratory, Bellvitge Biomedical Research Institute (IDIBELL), Barcelona, Spain
Center for Biomedical Research on Rare Diseases (CIBERER), ISCIII, Madrid, Spain

Marta Gut
CNAG-CRG, Centre for Genomic Regulation, Barcelona Institute of Science and Technology, Barcelona, Spain
Universitat Pompeu Fabra (UPF), Barcelona, Spain

Aurora Pujol
Neurometabolic Diseases Laboratory, Bellvitge Biomedical Research Institute (IDIBELL), Barcelona, Spain
Center for Biomedical Research on Rare Diseases (CIBERER), ISCIII, Madrid, Spain
Catalan Institution of Research and Advanced Studies (ICREA), Barcelona, Spain

Sergio Aguilera-Albesa
NavarraBioMed and IdiSNA, Health Research Institute, Pamplona, Spain
Pediatric Neurology Unit, Department of Pediatrics, CHN, Navarra Health Service Hospital, Pamplona, Spain

Shinji Itamura, Shimpei Baba and Hideo Enoki
Department of Child Neurology, Seirei-Hamamatsu General Hospital, Shizuoka, Japan

Yoshifumi Arai and Yoshiro Otsuki
Department of Pathology, Seirei-Hamamatsu General Hospital, Shizuoka, Japan

Mitsuyo Nishimura
Department of Clinical Laboratory, Seirei-Hamamatsu General Hospital, Shizuoka, Japan

Naoki Ichikawa and Ayataka Fujimoto
Epilepsy Center, Seirei-Hamamatsu General Hospital, Shizuoka, Japan

Yoshimichi Hirayama
Department of Pediatrics, Naha City Hospital, Okinawa, Japan

Naoko Ishihara
Department of Pediatrics, Fujita Health University School of Medicine, Toyoake, Japan

Takuya Hiraide, Hidetoshi Ishigaki and Tokiko Fukuda
Department of Pediatrics, Hamamatsu University School of Medicine, Hamamatsu, Japan

Greta Amore, Ambra Butera, Giulia Spoto, Giulia Valentini, Maria Concetta Saia, Gabriella Di Rosa and Antonio Gennaro Nicotera
Department of Human Pathology of the Adult and Developmental Age "Gaetano Barresi", Unit of Child Neurology and Psychiatry, University of Messina, Messina, Italy

Vincenzo Salpietro
Department of Neuromuscular Disorders, Institute of Neurology, University College London, London, United Kingdom
Pediatric Neurology and Muscular Diseases Unit, Scientific Institute for Research, Hospitalization and Healthcare (IRCCS) Istituto Giannina Gaslini, Genoa, Italy
Department of Neurosciences, Rehabilitation, Ophthalmology, Genetics, Maternal and Child Health, University of Genoa, Genoa, Italy

Francesco Calì
Oasi Research Institute-Scientific Institute for Research, Hospitalization and Healthcare (IRCCS), Troina, Italy

Robertino Dilena, Eleonora Mauri and Cristina Bana
Neurophysiopathology Unit, Department of Neuroscience and Mental Health, Foundation IRCCS Ca' Granda Ospedale Maggiore Policlinico, Milan, Italy

Alessio Di Fonzo
Neurology Unit, Department of Neuroscience and Mental Health, Foundation IRCCS Ca' Granda Ospedale Maggiore Policlinico, Dino Ferrari Centre, University of Milan, Milan, Italy

Paola Francesca Ajmone and Claudia Rigamonti
Child and Adolescent Neuropsychiatic Unit (UONPIA), Foundation IRCCS Ca' Granda Ospedale Maggiore Policlinico, Milan, Italy

Tamara Catenio
Grioni Center, Danelli Onlus Foundation, Lodi, Italy

Silvana Gangi and Monica Fumagalli
Foundation IRCCS Cà Granda Ospedale Maggiore Policlinico, University of Milan, Neonatology and NICU, Milan, Italy

Pasquale Striano
Pediatric Neurology and Muscular Diseases Unit, IRCCS 'G. Gaslini' Institute, Genoa, Italy
Department of Neurosciences, Rehabilitation, Ophthalmology, Genetics, Maternal and Child Health, University of Genoa, Genoa, Italy

Yujun Yuan, Fenghua Yang, Liang Huo, Yuying Fan, Xueyan Liu, Qiong Wu and Hua Wang
Department of Pediatrics, Shengjing Hospital of China Medical University, Shenyang, China

Mostafa Hotait, Maya Dirani, Tarek El Halabi and Ahmad Beydoun
Department of Neurology, American University of Beirut Medical Center, Beirut, Lebanon

Index

P

R

S

T

V

W

www.ingramcontent.com/pod-product-compliance
Lightning Source LLC
LaVergne TN
LVHW082213200926
848484LV00008B/2247